Quick Reference Guide to Strategies

Note: Also refer to the last page of the book and the inside back cover.

SAUNDERS
2022–2023

7 EDITION

CLINICAL JUDGMENT *and*
TEST-TAKING STRATEGIES

Passing Nursing School *and the* NCLEX® Exam

Linda Anne Silvestri, PhD, RN, FAAN

Nursing Instructor
University of Nevada, Las Vegas
Las Vegas, Nevada

President
Nursing Reviews, Inc. and Professional Nursing Seminars, Inc.
Henderson, Nevada

Elsevier
Next Generation NCLEX® (NGN) Consultant and Thought Leader

Angela E. Silvestri, PhD, APRN, FNP-BC, CNE

Assistant Professor and *BSN Program Director*
University of Nevada, Las Vegas
Las Vegas, Nevada

President
Nurse Prep, LLC
Henderson, Nevada

Associate Editor

Eileen H. Gray, DNP, RN, CPNP

Nursing Instructor
University of Nevada, Las Vegas
Las Vegas, Nevada

Consultant
Nursing Reviews, Inc.
Henderson, Nevada

ELSEVIER

Elsevier
3251 Riverport Lane
St. Louis, Missouri 63043

SAUNDERS 2022-2023 CLINICAL JUDGMENT AND TEST-TAKING STRATEGIES,
SEVENTH EDITION

ISBN: 978-0-323-76388-2

Notice

Practitioners and researchers must always rely on their own experience and knowledge in evaluating and using any information, methods, compounds or experiments described herein. Because of rapid advances in the medical sciences, in particular, independent verification of diagnoses and drug dosages should be made. To the fullest extent of the law, no responsibility is assumed by Elsevier, authors, editors or contributors for any injury and/or damage to persons or property as a matter of products liability, negligence or otherwise, or from any use or operation of any methods, products, instructions, or ideas contained in the material herein.

Previous editions copyrighted 2020, 2018, 2016, 2014, 2010, and 2005

Library of Congress Control Number: 2021934297

Content Strategist: Heather Bays-Petrovic
Content Development Specialist: Sara Hardin
Publishing Services Manager: Julie Eddy
Senior Project Manager: Cindy Thoms
Designer: Bridget Hoette

Printed in India

Last digit is the print number: 9 8 7 6 5 4 3 2 1

Working together
to grow libraries in
developing countries

www.elsevier.com • www.bookaid.org

To all nursing students,
your commitment to becoming successful
and your dedication to the profession of nursing
will bring never-ending rewards!

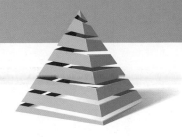

About the Authors

Linda Anne Silvestri, PhD, RN, FAAN

As a child, I always dreamed of becoming either a nurse or a teacher. Initially I chose to become a nurse because I really wanted to help others, especially those who were ill. Then I realized that both of my dreams could come true: I could be both a nurse and a teacher. So, I pursued my dreams.

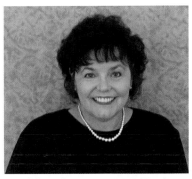

(Photo by Laurent W. Valliere)

I received my diploma in nursing at Cooley Dickinson Hospital School of Nursing in Northampton, Massachusetts. Afterward, I worked at Baystate Medical Center in Springfield, Massachusetts. While there, I cared for clients in acute medical-surgical units, the intensive care unit, the emergency department, pediatric units, and other acute care units. Later I received an Associate Degree from Holyoke Community College in Holyoke, Massachusetts; my BSN from American International College in Springfield, Massachusetts; and my MSN from Anna Maria College in Paxton, Massachusetts, with a dual major in Nursing Management and Patient Education. I received my PhD in Nursing from the University of Nevada, Las Vegas, and conducted and published research on self-efficacy and the predictors for NCLEX® success. I am also a member of the Honor Society of Nursing, Sigma Theta Tau International, Phi Kappa Phi, the American Nurses Association, the National League for Nursing, the Western Institute of Nursing, the Eastern Nursing Research Society, and the Golden Key International Honour Society. Additionally, I am a Fellow in the American Academy of Nursing. In 2012, I received the Alumna of the Year/Nurse of the Year Award from the University of Nevada, Las Vegas (UNLV), School of Nursing.

As a native of Springfield, Massachusetts, I began my teaching career as an instructor of medical-surgical nursing and leadership-management nursing at Baystate Medical Center School of Nursing in 1981. In 1989, I relocated to Rhode Island and began teaching medical-surgical nursing and psychiatric nursing to RN and LPN students at the Community College of Rhode Island. Later in 1994, I began teaching nursing at Salve Regina University in Newport, Rhode Island. Currently, I am a part-time nursing instructor at UNLV.

I established Professional Nursing Seminars, Inc. in 1991 and Nursing Reviews, Inc. in 2000. Both companies are located in Henderson, Nevada, and are dedicated to helping nursing graduates achieve their goals of becoming registered nurses, licensed practical/vocational nurses, or both.

Today, I am the successful author of numerous NCLEX review products published by Elsevier. I also work with Elsevier as a Consultant and Thought Leader for the Next Generation NCLEX® (NGN). I am so pleased that you have decided to join us on your journey to success in testing for nursing examinations and for the NCLEX examination!

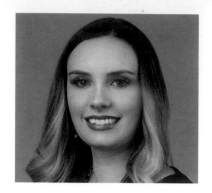

Angela E. Silvestri, PhD, APRN, FNP-BC, CNE

When asked what I wanted to do with my life and as a career, I always answered that I wanted to work in the medical field. At first my ambition was to become a physician; however, learning that nurses interact with their patients more often than physicians do swayed me to pursue nursing. While in nursing school, I worked as a tutor for my peers. I realized how much I enjoyed doing this and how much of a difference my help made in these students' college careers and ultimately their lives. I received my baccalaureate degree in Nursing and Sociology at Salve Regina University in Newport, Rhode Island. After earning my degree, I worked in long-term care, rehabilitation, and acute care settings. I then went on to earn my master's degree and PhD in nursing. I completed my family nurse practitioner post-master's graduate certificate program and am practicing as a family nurse practitioner on a college campus. I am a member of the Nevada Nurses Association, Sigma Theta Tau International, Golden Key International Honour Society, American Association of Colleges of Nursing, and American Association of Nurse Practitioners. I am an Assistant Professor and the BSN Program Director at the University of Nevada, Las Vegas, and teach Leadership and Transition into Practice. My short-term goals include conducting research focused on nursing education and nursing student success to help students transition to successful nurses in practice. Working with students while having been a student for quite some time helped me understand and realize the individual needs students have, both academic and non-academic. I am very excited to be a part of this opportunity to further assist nursing students in their ultimate goal: passing nursing school and the NCLEX exam and making substantial contributions to the profession of nursing!

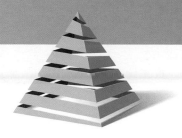

Contributors

Associate Editor

Eileen H. Gray, DNP, RN, CPNP
Nursing Instructor
University of Nevada, Las Vegas
Las Vegas, Nevada
Consultant
Nursing Reviews, Inc.
Henderson, Nevada

Consultants

Allison E. Bowser, MEd, BSB
Consultant
Nursing Reviews, Inc.
Henderson, Nevada

Dianne E. Fiorentino
Research Coordinator
Nursing Reviews, Inc.
Henderson, Nevada

James Guilbault Jr., BS, PharmD
Clinical Pharmacist
Wilbraham, Massachusetts
Pharmacology Consultant
Nursing Reviews, Inc.
Henderson, Nevada

Previous Item Writers

Linda Ann Aubrey, MSN, RN, CMSRN, CNE
Martha Barry, RN, CNM, MS
Jacqueline Rosenjack Burchum, DNSc, FNP-BC, CNE
Reitha Cabaniss, MSN
Mary C. Carrico, MS, RN
Mary L. Dowell, PhD, RN, BC
Kimberly R. Foisy, RN, MSN, CMSRN
Lena R. Greene, MSN, RN
Rebecca Russo Hill, DNP, FNP-C
Tiffany Jakubowski, RN
Christina Keller, RN, MSN
Lynn M. Korvick, PhD, RN, CNE
Terri Peterson, RN, BSN, MSNEd
Donna Russo, RN, MSN, CCRN, CNE
Julie S. Snyder, MSN, RN-BC
Bethany Hawes Sykes, EdD, RN, CEN, CCRN
Linda Turchin, MSN, RN, CNE
Koni J. Utley, MSN, RN
Polly Gerber Zimmermann, RN, MS, MBA, CEN, FAEN

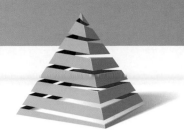

Previous Reviewers

Rita R. Armstrong, DNP, MSN Ed, RN
Professor
Dallas Nursing Institute
Dallas, Texas

Anna M. Bruch, RN, MSN
Nursing Professor
Illinois Valley Community College
Oglesby, Illinois

Lisa Hollett, RN, BSN, MA, MICN, TCRN, CFN, DABFN
Trauma Performance Improvement Coordinator
MedPartners
Ennis, Texas

Peter D. Smith, BA, MSN, RN
Instructor & Clinical Lead/Critical Care Nurse
Otolaryngology/Plastics & Cardio-Thoracic Acute Care
Goldfarb School of Nursing at Barnes-Jewish College
Barnes-Jewish Hospital
St. Louis, Missouri

Elaine Kay Strouss, MSN, RN, CNE
Professor—Nursing
Community College of Beaver County
Monaca, Pennsylvania

Elizabeth Wright, MSN, RN, CNE
Assistant Professor of Nursing
Indiana Wesleyan University
Marian, Indiana

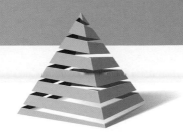

Preface

Welcome to Saunders Pyramid to Success!

Saunders 2022-2023 Clinical Judgment and Test-Taking Strategies: Passing Nursing School and the NCLEX® Exam is one in a series of products designed to assist you in achieving your goal of passing your nursing courses and becoming a licensed nurse. This product provides you with test-taking strategies that will help you pass your nursing examinations and the NCLEX examination.

Organization

Saunders 2022-2023 Clinical Judgment and Test-Taking Strategies: Passing Nursing School and the NCLEX® Exam contains three parts and 20 chapters. The chapters in Part I include information on test preparation and the NCLEX exam. The chapters in Part II describe the test-taking strategies and include several sample questions that illustrate how to use each test-taking strategy. The sample questions represent all types of question formats, including multiple choice and alternate item formats. The Next Generation NCLEX® (NGN) Item Types are described; samples of these item types can be located both in the book and on the accompanying Evolve site. In Part III of the book, there are practice questions, and the accompanying Evolve site contains the practice questions from the book along with additional practice questions for a total of 1200 practice questions. All of the practice questions reflect the framework and the content identified in the most current NCLEX test plans. The practice questions in this resource relate to each Client Needs category, each Integrated Process of the NCLEX exam, and the Cognitive Skills identified in the National Council of State Boards of Nursing (NCSBN) Clinical Judgment Measurement Model (NCJMM). The Client Needs categories include Safe and Effective Care Environment, Health Promotion and Maintenance, Psychosocial Integrity, and Physiological Integrity. The Integrated Processes include Caring, Communication and Documentation, Culture and Spirituality, Nursing Process (Clinical Problem-Solving Process), and Teaching and Learning. The Cognitive Skills include Recognize Cues, Analyze Cues, Prioritize Hypotheses, Generate Solutions, Take Action, and Evaluate Outcomes.

Part I: Study and Test Preparation

Chapter 1: Clinical Judgment and Nursing Examinations

The information in this chapter describes Clinical Judgment, the NCJMM and the Cognitive Skills of the Model, case studies and the NGN Item Types. The chapter also focuses on the exams that you will take during your nursing program and provides you with information on how to prepare for these exams. Topics include the purpose of nursing exams, what you can expect on nursing exams, how nursing exams are different from other exams, and the types of questions on nursing exams. Additional topics include preparing for a nursing exam using your syllabus, textbook, classroom notes, flash cards, study guides, and study groups.

Chapter 2: Developing Study Skills

This chapter discusses several topics related to study skills and study habits. It provides you with information on how to develop or refine study skills and how to develop good study habits so that you will be well prepared for your nursing exams. Included are the top 10 Pyramid Points and study habits. Also, study skills such as listening, note-taking, reading, remembering content, and critical thinking skills are discussed.

Chapter 3: Reducing Test Anxiety

This chapter focuses on the important points related to test anxiety. In this chapter, you are provided with self-assessment points to determine if you experience test anxiety. Additionally, the causes of test anxiety, how to prevent test anxiety, and how to control test anxiety before and during an exam are discussed. Points about maintaining a positive attitude and what you can do when you experience test anxiety are presented in this chapter.

Chapter 4: NCLEX® Preparation

This chapter focuses on preparing for the NCLEX exam—the exam that you must take and pass after you graduate from nursing school in order to become a licensed nurse. This chapter emphasizes the important point that NCLEX preparation begins the moment you enter your nursing program. Specific to the NCLEX, it provides you with the steps for preparing for the NCLEX, self-assessment points to determine your readiness, and a plan for preparation.

Part II: Strategies for Success

Chapter 5: Alternate Item Formats and the Next Generation NCLEX® (NGN) Item Types

Alternate item format questions and NGN items are designed to test competency in nursing skills and clinical judgment abilities. This chapter describes the various types of alternate item format questions that you may encounter on the NCLEX examination and on nursing school examinations and provides you with test-taking strategies to answer them correctly. Additionally, strategies for answering NGN item types are presented. Sample alternate item formats and NGN items are illustrated.

Chapter 6: How to Avoid "Reading into the Question"

One of the pitfalls that can cause a problem when answering a question is "reading into the question." This means that you are considering issues beyond the information presented in the question. This chapter describes the strategies to use when answering test questions to prevent this from happening and includes topics such as how to read a question, using strategic words, identifying the subject of the question, recognizing and analyzing cues and determining if an abnormality exists, focusing on the client of the question, considering available resources, and using nursing knowledge and the process of elimination.

Chapter 7: Positive and Negative Event Queries

This chapter describes the differences between a positive and a negative event query in a question. Reading the question carefully and noting the type of query used are important to assist in answering a question correctly. This chapter also identifies the strategic words or phrases that indicate whether the question contains a positive or negative event query.

Chapter 8: Questions Requiring Prioritization

Some of the test questions on your nursing exams and on the NCLEX will require you to use the skill of prioritizing nursing actions. These types of questions can be difficult because when a question requires prioritization, all of the options may be correct, and you will need to determine the correct order of importance. This chapter describes the test-taking strategies that you can use to answer prioritizing questions correctly. Some of these strategies include the ABCs—airway, breathing, and circulation   Maslow's Hierarchy of Needs theory, and the steps of the nursing process (clinical problem-solving process). Also included in this chapter are the strategies for determining the need to contact the primary health care provider.

Chapter 9: Leading and Managing, Delegating, and Assignment-Making Questions

Some test questions that you will need to answer will relate to the nurse's responsibilities regarding delegating care and assignment-making and the supervisory role of these responsibilities. This chapter reviews the guidelines and principles related to delegating and assignment-making, two very important roles of the nurse as a leader and manager. It also provides you with information about the tasks and activities that can be delegated and assigned to assistive personnel (AP), licensed practical/vocational nurses, and registered nurses. Guidelines for time management are also reviewed, because managing time efficiently is a key factor for completing activities and tasks within a given time period.

Chapter 10: Communication Questions

Communication is a process through which information is exchanged, either verbally or nonverbally, between two or more individuals and is an extremely important role of the nurse. This chapter reviews the guidelines to follow when answering communication questions and identifies various aspects to consider when communicating and caring for clients. Additionally, therapeutic and non-therapeutic communication techniques are presented.

Chapter 11: Pharmacology, Medication, and Intravenous Calculation Questions

Pharmacology is one of the most difficult nursing content areas to master and feel comfortable with. One reason that it is so difficult is because of the enormous number of medications available. Another reason is that there is a vast amount of information to know about each medication. It is important for you to spend ample time studying and reviewing pharmacology in preparation for your nursing exams and for the NCLEX and to use this knowledge to answer pharmacology questions. However, you may be presented with pharmacology questions on your exams that present medications you are unfamiliar with, in which case you will need to make an educated guess to answer the question. This chapter provides you with the strategies and general guidelines to use for making an educated guess to answer pharmacology questions correctly. This chapter also includes medication and intravenous calculations strategies and examples.

Chapter 12: Additional Pyramid Strategies

This chapter reviews additional helpful strategies that will assist in answering a test question correctly. Also included in this chapter are strategies that are useful for answering questions related to laboratory values, client positioning, and therapeutic diets. Strategies that will be helpful when answering questions related to disasters are also presented in this chapter.

Part III: Practice Tests

Part III is composed of eight practice tests that provide you the opportunity to practice answering exam questions using various test-taking strategies. These tests include Chapter 13, Foundations of Care Questions; Chapter 14, Adult Health Questions; Chapter 15, Mental Health Questions; Chapter 16, Maternity Questions; Chapter 17, Pediatrics Questions; Chapter 18, Pharmacology Questions; Chapter 19, Delegating/Prioritizing Questions; and Chapter 20, Leadership/Management Questions. The correct answer, rationales for correct and incorrect options, a test-taking strategy, a tip for the nursing student, and question codes including cognitive skills codes are provided.

Special Features of the Book

Pyramid Points

Pyramid Points are the bullets that are placed at specific areas throughout the chapters. The Pyramid Points identify content and strategies that are important in preparation for the NCLEX examination.

ⅠⅠ▶ Tip for the Nursing Student

A tip for the nursing student is provided for each sample question in the book. Additionally, a tip for the nursing student accompanies each question in the practice tests located in Part III and on the accompanying Evolve site. This tip provides the nursing student with a description of the content or health problem addressed in the question.

NCLEX® Tip

NCLEX tips are located throughout Parts I and II of the text. These tips relate to NCLEX information and detail important points associated with the content addressed and with the NCLEX exam.

Lifestyle Planning Tip

Lifestyle planning tips are located throughout Parts I and II of the text. These tips provide information about healthy lifestyle choices that will help you live a well-balanced life, leading to success in nursing school.

Scope of Practice Tip

Scope of practice tips are located throughout Parts I and II of the text. These tips provide information about what you, as a nurse or nursing student, are able to do in your practice settings. These tips will also help you answer questions related to delegation and assignment-making.

Student-to-Student Tip

Student-to-student tips provide information from a student's perspective on various topics that you will encounter during nursing school, such as tips for answering certain types of questions encountered on your nursing exams. These tips are located throughout Parts I and II of the text.

Preparing for Clinical Tip

Preparing for clinical tips are located throughout Parts I and II of the text. These tips provide information particularly related to working in the clinical setting and ways to be the most prepared when you start your clinical rotations.

Practice Test Questions

The chapters in this book contain several sample practice questions that illustrate specific test-taking strategies. In addition to the sample practice questions integrated into the chapters, there are practice test questions in the book. The accompanying Evolve site contains a total of 1200 questions (practice questions from the book and additional questions). The practice test questions in the book and all of the questions on the Evolve site provide the correct answer, rationales for correct and incorrect options, a test-taking strategy, a tip for the nursing student, and question codes including cognitive skill codes.

Alternate Item Format Test Questions

In addition to multiple choice questions, alternate item format test questions are included throughout the book, the practice tests located in Part III, and on the accompanying Evolve site. These alternate item format types include fill-in-the-blank, multiple response, prioritizing (ordered response), figure or illustration (hot spot), chart/exhibit, graphic item options, and audio.

Case Studies and Next Generation NCLEX® (NGN) Item Types

In addition to the sample questions in the book, case studies are presented on the Evolve site and are accompanied by NGN format practice questions. Refer to www.ncsbn.org for information on these question types and the plan for inclusion in the NCLEX exam.

Answer Section for Practice Test Questions

The answer sections for each practice test question in Part III and on the accompanying Evolve site include the correct answer, rationale, tip for the nursing student, test-taking strategy, and question categories. The structure for the answer section is unique and provides the following information:

Rationale: The rationale provides you with the significant information regarding both correct and incorrect options.

Tip for the Nursing Student: The tip provides you with a description of the content or health problem addressed in the question.

Test-Taking Strategy: The test-taking strategy provides you with the logical path in selecting the correct option and assists you in selecting an answer to a question on which you must guess. This feature reinforces what you learned in the book about the use of test-taking strategies. The specific strategy is colored in blue. Each test-taking strategy also provides a "suggestion for review." Content to review is colored in magenta.

Question Categories: Each question is identified based on the categories used by the NCLEX test plan. Additional content categories are provided with each question to help you identify areas in need of review. The categories identified with each practice question include Level of Cognitive Ability, Client Needs, Integrated Process, Clinical Judgment/Cognitive Skill, Priority Concepts, Level of Nursing Student, and the specific nursing Content Area. All categories are identified by their full names so that you do not need to memorize codes or abbreviations.

Evolve Site

The accompanying Evolve site contains 1200 practice questions in the multiple choice format or in the alternate item format such as fill-in-the-blank, multiple response, prioritizing (ordered response), figure or illustration (hot spot), chart/exhibit, graphic item options, and audio. Case Studies and NGN type questions are also presented in the Evolve site. This Windows- and Macintosh-compatible program offers two testing modes for review:

Study: All questions in a selected Cognitive Level, Strategies, Client Needs, Integrated Process, Priority Concepts, Clinical Judgment/Cognitive Skill, or specific Content Area. The answer, rationale, tip for the nursing student, test-taking strategy, and question categories appear after answering each question.

Exam: This is customizable for your time and study needs. You may take 10, 25, 50, or 100 randomly chosen questions from selected Cognitive Level, Strategies, Client Needs, Integrated Process, Priority Concepts, Clinical Judgment/Cognitive Skill, or specific Content Area from the entire pool of questions. The answer, rationale, test-taking strategy, tip for the nursing student, question categories, and results appear after you finish the exam.

Category Selection on the Evolve Site

When you use the software, you will be able to select practice questions based on your personal review needs. If you would like to focus on a specific area, you can select your preference from the categories. Otherwise, you can choose to review all of the questions to practice on a broader scale.

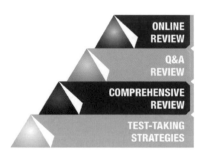

How to Use This Book

Saunders 2022-2023 Clinical Judgment and Test-Taking Strategies: Passing Nursing School and the NCLEX® Exam is especially designed to help you with your successful journey to the peak of the Saunders Pyramid to Success: becoming a licensed nurse. This book focuses on test-taking strategies that will help you pass both the nursing examinations that you need to take in nursing school and the NCLEX examination. You should begin your process through the Saunders Pyramid to Success by reading all of the chapters in this book to learn the strategies that you can use to answer test questions. Be sure to read all of the tips provided for you that are located throughout the chapters and the tip for the nursing student located with each sample question. While in nursing school, answer the questions in the practice tests located in Part III and on the accompanying Evolve site that relate to the content area you are studying.

When using the Evolve site, it is best to begin by selecting the study mode because you will receive immediate feedback regarding the answer, rationale, tip for the nursing student, test-taking strategies, content to review, and question codes. Therefore you will be provided with immediate information about your strengths and weaknesses. A self-check button is included to help you determine if you are thinking strategically. When you submit your answer to a practice question on Evolve, a window appears (if you have this feature turned on). Click on the strategy you used to help you answer the question. Then, click on *Strategy* to receive immediate feedback to help determine if you are on the right track! Once you have answered the practice test question, read the rationale, tip for the nursing student, and the test-taking strategy. The rationale provides you with the significant information regarding both the correct and incorrect options. The tip provides you with a description of the content or health problem addressed in the question. The test-taking strategy offers you the logical path to selecting the correct option. The strategy also identifies the content area you need to review if you had difficulty with the question.

It is very important to identify your strengths and weaknesses with regard to nursing content areas. Additionally, it is important to strengthen any weak areas in order to be successful on your nursing exams and on the NCLEX examination. Several products in Saunders Pyramid to Success can be used to strengthen any weak areas. These additional products in Saunders Pyramid to Success can be obtained by calling 1-800-545-2522 or visiting www.elsevierhealth.com. These products are described next.

RN Products

Saunders Comprehensive Review for the NCLEX-RN® Examination

This is an excellent resource to use, both while you are in nursing school and in preparation for the NCLEX examination. This book contains 20 units with 69 chapters and a comprehensive test, and each chapter is designed to identify specific components of nursing content. The book and accompanying software contain more than 5200 practice questions and include alternate item format questions. The software also contains a 75-question pre-assessment test that generates an individualized study calendar. A post-assessment test is also included as well as case studies and accompanying NGN item type practice questions.

Saunders Q&A Review for the NCLEX-RN® Examination

This book and accompanying Evolve site provide you with more than 6000 practice questions based on the NCLEX-RN test plan. Each practice question includes a priority nursing tip that provides you with a piece of important information to remember that will help you answer questions on nursing exams and on NCLEX. The chapters in this book are uniquely designed and are based on the NCLEX-RN examination test plan framework, including Client Needs and Integrated Processes. Alternate item format questions as well as case studies and accompanying NGN item type practice questions are included. With practice questions focused on the Client Needs, Integrated Processes, and Clinical Judgment/Cognitive Skills, you can assess your level of competence.

HESI/Saunders Online Review Course for the NCLEX-RN® Examination

The online NCLEX-RN review course addresses all areas of the test plan identified by the National Council of State Boards of Nursing, Inc. This self-paced online review contains 10 interactive, multimedia-rich modules and videos, practice questions, end-of-lesson case studies, and much more! A diagnostic pretest generates a study calendar to guide your review. Thousands of NCLEX-style questions—including every type of alternate item format question—are provided, concluding with a comprehensive examination that will sharpen your test-taking skills. Unique videos that simulate a live review course focus on difficult subjects such as dysrhythmias and making them easier to understand, along with case studies to apply learned material. By taking a systematic and individualized approach, this online review will prepare you for the NCLEX like nothing else can!

Saunders Q&A Review Cards for the NCLEX-RN® Examination

The Saunders Q&A Review Cards for the NCLEX-RN Exam provides you with 1200 NCLEX-RN review questions, including alternate item format questions, in a convenient flash card format. This is the perfect portable study resource that you can use anytime, anywhere. Review questions are on the front of each card and are organized by content areas. Client Needs categories, consistent with the current NCLEX-RN test plan, are also identified. Answers are included on the back of the card, along with rationales and test-taking strategies.

HESI Compass for the NCLEX-RN®

Getting close to taking the NCLEX? HESI Compass is available through your institution or instructor. It is a virtual NCLEX review course that provides a personalized study plan alongside a live nurse Coach who is dedicated to answering your questions and providing guidance in the final weeks before you take the NCLEX. In addition to content review modules, case studies, and practice questions, two full HESI Exit exams are provided as built in checkpoints at the midcourse and final to gauge your NCLEX readiness as you progress towards your testing date. Ask your instructor about this course!

PN Products

Saunders Comprehensive Review for the NCLEX-PN® Examination

This is an excellent resource to use both while you are in nursing school and in preparation for the NCLEX examination. This book contains 19 units and 65 chapters, and each chapter is designed to identify specific components of nursing content. The book and accompanying Evolve site contain more than 4500 practice questions and include alternate item format questions. The software also contains a 75-question pre-assessment test that generates an individualized study calendar. A post-assessment test is also included as well as case studies and accompanying NGN item type practice questions.

Saunders Q&A Review for the NCLEX-PN® Examination

This book and accompanying Evolve site provide you with more than 5500 practice questions based on the NCLEX-PN test plan. Each practice question includes a priority nursing tip that provides you with a piece of important information to remember that will help you answer questions on nursing exams and on NCLEX. The chapters in this book are uniquely designed and are based on the NCLEX-PN examination test plan framework, including Client Needs and Integrated Processes. Alternate item format questions as well as case studies and accompanying NGN item type practice questions are included. With practice questions focused on the Client Needs and Integrated Processes, you can assess your level of competence.

Saunders Review Cards for the NCLEX-PN® Examination

The Saunders Review Cards for the NCLEX-PN® Examination provide you with 1200 practice test questions, including alternate item format questions, in a convenient flash card format. This is the perfect portable study resource that you can use anytime, anywhere. Review questions are on the front of each card and are organized by content areas. Client Needs categories, consistent with the current NCLEX-PN test plan, are also identified. Answers are included on the back of the card, along with rationales and test-taking strategies.

HESI/Saunders Online Review Course for the NCLEX-PN® Examination

The online NCLEX-PN review course addresses all areas of the test plan identified by the National Council of State Boards of Nursing, Inc. This self-paced online review contains 10 interactive, multimedia-rich modules and videos, practice questions, end-of-lesson case studies, and much more! A diagnostic pretest generates a study calendar to guide your review. Thousands of NCLEX-style questions—including every type of alternate item format question—are provided, concluding with a comprehensive examination that will sharpen your test-taking skills. Unique videos that simulate a live review course focus on difficult subjects such as shock and make them easier to understand. By taking a systematic and individualized approach, this online review will prepare you for the NCLEX like nothing else can!

Good luck with your journey through the Saunders Pyramid to Success. We wish you continued success throughout your nursing program and in your new career as a nurse!

Linda Anne Silvestri, PhD, RN, FAAN and
Angela E. Silvestri, PhD, APRN, FNP-BC, CNE

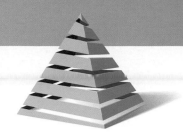

Acknowledgments

Sincere appreciation and warmest thanks are extended to the many individuals who in their own way have contributed to the publication of this book.

First, we thank our family for all of their support during the writing and publication of this book, and a special thank you to our husbands: my husband, Larry, and Angela's husband, Brent.

Both Angela and I sincerely acknowledge and thank some very important individuals from Elsevier who are dedicated to our work in creating NCLEX products for nursing students. We thank Heather Bays-Petrovic, Content Strategist, for her continuous assistance, enthusiasm, ideas, and tremendous support as we prepared this publication. And we thank Sara Hardin, Content Development Specialist, for her enormous amount of support and assistance, ideas for the product, and maintaining organization for manuscript production. Thank you, Heather and Sara!

We also want to acknowledge and thank all of the staff at Elsevier for their tremendous assistance throughout the preparation and production of this publication, and we especially thank Cindy Thoms, Senior Project Manager, for keeping all of the manuscript and questions for the Evolve site in order and moving through production so seamlessly – thank you, Cindy! We also thank Julie Eddy, Publishing Services Manager and Bridget Hoette, Designer. We offer a special thank you to all of you.

Angela and I extend a sincere thank you to our Associate Editor of this publication, Dr. Eileen Gray. Thank you, Eileen, for your superb work and expert contributions!

We also want to thank all of our past and current reviewers and item writers for their expert assistance and contributions to this review product. We thank Dianne E. Fiorentino for researching content for each practice question; Allison Bowser for her editorial suggestions and expertise; and James Guilbault for researching and updating medications. Angela and I also thank our Evolve site review team for their assistance in reviewing question components and functionality; so, thank you, to our AWESOME review team!

We wish to acknowledge and thank Dr. Brandy L. Lehman, Assistant Professor, College of Nursing, from the University of South Florida in Tampa, Florida. Dr. Lehman took the time to share her thoughts and ideas about the reorganization of the content of the first edition and additions that could be made that would enhance the learning experience for the student. It is apparent that she is dedicated to educating nursing students. Thank you, Dr. Lehman!

Lastly, we extend a very special thank you to all of our nursing students, past, present, and future. You light up our lives! Your curiosity, enthusiasm for learning, and desire to become successful are so inspiring.

Linda Anne Silvestri, PhD, RN, FAAN and
Angela E. Silvestri, PhD, APRN, FNP-BC, CNE

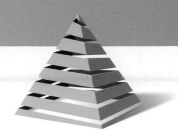

Contents

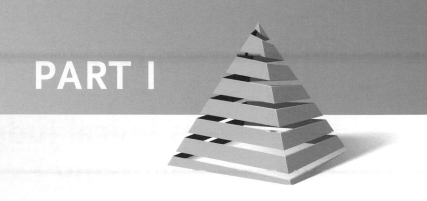

Study and Test Preparation

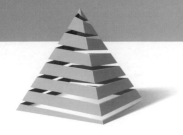

CHAPTER 1

Clinical Judgment and Nursing Examinations

Clinical Judgment and Next Generation NCLEX® Items

Clinical judgment is the observed outcome of critical thinking and decision-making (Dickison, Haerling, and Lasater, 2019). A priority focus in nursing education is on the development of clinical judgment in nursing students through targeted teaching, assessment, and testing. Sound clinical judgment skills are a critical component of competency and proficiency in nursing. Additionally, the National Council Licensure Examination (NCLEX) requires candidates to demonstrate the ability to use clinical judgment in the delivery of client care.

Clinical Judgment Measurement Model and Cognitive Skills

The National Council of State Boards of Nursing (NCSBN) has created an NCSBN Clinical Judgment Measurement Model (NCJMM) that consists of applying six cognitive skills or processes. These skills or processes include (1) recognize cues; (2) analyze cues; (3) prioritize hypotheses; (4) generate solutions; (5) take action; and (6) evaluate outcomes (Dickison et al., 2019). Table 1-1 provides a description of these six cognitive skills/processes. The measurement model also serves as a guide for nursing faculty and for the NCSBN to create Next Generation NCLEX (NGN) test items. Nursing students can apply these six cognitive skills/processes along with traditional test-taking strategies to answer test questions. Refer to Chapter 5 for these strategies.

Table 1-1 Cognitive Skills/Processes and Descriptions	
Cognitive Skill/Process	**Description**
Recognize cues	Identify significant (relevant) data; data can be from many sources (assessment/data collection)
Analyze cues	Connect data to the client's clinical presentation; determine whether the data are expected or unexpected and what the data means (analysis)
Prioritize hypotheses	Rank hypotheses (client needs or problems); determine the concerns or client needs and their priority (analysis)
Generate solutions	Use hypotheses to determine interventions for an expected outcome (planning)
Take actions	Implement the generated solutions, addressing the highest priorities or hypotheses (implementation)
Evaluate outcomes	Compare observed outcomes with expected ones (evaluation)

From Dickison, P., Haerling, K.A., & Lasater, K. (2019). Integrating the National Council of State Boards of Nursing Clinical Judgment Model into nursing educational frameworks, *Journal of Nursing Education, 58* (2), 72-78.

NGN Item Types

The NCJMM and the NGN item types that will be presented in the exam continue to develop as the NCSBN progresses in its research to determine the best ways to measure clinical judgment. The NCSBN plans to start to include these item types as scored test items in the spring of 2023. Currently, the major types of test items that will be used are highlight, drop-down, multiple response, multiple choice, and drag and drop (Table 1-2). There are variations of these types; for example, highlight item types may present as *highlight text* or *highlight table*. The variations of drop down include *drop down cloze*, *drop down rationale*, and *drop down table*. Variations of multiple response include *multiple response select N, multiple response select all, multiple response grouping*, and *matrix multiple response*. Variations of the multiple choice include the *single response multiple choice* and the *matrix multiple choice*. Variations of the drag and drop include *drag and drop cloze* and *drag and drop rationale*. Two additional item types include the *bow-tie* and the *trend item*. However, the NCSBN research is still in progress, so additional variations may be added.

Types of Case Studies

NGN test items will be accompanied by case studies. Test-takers may encounter standalone case studies or unfolding case studies. An *NGN standalone case study* presents a client scenario *at one point in time* or *multiple points over time*. The client scenario will be followed by an NGN test item that measures one or more of the cognitive skills/processes. Currently, the NCSBN indicates that the item types that will accompany the standalone case study will be the bow-tie (presents a client scenario at one point in time) or a trend item (presents a client scenario at multiple points over time). Research is continuing on these two innovative item types.

An *NGN unfolding case study* presents a client scenario that *changes over time through multiple phases of care*. The unfolding case will begin with a one- to two-sentence introductory statement. Then, the client situation data will be presented as part of the medical record for most items. The medical record presented for each item within an unfolding case will have one or more tabs that will be accessible for the test-taker. The data in this type of client scenario are more comprehensive than in the standalone case study as the "story" unfolds. All six of the cognitive skills will be measured in an unfolding case using the NGN test item formats.

Table 1-2 Next Generation NCLEX® (NGN) Item Types and Descriptions	
NGN Item Type	**Description**
Multiple Response	Items allow the test-taker to select one or more answer options at a time, depending on the item type presented. Options may be presented in a list or presented in a row as part of a table.
Drag and Drop	Items allow the test-taker to move or place response options into answer spaces.
Drop down	Items allow the test-taker to select option(s) from a drop-down list or table, depending on the item type presented.
Highlight	Items allow the test-taker to select an answer by highlighting predefined words or phrases in text or a table. These types of items allow an individual to read a portion of a client medical record, such as a nursing note, health history or physical exam, lab values, or medication record, and then select the words or phrases that answer the item.
Multiple Choice	Items allow the test-taker to select one answer from either a list of options or from options presented in a row as part of a table.

From Petersen, E., Betts, J., Muntean, W. (December 2020). *Next Generation NCLEX® (NGN) Webinar*. Chicago, NCSBN.

It is expected that the NGN test items will be scored items in the new test plan implemented in 2023. Some of these NGN item types can be found on the Evolve site accompanying this book. We highly encourage you to become familiar with these NGN item types found on the Evolve site and to frequently access the NCSBN website at www.ncsbn.org for a visual of the clinical judgment measurement model and for updates regarding the NGN item types.

When and Why Are Nursing Exams Administered?

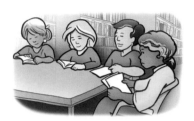

Nursing exams are administered at various points throughout each nursing course. Nursing faculty members administer these exams for several purposes. Exams test your knowledge of the content taught in a current course; your retrieval knowledge, which is knowledge gained in previous courses; and your clinical judgment, or the ability to analyze, apply, and synthesize concepts to care for clients in various situations. The exams you take in nursing courses are also designed to prepare you for the NCLEX exam, the examination that you need to pass after you graduate to become a licensed nurse. These and additional purposes for administering exams are listed in the following box.

Purposes for Administering Exams

1. To test your knowledge of the content taught in a course
2. To test retrieval knowledge, which is knowledge gained in previous courses that you took
3. To test your clinical judgment ability and to measure the six cognitive skills/processes of the NCJMM
4. To test your ability to analyze and apply concepts learned to care for clients in various situations
5. To ensure the development of a critical thinker who can make sound clinical judgments and decisions based on evidence-based practice
6. To ensure the development of a professional nurse who can safely and competently care for clients served in the profession
7. To make certain that you are a successful NCLEX exam candidate who will pass the NCLEX exam on his or her first sitting

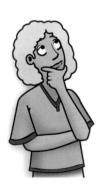

The Beginning Nursing Student: What Should You Think About?

What Is a Beginning Nursing Student?

If you have just completed your support courses (e.g., anatomy and physiology, microbiology, chemistry, pathophysiology, nutrition, and genetics) and are entering your first nursing course, then you are a beginning nursing student. Your first nursing course is most likely titled "Foundations in Nursing" or something similar. In this course you will learn the basic concepts necessary to safely care for clients.

❓ The NCLEX Exam: Why Do You Need to Think About It Now?

You may think that the NCLEX exam is far off, and it is; however, it is critical that you think about it the moment you enter your first nursing class. Why is this important? To be successful on the NCLEX exam, you need to become familiar with what this exam is all about as early as possible in the nursing program.

Taking the NCLEX exam will be a reality once you graduate, and you must pass this exam to become a licensed nurse. Often, students are concerned with the "here and now" of what they need to accomplish and are unconcerned about the future. Students say, "I will worry about the NCLEX exam when the time comes." At this point, it is much too late. So think about this exam early; visit the NCSBN website at www.ncsbn.org, and download the detailed test plan for the NCLEX exam. This test plan lists the content areas and activities that will be tested on the exam. Use these activity lists as your study guides for preparing for exams for each nursing course. By doing this, consider that you are not only preparing for your nursing exams but also preparing for the NCLEX exam. You will be ready when the NCLEX exam becomes a reality for you!

❓ Planning: Why Is It So Important?

Much of your success in nursing school has to do with how you organize your time. You will have a busy schedule and will need to plan ahead to best prepare for exams, clinical experiences, and other assignments. Get an organizer with a calendar or use another type of calendar, such as a calendar on a mobile device, and use this as your planning guide for everything you need to do. Your e-mail account linked to your institution often includes an electronic calendar. With this type of electronic calendar, important events can be marked for an entire group, and invitations can be sent using this platform. In addition, social media accounts are commonly used as organizers for student and school events.

In your calendar, make notes about your short-term and long-term goals. For short-term goals, note your classes and times, school meetings and appointments, study session times, assignment due dates, date and exam times, and other obligations related to school. For your long-term goals, note what you plan to accomplish each year until your projected graduation date. Look at your calendar daily to meet any day to day obligations, and look ahead at your long term goals to be sure that you are ready for graduation.

What Can You Expect on Nursing Exams?

❓ How Do Nursing Exams Differ From Other Exams?

When you enter your first nursing course, you need to remember that your exam experience in college up to this point has related to testing in support courses, such as anatomy and physiology, microbiology, chemistry, pathophysiology, nutrition, and genetics. In these courses, test questions have been primarily at the cognitive level of remembering or understanding. These support courses have required not only a great deal of reading but also memorization to answer exam questions correctly. So basically, your test-taking skills to this point may be quite good but are based on remembering, some understanding, and memorization.

Nursing exams differ greatly from the exams you are used to taking. Memorization alone will not get you through a nursing exam, although you will need to memorize certain laboratory values or formulas for calculating a medication dosage or intravenous flow rate. The questions on a nursing exam are at a higher cognitive level and will require you to analyze or synthesize information and apply it to a situation. Your exams will require you to demonstrate clinical judgment in the delivery of client care and will measure the six cognitive skills/processes noted in the NCJMM. You will not be able to rely only on recall to answer test questions. Instead, you will need to understand pathophysiology related to certain nursing content and disease processes and use critical thinking and clinical judgment to make decisions. Do not let that first nursing exam

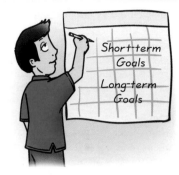

Beware of Nursing Exams!

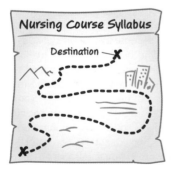

Nursing Course Syllabus

Destination ✗

"blow you away" or "throw you for a loop," as some may say. Be ready for it, and you will do great and pass!

What Types of Questions Can You Expect on Nursing Exams?

Many questions you will encounter on nursing exams will be multiple choice—a question and four possible options. Other types of questions, known as alternate item formats or NGN item types, may be included because these types of questions also are used in the NCLEX exam and require higher-level thinking. The alternate item formats include multiple response (select all that apply), fill-in-the-blank, prioritizing (ordered response), chart/exhibit, graphic item options (images as the options), questions that include a picture or illustration, and audio questions. The major NGN item types include highlight, drop-down, multiple response, multiple choice, and drag and drop. As noted previously, variations of these types may be a part of the NCLEX, in addition to other types, such as the bow-tie and trend items (see Table 1-2).

The total number of questions on a nursing exam varies, depending on the content being tested and the amount of time for testing, among other factors. Your nursing instructor determines the number of questions that will be included.

❓ Are Test-Taking Strategies Important?

The use of traditional test-taking strategies and the application of clinical judgment/cognitive processes and skills will help you determine what the question is asking, how to select the correct answer, or how to narrow your choices when you must make an educated guess at an answer. The use of strategies is critical when taking a nursing exam because in many of the exam questions, all options may be correct, but depending on the way the question is worded, you may need to prioritize to select the correct answer(s). In addition, many times you may be able to narrow your choices to two options but then struggle to make a selection. In these situations, using test-taking strategies and applying clinical judgment/cognitive processes and skills are essential. Chapters 5 through 12 of this book focus on traditional test-taking strategies and clinical judgment/cognitive skills for answering nursing exam questions. In addition, a guide to test-taking strategies for answering nursing exam questions can be found on the inside back cover.

Your Course Syllabus: Why Is It Important?

Your course syllabus is your map of the course. It provides your course objectives, course and program policies and procedures, required readings and other activities, class schedule (including your exam schedule), and other information related to the course. Your course outcomes (objectives) are the goals that you need to meet to pass the course, so be sure to read and understand them. They are also important because they are mapped specifically to program outcomes and other guiding standards, including the NCLEX exam. They serve as a road map in navigating course content. In addition, your exam questions directly reflect your course outcomes. Your required reading and other activities and your class and exam schedule are important to note because you need to plan ahead and prepare for these requirements. So be sure to pay attention to what is stated in your course syllabus, as there is a link between everything noted that in the long run will help you become a professional nurse.

What "Smart Study" Tips Can You Use for Your Nursing Courses and to Get Ready for a Nursing Exam?

"Smart Study" tips provide you with direction to prepare you for your nursing course, help you to become familiar with your course textbook, and give you guidance with how you should prepare for an exam. These "Smart Study" tips are listed below.

Required Reading

In a nursing program, you can expect to do a tremendous amount of reading. Your course syllabus lists the required reading, and it is important to do the reading before the scheduled class. For example, if a class is scheduled and the content listed is "Standard and Transmission-Based Precautions," you need to complete the associated reading assignment before class. Reading the material before class is vital for a number of reasons. First, faculty members expect you to read the material before class so that you are prepared for any in-class activities. Some instructors use case studies and other active learning strategies in their teaching. These methodologies require students to have an introduction to the material being covered for the method to be effective. Next, reading before class helps you to identify areas that you do not understand. If you jot down questions that come to your mind as you are reading, you can bring this list of questions to class. Finally, many faculty members give pop quizzes, which are unannounced quizzes administered at the beginning of class that include questions about the material that was to be read. So to be best prepared, read before class!

It is important to keep current with reading assignments because if you fall behind, it will be difficult to catch up; however, taking breaks while reading is important, too. During a reading session you may find that you get to the bottom of a page and cannot remember what you just read. This happens to everyone when concentration fades. This is the time to stop reading and take on another activity. Get out of your chair, move around, and take deep breaths. Taking a walk or some other form of exercise will help clear your mind and get you back on track. You will learn what your individual concentration tolerance is and which activities help you refocus; use this as a guide for planning your reading sessions. If you find that after 45 minutes your concentration level diminishes, plan on breaks and a different activity every 45 minutes.

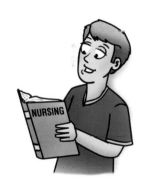

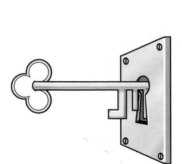

As you read your chapters, try to identify what you think will be asked on your nursing exams. Note the chapter headings and boldface vocabulary, and read the information in boxes, charts, tables, and graphs throughout your textbook. In addition to highlighting key points, make margin notes for yourself for study.

Reading the Preface of the Textbook

Many students skip over the preface in a textbook because they are eager to get started with Chapter 1 and the learning it will provide. But reading the preface can help acquaint you with the contents of the textbook and help you make the best use of your time. The preface also may provide information on special student resources available for preparing for exams. You may find that a website is available that provides practice exam questions of all types that correlate with each chapter in your textbook. Other types of resources commonly used include adaptive learning and quizzing technology, case studies, animations, and virtual simulation experiences or simulations in a laboratory setting that will enhance your understanding of new material. Take advantage of these valuable resources. Practice as many study questions as you can in preparation for exams, and look at any results reports provided to you on your level of preparation. This will give you data on your strengths and weaknesses.

❓ Practice Exam Questions

The questions on nursing exams are written in identifiable and structured ways, which are outlined in later chapters of this book. Remember that "practice makes perfect!" So practice as many questions as you can in preparation for your exams. Simply knowing how the questions are structured and becoming familiar and comfortable with what you will encounter will assist you in passing an exam. Get your hands on as many study questions as possible because this will help you be successful not only on nursing examinations but also on the NCLEX exam!

Many nursing textbooks provide practice exam questions at the end of a content chapter and provide a website that contains practice exam questions. Look for these in your textbook, and practice on these questions. Next, check the preface in your textbook to locate the website for access to additional practice questions. Finally, use your NCLEX review book, and review content and practice questions that correlate with the content and health problem you will be tested on. After answering practice questions, be sure to read the accompanying rationale and test-taking strategy for each question to understand the content and the logical path for answering correctly. Review any reports generated after taking a practice test so that you can gauge your progress as you learn new content.

Practice makes perfect!

Highlighting Key Points in the Chapter

As you read, highlight key points. Key points include any information in the text that has to do with the nurse caring for the client. For example, key points would include signs and symptoms of a disorder and nursing interventions. Highlighting key points is especially helpful when it is time to review before an exam, because you can reread only what you have highlighted rather than the entire chapter. Highlighting is also helpful to identify points that may require clarification from your instructor.

Flash Cards

Once you have highlighted key points, make flash cards. Flash cards serve as a study guide, are portable and easy to carry in your backpack, and will help you with studying and reviewing for exams. For example, you can list signs and symptoms of a disorder or various laboratory values on flash cards. You can also make electronic flash cards and review them on a smartphone or tablet. You may need an Internet connection to review them electronically.

 ## Classroom Notes: How Can You Best Use Them?

How to Take Notes in Class

Taking good notes is an important part of preparing for an exam. How you take notes in college may differ greatly from how you took them in high school. For example, you may be accustomed to copying notes from a blackboard or other platform because this was how that information was presented. This will differ in college, where notes are not written on a site for you to copy. Now you will need to take note of the significant points made by your instructor during in-class activities. Some instructors may provide handouts or other materials to be used as guides during class; even so, these do not replace the need for you to take notes during a learning session. However, regardless of whether handout materials are provided, one important point to remember is that you will not be able to write down every word the instructor says. Work at developing a personal method of shorthand and abbreviations that you will understand. Some faculty members may allow you to record the class. This can be helpful, but get permission first. Reading your textbook assignments before class will help with note-taking because you will be familiar with the significant points. Some teachers also record lectures for students to listen to before class. If this is available, listen to the lecture before coming to class but *after* reading your assigned chapters. During class, you can take notes on the significant points made by your instructor, and you will know what these points are if you read the assigned content before class. You also will be able to participate more effectively in any class activity if the preparation is done beforehand.

Using Nursing Class Notes to Prepare for an Exam

After your class, read and organize your class notes. Combine your class notes with the reading notes that you made when you read your chapters. You will better understand the information if you merge the key points. You can make flash cards for any content area that seems difficult; for example, make a flash card that lists the steps in a procedure or the signs and symptoms of a disease. The worst thing you can do is to put your class notes aside until it is time for an exam. Read your class notes daily so that you are learning and understanding as the course progresses. Plan a time for your own mini–study sessions each day to read your notes. One week before the exam, spend more time in your mini–study sessions so that you will be ready. You never want to cram content into your head the night before an exam!

Study Guides

Three types of study guides may be available in nursing courses. The first is an ancillary book that accompanies your textbook. This study guide correlates with the chapters of your textbook and provides practice exercises and questions designed to reinforce content. You should complete the study guide even if your instructor does not monitor the completion of the work and even if you receive no credit for doing it. Using the study guide will reinforce content from

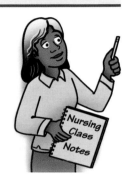

SMART STUDY TIP

Scope of Practice

When preparing for nursing exams, recall that all answers you choose will be *nursing related*. Note that as the nurse, it is beyond the scope of practice to prescribe treatments or medications or to alter current prescriptions. Keeping this in mind while taking nursing exams will assist you in eliminating incorrect options.

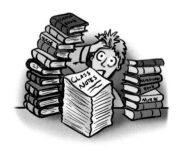

the textbook and help with retrieving knowledge in future courses. In addition, some questions and information in the study guide often will be placed on your exams as test questions.

The second type of study guide that may be available is provided by your course instructor. This type of study guide lists content areas that you need to be sure you understand. In nursing studies, you will receive a vast amount of information from class handouts, class notes, and your textbooks. It can be overwhelming to weed through the information and determine what is important. Study guides provide you with a focus or direction for study and review. If your instructor lists a certain point in the study guide, then it must be important!

If your course instructor does not provide a study guide, then make your own. As you read the assigned chapters in your textbook, list the important points that you are highlighting. Also, as you review your class notes, add the important points to your self-created study guide. These will be the points that your instructor emphasized or may have said in class, "Be sure that you remember this!"

The third type of study guide is based on electronic learning, through adaptive quizzing or an alternate type of questioning resource that provides you with a report to indicate your progress. The reports generated from these types of resources can be helpful to both faculty and students to understand where students need to improve. Work with your instructor to best utilize these resources in reinforcing content and learning new content, as well as in exam preparation.

Study Groups

Study groups are helpful for some students, but not all students, so think about whether they will be helpful to you. Knowing your personal learning style will guide you in deciding whether a study group will work for you. You may be the type of learner who requires quiet and alone time to absorb the material, or you may be the type who learns best by reviewing content aloud with others. One strategy to consider is to do your quiet and alone studying first; then, once you feel that you have mastered the content, join a study group to reinforce information. Just be sure that you meet your needs, and do not be persuaded to join a study group if it will not work for you. Whether you study alone or with a group, try to anticipate what the instructor may ask on the exam. Also, it is helpful to create your own exam questions for review.

Standardized Testing: Why Is It So Important?

You may be given a standardized test at the end of each nursing course. This depends on the preference of your nursing program. These tests are administered primarily to assess your mastery of the content. Another purpose of standardized tests is to provide detailed reports on your strengths and weaknesses and on content areas you need to improve on. These reports will help you plan both short-term and long-term goals and provide you with valuable information for planning for the NCLEX exam. Some standardized exam proprietors have demonstrated through research that scores on standardized exams are predictive of NCLEX success. So take these standardized exams seriously and prepare for them even if they carry no weight with regard to course grading. These are your individualized study guides for future nursing courses and the NCLEX exam. Get a three-ring binder, label it "My NCLEX Study Guide," and place all your detailed standardized reports in this binder. When it comes time to focus on future exams, primarily the NCLEX exam, you will have what you need to direct your review and study.

NCLEX EXAM TIP

Use the NCLEX Test Plan as a study guide. Highlight the NCLEX Test Plan content and activities that you have learned and mastered as you proceed through your nursing courses.

CHAPTER 2

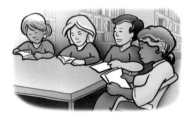

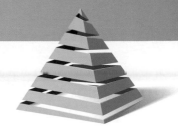

Developing Study Skills

What Are Good Study Skills?

Having good study skills means you have developed conscious and skillful study habits, devised a consistent study schedule that incorporates methods for learning and understanding nursing content, and established a routine that promotes use of clinical judgment and synthesis of client information. Good study habits develop through time management and discipline. It is important to remember that success comes from working hard, so you should think beyond the task of studying; instead, incorporate study into your daily routine. Time management is an important factor in developing good study habits and skills. In the nursing program, you will be very busy with classes, simulation and skills lab, and clinical experiences. You will need to complete a great deal of reading and assignments and take and pass exams. There are only 24 hours in a day, and you will have a limited number of hours in each day to spend on studying, so you need to use this time as effectively and as efficiently as possible. To help you get started, this chapter discusses some important points for developing these habits and skills. Chapter 1 gives additional study habits and skills as they relate specifically to nursing exams.

How Do You Identify and Plan Your Study Times?

An important part of identifying time for study is using a calendar. The calendar can come in the form of an electronic calendar or the more traditional paper type of calendar. Choose the type that best fits your needs, and let it be your academic life-guide.

At the beginning of each semester, enter your class schedule into your calendar. Once you receive your course syllabus for each course, read it carefully and pay close attention to due dates for assignments and exam dates. Enter these dates in the calendar. In addition, enter into your calendar any other important dates, such as extracurricular activities or other personal activities you have scheduled. Carry your calendar with you when you go to class. The instructor may change an assignment due date or an exam date, so you want to be sure that you can make that change in your calendar. Once all this information has been added to your calendar, you can plan your study times.

Your calendar or academic life-guide is critical to your success in effectively managing your time and developing a study plan for the semester. Be sure to look at your calendar every day to plan for the following day. Look ahead to the next week, and note what is scheduled (e.g., an exam) or due (e.g., an assignment). If you are diligent about entering your semester schedule and course requirements into your calendar and reviewing your calendar daily, you can easily manage your time in a busy semester.

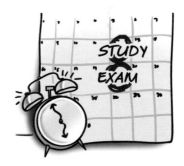

What Smart Study Habits Do You Need to Develop?

A habit is a pattern of behavior an individual establishes through repetition of the behavior. Habits can be good or bad, and you need to focus on developing good habits for studying. If you develop good habits and stick to them, you will be successful in the nursing program. You can develop many smart study habits for yourself, and you may already have some smart study habits in place that you developed while in high school. If you do, and if these worked, integrate these smart study habits into your college study plan. In addition, use the following top-10 pyramid points and smart study habits to help plan your study sessions.

Top-10 Pyramid Points and Smart Study Habits

Pyramid Point and Smart Study Habit 1: Plan Daily Specific Times for Studying

Look at your calendar to identify daily times that are free of any other commitments, such as class or clinical obligations, and make these your study times. Block these times off in your calendar as your study times. If you have breaks between classes, use them for study. For example, if you have a class from 8:00 AM to 10:00 AM and do not have another class until 1:00 PM, block out the time between these classes as study time. Set regular study time sessions for each day because this will help establish a routine that becomes part of your school life, and remember that it is acceptable to revise your study time sessions if necessary. In other words, if you find a particular study time is not working, select another time to take its place. During your study time be sure your time is spent on something related to your nursing course work.

Pyramid Point and Smart Study Habit 2: Try Not to Do Too Much Studying at One Time

It is better to plan more than one study time per day rather than to plan a lengthy block of study time. In other words, plan more than one study session daily. If you try to do too much studying at one time, you will easily tire and will not be able to concentrate and retain the information. Your study time will be more effective if you space it over shorter periods of time. Always maintain a positive attitude that you will be successful; you are studying and adequately preparing.

Pyramid Point and Smart Study Habit 3: Set Goals for Your Study Time

Think about what you want to accomplish during each study time. Set your goal in writing. This will help you keep focused and concentrate on your task at hand. Then work at meeting your goal. If for whatever reason you are unable to meet your set study time goal, do not become discouraged. Just look at where you left off, revise your goals for your next study session, and keep moving forward on your plan!

Pyramid Point and Smart Study Habit 4: Avoid Procrastination

Stick to your study schedule, and start studying as you planned to do. It is very easy to get off track and procrastinate because "I just do not feel like studying" or "the content or assignment is difficult" or "I would rather be doing something else." If you procrastinate, you will not meet your goals and will need to rush at a later time to complete your work. This places unnecessary stress on you and then you will end up having to cram, so start studying when you planned to. You will feel great after your study session knowing you accomplished a goal.

Pyramid Point and Smart Study Habit 5: Study the Most Difficult Material When You Are Most Alert

Some students do best with studying in the early-morning hours, some do better during the daytime hours, and some do best during the evening hours. You need to determine which time is best for you and when you are most rested, are alert, and have the most mental energy. Once you have determined this, use this time to work on your most difficult material. If you have the mental energy and stamina, this difficult material will be easier to grasp.

Pyramid Point and Smart Study Habit 6: Find a Special Study Place That Is Free of External Distractions

Your special study area should be quiet and comfortable. It can be your dormitory room, a study lounge, the library, a special room at home, or any other quiet area that works for you. Do not plan to study in a crowded or noisy room, such as a student social lounge, cafeteria, or cafe. Find your special area of tranquility, and post a "do not disturb" sign. Be sure that your cell phone is silenced and that any other phone or the television is off or far enough away from you so that you will not be distracted. Your study area should be adequate and roomy enough to support your necessary books, notes, and other essentials required to make the study session a success. The lighting in your special study area should be soft and provide the right amount of light to allow easy reading. Remember that temperature control is also critical to your comfort. If it is too hot, you may become sleepy. If it is too cold, you may begin to shiver and have difficulty concentrating. So find a room temperature that is comfortable for you.

Pyramid Point and Smart Study Habit 7: Seek Help When You Do Not Understand the Material

If you are having difficulty understanding the material, seek help. Remember that in many cases "two heads are better than one." You can ask another student to help explain a difficult content area that you do not understand, but do not ever hesitate to ask your instructor to explain the information to you. During your study session, if you are "stuck" and are not able to understand the information using the resources that are immediately available to you, move on to the next topic. Do not waste your valuable study time. Make note of the information that you do not understand, and seek clarification later. Start the next topic to make the most of the study time you have planned. Make your own "flash cards" to help you remember that difficult-to-learn information.

Pyramid Point and Smart Study Habit 8: Plan Study Breaks

Study breaks are important to keep your mind fresh and alert. All people differ in terms of the length of time that they can sit and study and maintain focus to concentrate, so don't compare your study needs to those of other students. How will you know when you need a study break? If you are having difficulty focusing and are moving through content but are not grasping the material, then you need a study break. If you read a page of content but at the end of the page you do not remember what you read, then you need a study break. If you are experiencing "mind chatter" or are thinking about things other than the task you are supposed to be focusing on, then you need a study break. If you are feeling sleepy or hungry, you need a study break.

Pyramid Point and Smart Study Habit 9: Eat a Healthy Diet, and Exercise Regularly

Eating a healthy diet will build and maintain your energy level and your stamina to meet your set goals. Did you know that eating fatty foods will slow you down? Yes they will; so you need to avoid fatty foods. As you will learn in nursing school,

> **SMART STUDY TIP**
>
> **Student-to-Student**
>
> When studying, if you find something you are having difficulty understanding, highlight it and make a note of it so you can ask your instructor for clarification during the next scheduled class or clinical time. In addition, take advantage of scheduled office hours for meeting with your instructor if you need extra help.

nutrition is important for the functioning of every cell in your body. A nurse is also a teacher, and you will be teaching your clients about the importance of eating healthy. So practice what you will be preaching!

Breakfast is an extremely important meal because it starts your day with the fuel that you need to think and perform all the activities ahead of you; however, be sure to eat a *healthy* breakfast. Stay away from bacon, sausage, and high-sugar syrups. Instead, for example, eat a bagel or toast with some peanut butter, cereal, or fruit, and drink plenty of water. Eat lighter meals and eat more frequently to keep your body fueled and energized. Include complex carbohydrates and protein in your diet for energy. In addition, carry snacks in your backpack for between meals or for your study breaks, but again, be sure that these snacks are healthy ones. Also, be careful not to include too much caffeine in your daily diet. Caffeine will make you jittery and nervous and cause you to have difficulty focusing and concentrating. Remember that a car needs gas or it will not run; so think about your body as the motor vehicle needing healthy food to move along and progress efficiently through the day!

Exercising regularly is another extremely important habit to develop. Exercise will enhance or maintain your *physical fitness* and strength and your overall *health.* Regular physical exercise also boosts the immune system, helps prevent disease, and improves your mental health. So get into the habit of exercising regularly. As with healthy eating, you will be teaching your clients about the importance of regular exercise. Again, practice what you will be preaching! What type of exercise should you do? That depends on what you like to do. It can be anything from walking or running to working out at a gym. Even simply getting into the habit of walking to class rather than driving to class will help. Exercise is also a great outlet when you take a study break; take a walk during your break. This will get your circulation flowing, and you will find that your mind will clear and you will be able to focus and concentrate.

Pyramid Point and Smart Study Habit 10: Get an Adequate Amount of Sleep Every Night

Sleep is like food, air, or water. You need it to think and function adequately, and you need it to survive. Lack of an adequate amount of sleep will cause mental, emotional, and physical fatigue and irritability. Think about it—do you want to go into a classroom to take an exam feeling irritable or mentally, emotionally, or physically fatigued? Of course not, because then you are placing yourself at risk for failure. If you develop a schedule for studying and stick to it, then you will not have to worry about being up all night preparing for an exam the next day. One of the worst things that you can do is to cram the night before an exam and stay up all night studying. If you do this, it will be very difficult to focus and concentrate while taking the exam. If you have developed a structured study plan and stuck to it, the night before the exam will require simply a review of the content. So get into the habit of going to bed at night at a specific time that will provide you with an adequate amount of quality sleep.

Do you have difficulty falling asleep? If you do, this is probably because you are lying in bed thinking about all sorts of things, such as everything that you need to get done over the next day, the next week, and the remainder of the semester; or you may have other sorts of things on your mind. Whatever it may be that is keeping you awake needs to be eliminated from your mind. How do you do this? This may be a trial-and-error sort of task that will require implementing various measures or strategies to help you fall asleep until you find the one that will work for you. Remember that a measure that works for someone else may not work for you; however, if you determine what will work for you and get into the habit of implementing this measure repetitively, you will find that you will easily be able to fall asleep at night. Some measures to help you fall asleep are listed in the following box.

Measures to Promote Sleep

Develop a time schedule for when you will go to bed at night.
Avoid taking naps during the day.
Avoid consuming caffeine-containing drinks and foods.
Eat healthy and exercise regularly (avoid exercise within 3 or 4 hours of bedtime because activity increases metabolism and alertness for a few hours).
Avoid eating heavily close to bedtime.
Adjust the room temperature to meet your physical needs; a cool environment is best.
Keep the lights off in the room at bedtime.
Ensure a quiet environment; place a "sleeping" sign on your door, and use comfortable earplugs if necessary.
Turn your device that displays a clock around or place it in a drawer so that you cannot see it.
Perform a relaxation technique, such as reading; slow, deep breathing; or meditating.
Use a natural sleep remedy, such as drinking a cup of warm caffeine-free tea.

NCLEX® EXAM TIP

When you graduate from nursing school and are preparing to take the NCLEX exam, remember that you have been successful up to this point. Therefore, the study habits and study skills that you used during your nursing education were effective. Use these same study habits and study skills to prepare for the NCLEX exam!

What Study Skills Are Important?

Effective study skills develop once you have your study schedule in place and begin to implement your plan of study. Effective study skills also develop from good smart study habits. You may already have effective study skills in place that you developed when you were in high school; if you do and these worked for you, continue with these study skills during your nursing education. Remember that everyone is different, and what may work for someone else may not work for you. So it is important to know what works for you! This chapter provides some of the many study skills that you can implement.

Good Listening Skills

It is vital to your success that you become a good listener. Listen, and get to know your instructor. Listen carefully for verbal indicators made by your instructor that will alert you to what is important to note. Some verbal indicators are statements that begin with the words: "Never forget …," "Please understand …," or "This is definitely on the NCLEX exam." Listen to the inflection of your instructor's voice, and if he or she suddenly accents some content area, take that note. If your instructor becomes more animated during part of the lecture, pay attention and take note of that content. Finally, whatever the instructor reviews in class is worth highlighting because it will likely be on the next exam as an exam question.

If you are going to succeed as a good listener, you must get your mind prepared before arriving to class. You must leave the daydreaming and "mind chatter" at home and come to class ready to pay close attention to every word the instructor speaks. You may not always find the content being discussed interesting, but keep in mind that you will be tested on the material, and it is your responsibility to listen and learn.

Always pay attention to what your instructor may write on a classroom board or provide in a handout. If the instructor takes the time to write or diagram something on a board or in a handout, you can be fairly certain that this information will turn up on the exam as an exam question.

Effective Note Taking

Be sure to bring everything you need, such as a notebook, computer, or tablet to class for note-taking. Highlight any key points during the lecture. If you are allowed to bring your computer or tablet to class for taking notes, be sure that your computer battery is fully charged and you have easy access to an electrical outlet for recharging. Many instructors will provide PowerPoint presentations.

You can take notes in the notes section of the PowerPoint as it is covered during class. If the instructor doesn't use PowerPoint presentations or doesn't lecture during class, notes should be taken during in-class activities such as case studies, group discussions, or simulation.

Good note taking is a talent that requires practice and good listening skills. First, remember that you are taking notes, not writing a novel. You cannot write down every word that the instructor says. Develop a personal shorthand that will help you transcribe the important points of your instructor's lecture. For example, the instructor may say, "The signs and symptoms include nausea, vomiting, and diarrhea." Your shorthand note could read, "S&S = N/V/D." With practice you can develop an abbreviated note-taking style that will work successfully for you. Also, most students find that rewriting their notes after class is a good smart study habit because it clarifies and reinforces what they have read and learned in class. You may find this strategy valuable to add to your study regimen. Some additional points related to effective note taking are provided in Chapter 1.

Reading Skills

In nursing, reading involves active involvement with your textbook. Plan to do detailed reading to extract information accurately. In other words, do not scan or skim the content in the textbook chapter. In addition, always have a medical/nursing dictionary with you when you study; when you come across a word that you never heard of (e.g., edema, which means swelling), look it up and make note of it in your notebook as a new vocabulary word. Chapter 1 provides strategies to implement when you are reading your textbook. Some additional strategies include the following:

1. Read one section at a time under each major heading. Highlight the key points. Develop some questions that come to mind and write these questions in your notebook. Find the answers to the questions and if necessary, plan to bring the question to class for further clarification.
2. After you finish reading some of the sections under major headings, look again at the questions that you developed and think about the answers. If you were not able to recall the answers, review these sections in the text again. Then continue reading the chapter.
3. After you have read the entire chapter, review all the highlighted key points and any notes that you made, and review the questions that you have developed to see if you can answer them. If you cannot, then review these areas in the chapter again. It may also be helpful to make a flash card for any information that is difficult.

Interactive Learning

Many textbooks are bundled with electronic interactive learning resources. It is recommended that you read the chapter first, then use the interactive learning and quizzing resources to reinforce what was learned. These resources typically utilize a questioning format and produce results reflecting student progress. Students can use this report to determine if more studying is required and what content they should focus on.

Remembering Content

Remembering what you have listened to in class and remembering what you read and study are essential for your success in passing exams, success in future nursing courses, and success on the NCLEX exam. If you are unable to remember what you learned, then you will be unable to apply the information in future nurs ing courses, in the clinical setting, or on the NCLEX exam. Some strategies for remembering content include rewriting class notes, reading your class notes every day, doing the required reading before coming to class, highlighting key points in your textbook as you read, completing study guides provided for you, and creating flash cards for the material that is difficult for you. Chapter 1 provides points related to these strategies.

An additional strategy that you can use to remember content is to develop an acronym; a mnemonic device; or easily remembered letters, words, or phrases for difficult information. Many times your instructor will identify ways to remember difficult information, but you can develop these on your own or with your classmates. Three examples of these are regular and NPH insulin, decorticate versus decerebrate posturing, and MAOIs.

Regular Insulin and NPH Insulin—RN

RN—Although NPH and regular insulin is used less frequently than in the past, when mixing regular and NPH insulin in the same syringe, draw up the **R**egular insulin first, followed by the **N**PH insulin. Remember the acronym **RN** when mixing both these types of insulin in the same syringe.

Tip for the nursing student: Insulin is a medication that is prescribed for some clients with diabetes mellitus. Many times it is necessary to administer both regular and NPH insulin, and these insulins may need to be mixed in the same syringe. There is a procedure for mixing these insulins, and it is important to draw the regular insulin into the syringe first. You will learn about this procedure when you study medication administration and in your medical-surgical nursing course when you study endocrine disorders.

Decorticate Posturing Versus Decerebrate Posturing

In de**cor**ticate (flexor) posturing, the upper extremities (arms, wrists, fingers) are flexed on the chest. In other words, the upper extremities are brought to the **core** of the body; whereas in decerebrate (extensor) posturing, the upper extremities are stiffly extended with internal rotation and pronation of the palms. Therefore, when trying to distinguish the characteristics of each type of posturing, remember that in de**cor**ticate, the upper extremities are brought to the **core** of the body.

Tip for the nursing student: Posturing is an abnormal position assumed by a client with a neurological disorder and indicates deterioration in the client's condition. You will learn about posturing in your medical-surgical nursing course when you study neurological disorders.

Monoamine Oxidase Inhibitors (MAOIs)

MAOIs are antidepressants and include the following medications:
Phenelzine sulfate
Tranylcypromine sulfate
Isocarboxazid
Selegiline

Remembering the acronym **PTIS** as meaning **P**lease **T**ake **I**t **S**eriously will assist in remembering the medications that belong in the MAOI classification.

Tip for the nursing student: MAOIs are medications that are used to treat depression. Adverse effects are associated with this classification of medications, and clients must follow specific dietary measures when taking them. Therefore, it is important to know which medications are in the classification of MAOIs. You will learn about MAOIs in your pharmacology and your psychiatric/mental health nursing courses.

SMART STUDY TIP

Scope of Practice

As a student in the clinical environment, you will create your own acronyms to use in certain situations, such as an acronym for an electrocardiogram (ECG) pattern and its interpretation. These acronyms will assist you in nursing practice, but remember that these cannot be used for documentation unless they are acceptable for use by the clinical agency.

Critical Thinking Skills

Critical thinking skills involve an intellectual process of actively analyzing information. It is essential that you develop good critical thinking skills because you will be making very important decisions and clinical judgments in the clinical setting when you care for clients. In the clinical setting, you will gather information and then will need to analyze, synthesize, and apply this information, make decisions, and evaluate the outcome.

Critical thinking skills take time to develop, but if you are mindful of the fact that you need to develop these skills, you can set some goals for yourself regarding becoming a critical thinker. So what can you do to develop critical thinking skills? One strategy that you can begin with is curiosity. Consistently ask yourself questions as you read nursing content. Write these questions in your notebook and then present them in class for discussion. This discussion will generate critical thinking among your classmates. Another strategy to develop critical thinking skills is to learn content from an analytical perspective. In other words, be creative. Look at a collection of information that you are learning, and instead of simply learning the facts, think about the information in an investigative manner. For example, if you are learning about standard precautions (a basic level of infection control that needs to be used in the care of all clients all of the time to reduce the risk of transmission of microorganisms), do not simply remember that handwashing must be done before and after contact with a client or that gloves are worn when coming in contact with blood or body fluid excretions and secretions. Think about this content critically, and question *why* these procedures need to be followed. Critical thinking takes more time and energy than simply learning facts and content, but it is an essential part of the learning process in nursing. So work at it, and make it a habit to be curious and creative and think about things critically.

SMART STUDY TIP

Preparing for Clinical

An integral part of your success as a student in clinical is your ability to think critically. You will be assigned to care for a client (or clients) and will be required to interpret pertinent information regarding the client's status and determine the important nursing considerations with regard to client care. Gather all of your client's information before the clinical session and think critically by determining why certain medications and treatments are prescribed for the client and why the client may have a certain laboratory result or diagnostic finding.

When Should You Start to Study for an Exam?

Studying for an exam begins the moment your course begins and you start reading your textbooks, attending class, and taking notes. Always pay close attention to the syllabus for upcoming test dates and use the syllabus as a planning guide. Plan and schedule daily study sessions for yourself, and read your class notes taken up to that point, with a particular focus on your new notes, the notes taken that day. This is an important part of preparing for an exam so that you will not be faced with cramming the night before. Procrastinating and waiting until the last minute to prepare for an exam are two of the worst things that you can do because these place unnecessary pressure on you and set the stage for developing test anxiety. So start preparing right away. One week before a scheduled exam, increase the time that you spend in your study session. The amount of time that you need to plan for your study sessions depends on the type of learner that you are and how quickly you are able to grasp the new content and material. A guideline that you may want to use to begin scheduling your study sessions is to plan 1 hour of study for every 3 hours of class time. So, for example, if your nursing class is scheduled for 3 hours, then plan for a 1-hour review of your notes after the class. Then 1 week before the exam, increase the time that you spend in each study session to 2 hours of study for every 3 hours of class time. This is only a guideline to help you think about planning and is not a rigid rule that needs to be strictly followed. Remember that everyone is different when it comes to learning needs, so think about what works best for you and plan accordingly. Chapter 1 provides additional information regarding using your class notes to prepare for an exam.

Will a Study Group Work for You?

This question is one that only you can answer. If the idea of studying in a group environment has worked for you in the past and you feel comfortable with this type of study arena, by all means continue this way of studying. If you are the type of learner who needs to be alone to study in order to master the content, then a study group will not work. Some combination of alone study time and group study time may also be an option for you. In other words, you can plan to study on your own, and once you are comfortable with the content and think that you have mastered it, join a study group to help reinforce content.

Study groups can be very helpful when preparing for an exam, but the study team needs to be motivated and stay on track with regard to the goal of the group. A study group can easily get off track and waste time discussing "outside of study" issues. If this happens, then the goals of the group may not be met. Be sure to join a study group that has the same goals as you, and be sure that your study partners have personalities that are compatible with yours so that you can easily work together. This will help with motivating and driving each other to meet group goals.

The size of the study group should be between three and five, and every group member needs to come to the study time prepared to participate. When the study group is initially created, group goals and expectations should be developed. Each study session should have established goals and work to achieve the study goals within the study time. Each group member should accept a task with regard to the contribution or role he or she will take as a member of the group. For example, if the content for a scheduled exam includes the medical-surgical areas of coronary artery disease, myocardial infarction, and heart failure, then each group member should accept a topic area or a part of it for presentation at the study group session. At the end of each study session, the group members should decide when the next study group session will be, what the goals for the session will be, and each member's assignment. Remember that study groups are made of individuals and each individual is a part of the team. If each team member contributes to the study session as planned, then the team will succeed. Chapter 1 provides additional information about study groups.

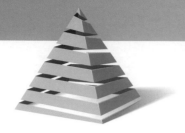

CHAPTER 3

Reducing Test Anxiety

What Is Test Anxiety?

Test anxiety can cause a significant amount of stress related to preparing for and taking an examination. Test anxiety is a type of performance anxiety because the individual is under pressure to do well in order to pass. A person with test anxiety experiences tension and stress before, during, and possibly after finishing an exam. Test anxiety can block the thinking processes and cause poor performance with testing, regardless of the amount of preparation for the exam. This chapter provides some tips and strategies to help you prevent test anxiety and to reduce the anxiety if it occurs. However, if you feel that your test anxiety is so overwhelming that you are unable to focus or concentrate, seek assistance. As a starting point, you may want to contact your advisor to discuss your test anxiety experiences.

How Can You Know If You Have Test Anxiety?

You have attended all your classes, you have done all your reading assignments, you have participated in class discussions, and you followed your study plan. Then the day of the test arrives, and you feel so nervous that you freeze up and are unable to focus, think, or concentrate. It is normal to feel a little nervous and stressed before a test, and actually a little anxiety can keep you sharp and alert during testing. But if the anxiety is overwhelming and you cannot control it, your thinking processes will be blocked, you will have difficulty focusing and concentrating, and you will forget the material that you learned.

Anxiety related to taking an examination can cause various symptoms. Test anxiety can bring on a feeling of "butterflies in the stomach," a stomachache, nausea, vomiting, or diarrhea. Test anxiety also can cause headaches, excessive sweating, a rapid heart rate (feeling like the heart is pounding), and rapid breathing. Some students may describe their physical feelings related to test anxiety as "I feel like throwing up" or "I feel like I might pass out." Test anxiety can also cause overwhelming feelings of helplessness and a sense of feeling out of control of the situation.

What Causes Test Anxiety?

Taking a test can be stressful because you know that you need to perform well to pass the exam. Physiologically, when you feel stressed, your body releases a hormone called *adrenaline*, which prepares you for the stressful situation. This is called the *fight-or-flight response* and is the same physiological response that occurs when someone encounters a dangerous situation. When the adrenaline is released, the physical symptoms of sweating, the heart pounding, and rapid breathing occur.

Someone who worries about everything or who thinks that he or she needs to achieve a perfect test score is likely to experience test anxiety. This person, who may be termed a *perfectionist,* may find it difficult to obtain anything less than a perfect score and may experience test anxiety because of the great pressure and stress being placed on oneself.

A person with negative thoughts about how he or she will perform promotes test anxiety. Previous experiences, such as poor performance on a previous test, can affect how one might feel about testing. Negative experiences can affect self-confidence and the belief that one can be successful. Focusing on the negative takes a lot of energy and drains the individual of energy needed to perform because it causes fatigue and makes the individual feel worse. This pessimistic view of how one might perform creates more intense feelings of anxiety and distracting thoughts, setting the stage for failure on the exam.

Another cause of test anxiety is a lack of preparation for the exam. If you are not prepared for an exam, then you will be worried about passing, and this will produce anxiety. Anxiety from lack of preparation occurs as a result of failing to organize and manage your time, poor study habits, not studying enough, or feeling tired because of being up all night and cramming for the test.

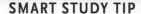

What Will Help Prevent Test Anxiety?

One important way to prevent test anxiety is to be as prepared as possible for the exam. Time management and a structured study plan also prevent test anxiety because you are planning ahead and working on preparing for a test and other assignments well in advance of the scheduled date. You cannot procrastinate. Procrastinating places unnecessary pressure on you, creating test anxiety or making test anxiety worse. If you study daily rather than cramming at the last minute, you will know the content well enough so that you can recall it even if you are stressed. Preparation also builds your confidence because you will feel more comfortable about knowing the material. Refer to Chapters 1 and 2, which provide specific tips and strategies on smart study habits, study skills, and time management that will help you prepare for an exam. Incorporating these tips and strategies on test preparation into your academic life will help prevent test anxiety.

What Can You Do When You Are Experiencing Test Anxiety?

Relaxation techniques can help when you experience test anxiety because they relax you and help you gain control. Several types of relaxation techniques that you can use include resting your eyes, muscle relaxation/tightening exercises, meditation, or breathing exercises. Use whatever technique works for you. Breathing exercises are a commonly used technique that can be done at any time, including during your testing. These exercises will not only help relax you but also oxygenate your body. Think about it: you would ask a postoperative client whose pulse oximetry reading is low to take slow, deep breaths. When the client takes the breaths, what happens? The pulse oximetry reading rises. This same effect will occur for you if you take slow, deep breaths, which will increase oxygenation throughout your body and tissues and help you relax and control your anxiety. In addition, the slow, deep breaths will give your body and brain an oxygen boost. And wouldn't you want your brain to be as oxygenated as possible when taking the exam?

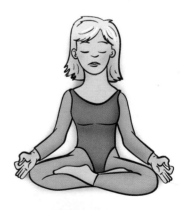

Now, how do you effectively take slow, deep breaths? If you become anxious before or during the exam or if you are having difficulty sleeping the night before the exam, sit or lie in a comfortable position, close your eyes, relax, inhale deeply through your nose, hold your breath to a count of 4, exhale slowly through your mouth, and, again, relax. Repeat this breathing exercise several times until you begin to feel relaxed and free from anxiety. During the exam, if you find that you are becoming anxious and distracted and are having difficulty focusing, sit back,

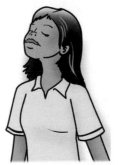

close your eyes, and perform your breathing exercises to help relax and get oxygen moving through your body. Remember that the slow, deep-breathing exercises will help you relax and gain control of the moment.

Breathing Exercises

Sit or lie in a comfortable position.
Close your eyes.
Relax.
Inhale deeply through your nose.
Hold your breath to a count of 4.
Exhale slowly through your mouth and relax.
Repeat until you begin to feel relaxed and free from anxiety.

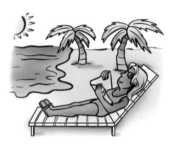

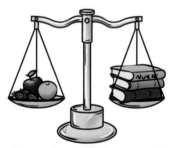

Remember, pamper yourself to maintain balance!

What Is Positive Pampering and Why Is It Important?

Positive pampering means that you take care of yourself from a holistic perspective. It helps maintain an academic and nonacademic balance as you prepare for any examination, which in turn will help alleviate some anxiety. You need to care for yourself by including physical activity, fun and relaxation, and a balanced and healthy diet in your preparation plan. You can implement several measures, identified next, to be sure that you are caring for you. Specific interventions for these measures are described in Chapter 2 under the heading "Top-10 Pyramid Points and Smart Study Habits." Be sure to read this section to help you incorporate positive pampering strategies into your daily academic life.

Just as you have developed a schedule for studying, you need a schedule that includes some fun and some form of physical activity. It is your choice—aerobics, running, weight lifting, bowling, a movie, a massage, going to the beach, or whatever makes you feel good about yourself. Time spent away from a hard study schedule and devoted to some form of fun and physical exercise pays its rewards 100-fold. You will feel more energetic and less anxious about your upcoming exam with a schedule that includes these activities.

Establish a balanced diet and healthy eating habits if you have not already done so. Eat lighter and well-balanced meals, and eat more frequently. Include complex carbohydrates and protein in your diet for energy. Avoid caffeine because it will make you jittery and anxious, and avoid eating fatty foods because they will slow you down and make you feel sleepy. If you are having difficulty planning a balanced and healthy diet, another resource is the MyPlate Food Guide, located at http://www.choosemyplate.gov.

 ## What Should You Do the Night Before the Exam?

Remember to avoid cramming the night before the exam because this will increase your test anxiety. Prepare ahead, and rest your body and your mind. Remember that the mind is like a muscle, and if it is overworked, it has no strength or stamina. Therefore, on the night before the exam, as long as you have prepared well and followed your study plan all along, put your textbook and notes away and get to bed early. At bedtime perform deep-breathing exercises and listen to soothing music to help you relax and fall asleep. Set your alarm clock and plan to get up 15 to 30 minutes earlier than usual to have some time to wake up and eat a healthy breakfast. If possible, walk to class on the day of the exam to get the circulation and oxygen moving throughout your body. Remember that you have prepared yourself well for the challenge of the day.

How Can You Control Your Test Anxiety Before the Exam?

Before the examination you may become anxious and think, "I am not ready!" As a nursing student, it is important to remember that it is very difficult to feel 100% prepared for an exam. This feeling is not necessarily caused by inadequate preparation and is usually caused by test anxiety. First, stay away from peers who are experiencing anxiety before the exam. These peers may be discussing content and what might be asked on the test, and this is going to cause confusion and fear about preparing well enough, contributing to anxiety. Next, stop whatever you are doing and reflect on all that you have accomplished in your preparation plan. Sit quietly somewhere where you can concentrate on relaxing and tell yourself that you indeed prepared adequately for the test and are ready. Smile, brush those negative feelings away, do your breathing exercises, and keep repeating to yourself, "I am going to do well. I am prepared." Repeating this statement will build the extra confidence that you need by helping you maintain a positive attitude, relax, and focus before the exam.

How Can You Control Your Test Anxiety During the Exam?

During the exam, if you begin to experience any anxious feelings, sit back in your chair, close your eyes, and perform a relaxation technique, such as breathing exercises. These will help relax you. The breathing exercises are also helpful if you begin to feel your mind wandering, if you feel distracted, or if you are unable to concentrate on the test question. Oxygenating your body will help you focus and concentrate on the exam question.

Structured Sequence for Taking an Exam

Place your name on the test and on any other required testing documents.*
Read the directions.
Skim through the pages in the test so that you have an idea of how to pace yourself.*
If you are allowed to write on the test, jot down data that you needed to memorize and may need as a reference, such as a laboratory value. Remember though that you will not be able to do this when you take the NCLEX. Jotting down data is known as *brain dumping* and is not allowed when you take the NCLEX.*
Read each question and all options slowly and carefully.
Take your time when answering a question.
Use nursing knowledge and test-taking strategies to help you answer the question.
Skip any questions that are difficult.*
Answer all the questions that you know and that are easy for you to answer.*
Once you have answered all the easy questions, go back to the questions that were difficult.*

Note: These tips relate specifically to pencil-and-paper tests.

NCLEX® EXAM TIP

On a pencil-and-paper nursing exam taken in nursing school, one strategy is to skip questions that are difficult and go back to them once you have answered as many as you can. On the NCLEX exam, you need to remember that you will not be able to skip a question and then go back to it. On the NCLEX exam, you must answer the question on the computer screen in front of you or the test will not advance. So be prepared for this type of testing when you take the NCLEX exam.

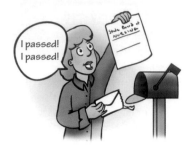

That Positive Attitude: How Can You Maintain It?

Maintaining a positive attitude will lead to success. It is natural to be a bit apprehensive about the path before you, especially if you are a beginning nursing student; but it is critical to your continued success that you believe in yourself and your ability to confidently conquer the challenges in your nursing program. Surround yourself with positive thoughts and positive people, and remember that your self-confidence in your ability to succeed is critical to your continued success.

SMART STUDY TIP

Preparing for Clinical

It is normal to become anxious before going to clinical. Actions you can take to decrease this anxiety include researching your client's condition, any related diagnostic tests, laboratory results, and prescribed medications and treatments. Researching in advance will best prepare you, thus making the experience less anxiety producing. If you are not anxious or nervous, you will be able to perform at your best, so use these tips to reduce your anxiety when preparing to care for clients.

"Yes, I can do this."

When you start to fall into the trap of negative thought, stop! Control the moment and believe in who you are! Step out of the negative and into the positive and do not allow anything to stand in your path to success. The one phrase that should become your mantra is "Yes, I can do this." When you open your eyes in the morning and need to face a difficult day, this positive phrase should be your first thought. Use visual reinforcement to help maintain your positive attitude. On a piece of paper write the words "Yes, I can do this," and keep this with you always. When you face a difficult challenge or need to take an exam and have test anxiety, place these written words in front of you so that you can see them. You will constantly be reminded of your self-confidence and ability to be successful.

CHAPTER 4

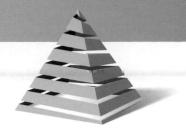

NCLEX® Preparation

 ## Where Does Preparation Begin?

NCLEX preparation began the moment you entered your nursing program. Your nursing courses, clinical experiences, reading and other assignments and activities, and any standardized examinations that may have been required to be taken prepared you for the NCLEX exam. In addition, all the practice questions that you reviewed from your course textbooks and NCLEX review book have reinforced content, refined your knowledge base and critical thinking and clinical judgment skills, and provided practice with test-taking strategies and how to answer a test question correctly. When you become an advanced student nurse and as you near the end of your program, NCLEX preparation will become your highest priority. At that time you need to fine-tune your nursing knowledge base, critical thinking and clinical judgment skills, and test-taking skills. You may feel overwhelmed and just not sure where to begin preparing for the NCLEX exam. You may even become more overwhelmed when you look at all the boxes of class notes that you have accumulated and all the textbooks that you have read during nursing school. Now you are saying to yourself, "Where do I start?" Let's look at some points about the NCLEX exam and your plan for preparation!

The NCLEX Test Plan: Why Is It So Important?

An important strategy for success is to become as familiar as possible with the NCLEX test plan. You can experience a significant amount of anxiety as you face the challenge of this examination. Knowing what the examination is all about will assist in alleviating your fear and anxiety.

The test plan for the NCLEX exam is developed by the National Council of State Boards of Nursing (NCSBN). This test plan is developed based on state laws and regulations, including nurse practice acts, and research studies done with newly licensed nurses to determine the nursing activities that they perform. Once this information is identified, the NCSBN formulates the test plan, and the test questions for the NCLEX exam are written. All the information that you will need about the test plan can be located at the NCSBN website at www.ncsbn.org. In fact, when you access this website, you are able to download a copy of the current test plan for your use. The test plan identifies the framework of the NCLEX exam and lists content areas and nursing activities that you will be tested on. This is an extremely valuable resource and can be used as one of your study guides for preparing for the NCLEX exam. Pearson Vue is the agency that delivers the examination provided by the NCSBN. Through this agency, you will schedule your NCLEX test date and testing center. An additional fee must be paid to Pearson Vue before testing can occur. See the following boxes for the NCSBN contact information and Pearson Vue contact information.

SMART STUDY TIP
Scope of Practice

When preparing for the NCLEX exam, as you begin to practice questions, always remember that the answer will most likely be something nursing related and within the scope of nursing practice. However, it is important to be familiar with the scopes of practice of other members of the interprofessional team so that appropriate consultations can be made; you may encounter questions on the NCLEX regarding consulting and making referrals.

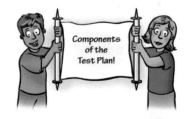

SMART STUDY TIP
Lifestyle Planning

When you download the NCLEX test plan, keep in mind that it is very lengthy. Download this test plan early on in your nursing program so you can plan your time around addressing all of the topics identified in the plan. You can make out a study calendar that will work for you to be sure that you address all areas.

In addition to the test plan, the NCSBN website provides information about the examination process, registering for the NCLEX exam, scheduling a test date, the testing center, and processing results. A tutorial is available to provide you with the experience of answering questions on the NCLEX exam. Multiple-choice questions and alternate-item format questions are also available for practice. Additionally, the NCSBN Clinical Judgment Measurement Model and the Next Generation NCLEX® (NGN) item types are presented on the website. So take the time to visit the NCSBN website and find out everything you need to know about the test plan and the testing experience. Remember that you want to face this challenge with as much information as possible, and knowing what the test is all about will help alleviate your anxiety!

What Are the Steps for Preparing?

Steps for Preparing for the NCLEX Exam

Step 1: Your Self-Assessment
Step 2: Your Preparation Plan and Goals
Step 3: Scheduling a Testing Date
Step 4: Implementing Your Preparation Plan
Step 5: Determining Your Readiness for the NCLEX Exam

Step 1: Your Self-Assessment

The first step in preparing for the NCLEX exam is a self-assessment. Your self-assessment is important because it will guide your development of a structured and individualized preparation plan. Open your "My NCLEX Study Guide" binder or computer folder and review any notes that you have taken about your strengths or weaknesses. Also review any detailed reports from standardized tests that you have taken, because these reports provide extremely valuable information about your areas of strength and the areas that you need to particularly focus on. If you have not yet set up your binder or computer folder labeled "My NCLEX Study Guide," you may want to do so to begin your preparation for the NCLEX exam. If you do not have copies of standardized test results or did not take standardized tests in your nursing program, then use your NCLEX review book to perform a self-assessment. Access the accompanying website in your NCLEX review book to take a pretest assessment exam or a 100-question comprehensive exam. Print out the results, place the printout in your "My NCLEX Study Guide" binder or computer folder, and identify your areas of strength and weakness to assist you in determining your preparation plan and goals.

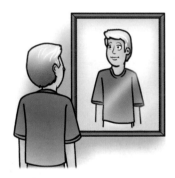

SMART STUDY TIP

Preparing for Clinical

Accessing the NCSBN website and reading the NCLEX test plan as early as possible in your nursing program can be of great benefit to you. Look at the learning activities listed in the test plan, and prepare to seek out these activities during your clinical experiences. This will also help prepare you for the NCLEX exam.

SMART STUDY TIP

Preparing for Clinical

Maintaining client confidentiality, build a portfolio of the clients for whom you cared and their diagnoses, noting the important aspects of nursing care you provided. You can then use this as a resource when preparing for your exams and for the NCLEX.

Step 2: Your Preparation Plan and Goals

Your self-assessment is an ongoing process. Your next step in your preparation plan and goals is to answer some specific self-assessment questions. The Top-10 Self-Assessment Questions are listed next with some pyramid points to consider as you develop a plan of preparation and goals.

The Top-10 Self-Assessment Questions and Pyramid Points

Question 1: What do I feel are my strong and weak areas in nursing content, and what strong and weak areas were identified in standardized testing or other assessment tests that I took?

Prioritize your plan of study, listing your weakest to your strongest area(s). You want to plan to begin your NCLEX preparation by reviewing your weakest content areas first; once you have demonstrated improvement in your weak area(s), proceed to review your stronger area(s).

Question 2: How do I normally study for exams: alone or in groups?

Study groups are very helpful for some students but not for all students. So you need to think about whether they will help you. You may be the type of learner who requires quiet and alone time to absorb the material, or you may be the type of learner who learns best by reviewing content aloud with others. Continue to do what you have done during your nursing program. If you studied alone, then this is what you should do to prepare for the NCLEX exam. You need to meet your needs, so do not be persuaded to join a study group if it will not work for you. You have been successful thus far, so keep doing what you were doing!

Question 3: Where is my special study place?

Think about how you have normally studied for your nursing exams and where you have studied. If you normally study alone in the early morning, then plan to study at this time. If you have a special study place, then continue to use it. Do not change these study habits, because they have worked for you in the past. Do what you normally do, and stick to that special study place that you used throughout nursing school!

Question 4: Am I comfortable with using a computer?

Most nursing students are quite comfortable using a computer. If this is not the case, then you need to use a computer so that when you take the NCLEX exam, any anxiety related to testing on a computer is eased. If you do not have a computer, then locate one that you can use, such as at your nursing school, school library, or a public library. Use the website that accompanies your NCLEX review book to begin studying by practicing test questions. In addition, while using the computer, access the NCSBN website and do the tutorial and any other NCLEX-related practice sessions provided.

Question 5: Do I complete exams within the allotted time?

Currently, for both the RN and the PN exam, there is a minimum of 75 questions and a maximum of 145 questions. Fifteen of these questions are pretest questions, which are unscored questions that are being analyzed for use on future exams. You do not know which questions are the pretest questions. You have 5 hours to complete the exam therefore, if each question on the NCLEX exam was individually timed, you would have approximately 2 minutes for each question on the exam. If you did not have a problem completing exams within the allotted time in nursing school, then you will probably not have a problem completing the NCLEX exam within the allotted time. If you had a problem completing exams on time in nursing school, then you need to work on picking up your speed with answering questions without jeopardizing the quality of how you are thinking through the question and answering it. You may ask, "How do I do this?" Practicing is the answer! Use an alarm clock, or set an alarm on your cell phone. Access the website that accompanies your NCLEX review book and select a 100-question exam. Allow approximately 2 minutes for each question. For example, set the alarm to ring in 200 minutes (or 3.3 hours). When the alarm rings, note how many questions you have completed. If you did not complete the 100 questions in the allotted time, note how many were unanswered. Then you need to work on picking up speed. Keep practicing until you are able to complete a 100-question test in the allotted time without jeopardizing the quality of how you are answering the questions. Keep in mind that the NCSBN plans to launch the NGN in April 2023. The number of questions and types administered, and the time for the test will change so we encourage you to access the NCSBN website at www.ncsbn.org for these updates.

Question 6: Do I have balance in life; do I exercise, have fun, relax, and eat a balanced and healthy diet?

Balance in life is extremely important if you want to be successful. Remember that all work and no play is not healthy. You cannot spend every hour of every day preparing for the NCLEX exam. You need to develop a study plan and stick to it, but you also need time to relax, have some fun, and eat healthy, because a healthy diet will build and maintain your energy level and your stamina to meet your set goals. Chapter 2 provides specific strategies related to exercise and eating healthy.

Question 7: Do I have test anxiety, and how do I control it?

Controlling your test anxiety is a must. Some anxiety is useful because it keeps your senses sharp and alert, and you definitely want to feel sharp and alert on the day of the NCLEX exam. However, overwhelming anxiety can block your thinking and become an obstacle. So think about what you did when you had to take exams during nursing school, and use these same strategies. Also, be sure to read Chapter 3 for strategies to reduce your test anxiety.

Question 8: Am I able to focus and concentrate during an exam?

If it is difficult to focus and concentrate during an exam, sit back in your chair and close your eyes. Inhale deeply through your nose, hold your breath to a count of 4, exhale slowly through your mouth, and relax. Repeat this breathing exercise four or five times, and then go back to the questions on the exam. These breathing exercises will fill your body and cells, including your brain cells, with oxygen. This will help you regain control, and you will be better equipped to focus and concentrate.

Question 9: Am I able to practice self-discipline and stick to a study plan?

Self-discipline is the ability to get yourself to do what you planned, such as adhering to a study plan, regardless of how you feel. It is very easy to get off track with your study plan because "I just do not feel like studying," or because "I would rather be doing something else." If you do not practice self-discipline, you will not meet your goals. Remember that every successful person works hard and has a great deal of self-discipline. If you want to be successful, practice self-discipline and stick to your study plan. You will feel great after your study session knowing that you accomplished your goal.

Question 10: Do I have a positive attitude?

A positive attitude will lead to success. You must stay positive about your ability to pass the NCLEX exam. Do not for one moment ever think that you will fail—

no negative thoughts! On a large piece of paper write your name in large letters across the top. Now underneath your name, in large letters, write the letters RN or LPN, depending on what your credentials will be when you become licensed. Now, doesn't that piece of paper with your name and credentials on it look great? Keep this with you always, especially during your study sessions. This visual will change any negative thoughts that you may have into positive ones!

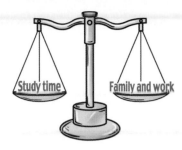

NCLEX® EXAM TIP

After you graduate from your nursing program, plan to spend at least 2 hours daily preparing for the NCLEX exam. Open your calendar and mark off days that you have obligations or commitments and will not be able to spend any time on NCLEX preparation. For the remaining days, set a 2-hour time schedule for NCLEX preparation time that will work for you considering your family and personal responsibilities. This is your time and needs to be uninterrupted, so shut off your cell phone and close off the world. This will help you concentrate and make the most of your preparation time. Remember, though, that you need to maintain balance in your life, so during your off-study hours, exercise, relax, and have fun.

Your NCLEX Preparation Plan

Do not change your study habits.
Review your weakest areas first.
Plan a 2-hour daily study session.
Practice a *minimum* of 4000 questions before taking NCLEX and be sure to practice NGN items.
Review all rationales and test-taking strategies accompanying your practice questions.
Learn ways to control your test anxiety.
Eat healthy and make time to relax, exercise, and have fun.

Step 3: Scheduling a Testing Date

Many nursing graduates ask the question, "How long should I wait to schedule an exam date for the NCLEX exam?" There is no easy or cut-and-dried answer to this question. This is a very individualized decision based on how much preparation you need to do, your goals, your preparation plan, and your time frame for implementation of your plan. You definitely need to prepare for this exam—this is critical. However, it is also extremely important that you do not wait too long. So, depending on your individual preparation needs, how much preparing you need to do, and how much time you have to prepare, schedule a date within 1½ to 2 months after graduation. Then, after graduation, get working on implementing your preparation plan. So get yourself ready and take that exam!

Step 4: Implementing Your Preparation Plan

Do not for a moment think that the way you will prepare for this exam is to read all your class notes and textbooks cover to cover. This is not the way to prepare for the NCLEX exam, and just the thought of doing this can exacerbate your sense of being overwhelmed. Place your boxes of class notes in a closet out of your sight. The information in them is much too detailed to assist in your preparation. Use your textbooks as a reference to review content areas that you find difficult when you are answering your practice test questions.

Practicing answering test questions is a must, and the best way to prepare for the NCLEX exam is to practice question after question after question on a computer. Practicing answering test questions yields a two fold reward: (1) you will strengthen

SMART STUDY TIP

Lifestyle Planning

When scheduling your study time, involve your family and friends in this planning. Make them aware of the fact that at this time you need their support in preparing for your exam. If they are involved in planning your study schedule, they will be supportive, and you will likely be better able to meet your goals successfully.

NCLEX® EXAM TIP

If for any reason you need to change your appointment to test, you can make the change on the candidate website or by calling candidate services. Refer to the NCLEX Examination Candidate Bulletin for this contact information and other important procedures for canceling and changing an appointment.

SMART STUDY TIP

Student-to-Student

Getting an NCLEX review book early on in your nursing program is important. You can review your course textbook and class notes to prepare for nursing exams, and then polish up your test preparation by using your NCLEX review book to answer as many practice questions as you can related to the content area that you will be tested on. This practice will ultimately help you in preparing for NCLEX as well!

Practicing answering test questions is a must!

your knowledge base of nursing content, and (2) you will become skillful in the use of test-taking strategies. The more you practice, the more prepared you will be for this exam. You should practice answering a *minimum* of 4000 NCLEX-style practice questions before taking the exam. You also need to practice answering NGN items; these will strengthen your clinical judgment abilities. This is very individualized, and to be proficient and skilled with answering exam questions correctly, many graduates need to practice answering even more than the minimum and need to practice between 4500 and 5000 NCLEX-style questions before taking the exam. You need to work at achieving a passing score on your practice tests. What is a passing score? Determine what you needed for a score to pass your nursing exams while in nursing school. You want to achieve at least that score and as a goal, an even higher score. It is important to remember that you also need to read the rationales and test-taking strategies that accompany each practice question because this will help you refine your nursing knowledge and critical thinking and clinical judgment skills. Remember that NCLEX questions will be presented at the cognitive levels of applying, analyzing, evaluating, synthesizing, and creating. Reading the rationales and test-taking strategies will improve your critical thinking and clinical judgment skills for answering future questions. Now, you may ask, "What do you mean by cognitive levels?" Table 4.1 provides a description of each level and an example.

You may have obtained a comprehensive NCLEX review book during your nursing program, and this book most likely contained both content review and practice questions. You can continue to use this book for NCLEX preparation, but you should also consider selecting a second resource that contains only practice questions. Be selective when deciding on a review book. Also, the preface of this book describes several different NCLEX review products available that will ensure your success on the NCLEX exam.

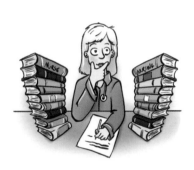

SMART STUDY TIP

Scope of Practice

When answering nursing course exam questions and when practicing questions from your NCLEX review book, remember that the answer is something that is within the scope of nursing practice. Usually, the answer that indicates notifying the primary health care provider is not the correct choice unless the situation presented is a life-threatening emergency. Your exams and the NCLEX exam seek to determine your clinical judgment ability about what you, as a nurse, would do in the presented client situation.

Selecting a Review Book

Make sure that your resource provides *at least* 4000 practice questions and case studies with accompanying NGN items.

Check to see if each question is accompanied by a rationale that provides an explanation for both the correct and incorrect options and a test-taking strategy.

Find out what other information accompanies each question, such as test plan codes, content area codes, health problem codes, cognitive skill codes, and concepts codes.

Be sure that a website with additional practice questions accompanies the book.

Be sure that the website accompanying the book offers a preassessment or assessment test and a generated study calendar based on your strengths and weaknesses.

Check to see what options for content selection are available for the practice questions on the website.

Note the modes for testing on the website, and look for a book that provides a study mode and exam mode.

Be sure that you are given detailed printouts of your performance on your practice tests.

Now that you have your NCLEX resource, start practicing questions. Begin selecting content areas that are your weakest, and select the study mode. The study mode will generate all possible available questions on the website in the content area selected and also provide the correct answer, rationale, and test-taking strategy as soon as you submit your answer. This is an important mode to use when you start your preparation, because you will learn as you go along. When you find that you have difficulty with answering a question, note the problem area in your NCLEX binder or folder, and after you have completed your study session, review this content in your textbooks or your NCLEX review book. Once you feel that you have strengthened your weak area by using the study mode, move to the exam mode and take an exam to note your improvement. This mode differs from the study mode in that it provides feedback after you answer all the questions rather than after each question. Continue with this pattern of review, moving from your weak areas to your strong areas.

Table 4-1

Level	Description and Example
Remembering	Recalling information from memorizing. Example: A normal blood glucose level is 70 to 99 mg/dL (4 to 5.5 mmol/L).
Understanding	Recognizing the meaning of information. Example: A blood glucose level of 60 mg/dL (3.4 mmol/L) is lower than the normal reference range.
Applying	Carrying out an appropriate action based on information. Example: Administering 10 to 15 g of carbohydrate, such as a half-glass of fruit juice, to treat mild hypoglycemia.
Analyzing	Examining a broad concept and breaking it down into smaller parts. Example: The broad concept is mild hypoglycemia and the smaller concepts are the signs and symptoms of mild hypoglycemia, such as hunger, irritability, weakness, headache, and blood glucose level lower than 70 mg/dL (4 mmol/L).
Evaluating	Making judgments, conclusions, or validations based on evidence. Example: Determining that treatment for mild hypoglycemia was effective if the blood glucose level returned to a normal level between 70 to 99 mg/dL (4 to 5.5 mmol/L).
Synthesizing/ Creating	Examining smaller parts of information, determining the broad concept, and creating a plan of care. Example: The smaller concepts are manifestations such as polyuria, polydipsia, polyphagia, vomiting, abdominal pain, weakness, confusion, and Kussmaul respirations. The broad concept is diabetic ketoacidosis (DKA). Creating a safe and individualized plan of care with the interprofessional health care team to treat DKA.

Adapted from: *Understanding Bloom's (and Anderson and Krathwohl's) Taxonomy, 2015,* ProEdit, Inc. http://www.proedit .com/understanding-blooms-and-anderson-and-krathwohls-taxonomy/
References: Ignatavicius, Workman (2016), pp. 1331–1333. Lewis (2017), Appendix C, Laboratory Reference Intervals.

Step 5: Determining Your Readiness for the NCLEX Exam

Remember that you are ready to take the NCLEX exam and that you were ready when you completed your nursing program. However, preparation for the NCLEX exam after graduation is a critical piece in being successful on this exam. At this point you have implemented your preparation plan, and now you need to determine your readiness and refine any remaining weak areas while waiting for your scheduled NCLEX date. How will you do this? Using the website accompanying your NCLEX review book, select the exam mode (100 practice questions), and select all content areas so that you generate an integrated content exam. Review your results and brush up on any weak areas. Continue to take these 100-question exams and follow this pattern until it is time to take the NCLEX exam. Remember that it is important to maintain momentum and a pattern when getting ready for this exam, so continue to practice questions every day.

It is time to take the NCLEX exam. Are you ready? Of course you are! As long as you followed your preparation plan and worked at strengthening any weak areas, you are ready for the challenge!

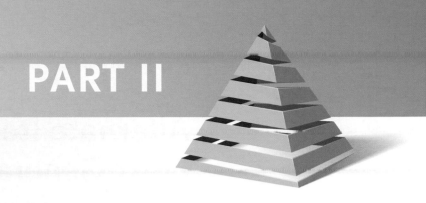

PART II

Strategies for Success

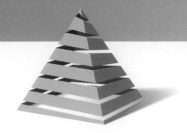

CHAPTER 5

Alternate Item Formats and Next Generation NCLEX® Item Types

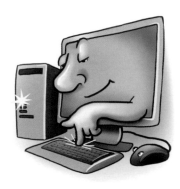

Introduction

An important strategy for success on examinations during your nursing program and for the NCLEX® is to become as familiar as possible with the types of questions that may appear on these examinations. Facing the challenge of achieving success on nursing examinations and the NCLEX may cause significant anxiety. Knowing what these examinations are all about will help alleviate that anxiety. This chapter describes the various types of alternate item format questions currently administered on nursing school examinations and on the NCLEX; it also describes test-taking strategies to assist in answering them correctly. Additionally, some Next Generation NCLEX (NGN) item types that may be on the NCLEX examination are also presented.

Clinical Judgment and Cognitive Skills

Clinical judgment is the observed outcome of critical thinking and decision-making (Dickison, Haerling, and Lasater, 2019). Sound clinical judgment skills are a critical component of competency and proficiency in nursing. The National Council of State Boards of Nursing (NCSBN) has created an NCSBN Clinical Judgment Measurement Model (NCJMM) that consists of applying six cognitive skills or processes to measure clinical judgment with an NGN item. These cognitive skills/processes include (1) recognize cues; (2) analyze cues; (3) prioritize hypotheses; (4) generate solutions; (5) take action; and (6) evaluate outcomes (Dickison et al., 2019). See Table 5-1 for the cognitive skills and their description. The NGN item types that will be presented in the NCLEX examination continue to develop as the NCSBN progresses in its research to determine the best ways to measure clinical judgment. The NCSBN plans to start to include these NGN item types as scored test items in the spring of 2023. Chapter 1 describes specific information about the measurement model for clinical judgment, the cognitive skills that measure clinical judgment, and NGN item types. We also encourage you to access the NCSBN website at www.ncsbn.org for the most up-to-date information about the NCSBN research, the measurement model, and the NGN item types that will be a part of the NCLEX examination.

What Is an Alternate Item Format?

Alternate item format questions are presented in a format other than a four-option multiple choice question. You will encounter these types of questions on nursing school examinations and the NCLEX examination. Therefore, it is critical to be familiar with these types of questions and the test-taking strategies for answering them correctly.

Table 5-1 Cognitive Skills/Processes and Descriptions

Cognitive Skill/Process	Description
Recognize cues	Identify significant (relevant) data; data can be from many sources (assessment/data collection)
Analyze cues	Connect data to the client's clinical presentation; determine whether the data are expected or unexpected and what the data means (analysis)
Prioritize hypotheses	Rank hypotheses (client needs or problems); determine the concerns or client needs and their priority (analysis)
Generate solutions	Use hypotheses to determine interventions for an expected outcome (planning)
Take actions	Implement the generated solutions, addressing the highest priorities or hypotheses (implementation)
Evaluate outcomes	Compare observed outcomes with expected ones (evaluation)

From Dickison, P., Haerling, K.A., & Lasater, K. (2019). Integrating the National Council of State Boards of Nursing Clinical Judgment Model into nursing educational frameworks, *Journal of Nursing Education, 58* (2), 72-78.

Alternate Item Format Questions

Fill-in-the-blank
Multiple response
Ordered response
Figure or illustration
Chart/exhibit
Graphic item options
Audio

The traditional alternate item format questions (those currently on the NCLEX) include fill-in-the-blank, multiple response, ordered response (also known as drag and drop); questions that contain a figure or illustration, chart/exhibit, or graphic option item; and audio formats.

A **fill-in-the-blank** question requires that you use the computer keyboard to type in a numerical answer. In a **multiple response** question you will need to use the computer mouse to click in a small box in front of the options to select the correct answers. In an **ordered response** question you will be asked to use the computer mouse to "drag and drop" the options from the left side of the screen (unordered options) to the right side of the screen in order of priority (ordered responses). In a **figure or illustration** question you may be asked to "point and click" (using the mouse) on a specific area (represented by a circle and also known as the *hot spot*), or you may be asked a question about the figure or illustration in a different type of question format. In a **chart/exhibit** question you will need to use the computer mouse to click on designated tab buttons to read client information in order to answer the question. In a **graphic item option** question, images will be presented as options, and you will need to select an image as an answer. The **audio** questions may require you to use a set of headphones. You will click on an icon to play the sound and then answer the question based on the content presented. You will be able to listen to the audio as many times as you need to.

The NCSBN provides specific directions for alternate item format questions to guide you in the testing process, and it is important to read these directions as they appear on the computer screen. The NCSBN provides a tutorial on their Web site to assist you in answering these types of questions. We encourage you to access the NCSBN website at www.ncsbn.org website to obtain additional information about the NCLEX examination and alternate item formats and to review the tutorial that the NCSBN provides for you.

SMART STUDY TIP

Student-to-Student

Before a pencil-and-paper exam in nursing school, make sure you have the materials you need, such as pens, pencils, scrap paper, and a calculator. For computerized exams, an on-screen calculator should be available for your use. Being prepared will help decrease your test anxiety!

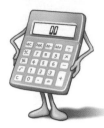

 ## What Test-Taking Strategies Are Helpful for Answering Fill-in-the-Blank Questions?

Fill-in-the-blank questions will ask you to perform a medication calculation, calculate a flow rate or infusion time for a specific intravenous solution, or calculate an intake or output record on a client. You will need to type in your answer, and the answer will be in a numerical format.

Test-Taking Strategies: Fill-in-the-Blank

Always follow the directions accompanying the question.
Use scrap paper (erasable noteboard on NCLEX) to perform the calculation.
Read the question and set up the formula you will use to solve the problem.
Think about the cognitive skill(s) being measured.
Be alert to the need to perform conversions.
Perform the calculation.
Verify your answer using a calculator (on-screen calculator for computer tests).
Record the answer using one decimal place or a whole number if asked to do so.
If rounding is necessary, perform at the end of the calculation.

In a medication calculation question, you need to record only the numerical component of the answer. In other words, if the answer to a question is 1.4 mL, type 1.4 only. Additionally, a medication calculation question may ask you to record your answer using one decimal place. If it so indicates, you must record the answer using one decimal place in order to answer correctly. For example, if the answer to a medication calculation is 2.33 and you are asked to record the answer to one decimal place, then you must type in the answer as 2.3.

In a question on intravenous flow rate or intravenous infusion time, the directions may indicate to round the answer to the nearest whole number. If this is indicated, then you must type in the answer as a whole number. For example, if the answer is 21.4 drops per minute, type the answer as 21. Remember that it is not possible to infuse 4/10 (0.4) of a drop.

In an intake and output calculation question, read the data carefully. These types of questions may require that you convert ounces (oz) to milliliters (mL). If you read the data carefully, you will note specifically what the question requires and will answer correctly.

Fill-in-the-blank questions will require you to use clinical judgment and generate solutions. Carefully consider each factor in the fill-in-the-blank question, and determine relevant and irrelevant data before solving the problem.

 ### SAMPLE QUESTION: Fill-in-the-Blank

A client drank 6 oz of juice and 8 oz of tea for breakfast, 4 oz of water to swallow medications at 0900 and 1300, and 8 oz of milk and 8 oz of coffee for lunch. The nurse determines that the client consumed how many mL of fluid?

ANSWER:
☐ mL

ANSWER: 1140

TEST-TAKING STRATEGY
Note the *subject*, a fill-in-the-blank question that requires that you calculate the total intake. Apply the cognitive skill, *generate solutions*. Read the data in the question carefully, and note that the client drank 4 oz of water at both 0900 and 1300. Also note that the question uses data expressed in ounces, and you are required to convert ounces to

milliliters. Use the erasable noteboard to add the total ounces and verify the amount using the on-screen calculator. Next convert the total amount of ounces to milliliters, recalling that there are 30 mL in 1 oz. Therefore, 6 oz of juice, 8 oz of tea, 4 oz of water at 0900, 4 oz of water at 1300, 8 oz of milk, and 8 oz of coffee total 38 oz. Next, to convert ounces to milliliters, multiply 38 by 30 to yield 1140 mL.

TIP FOR THE NURSING STUDENT

As the nurse, you will be required to monitor intake and output on clients, and you will need to demonstrate this skill before moving to clinical experiences. Intake and output measurements are used for a variety of reasons in the care of clients, including the monitoring of renal (kidney) function. The kidneys are primarily responsible for ridding the body of waste and play a major role in maintenance of fluid balance in the body. If a client's intake is proportionately different from his or her output, it can provide information about what is going on in the body and what disease processes may be occurring. You will learn more about medication calculations and intake and output measurements in your foundations nursing course.

SMART STUDY TIP

Preparing for Clinical

Read your assigned client's medication list before clinical and determine whether a calculation will need to be performed before administering a medication. When in clinical settings, be careful when administering medications and be aware of high-risk medications.

What Test-Taking Strategies Are Helpful for Answering Multiple Response Questions?

In a multiple response question, you will be asked to select or check all of the correct options that pertain to the question. The number of correct responses will vary; only one option could be correct or all of the options presented could be correct. These questions require you to use the computer mouse and click in a small box placed in front of the options that you select. Multiple response questions are used for various nursing content areas, including, but not limited to, nursing interventions, expected assessment findings, intended medication effects, medication side effects or adverse effects, or expected responses to treatment. Multiple response questions will require you to use clinical judgment and may address any of the six cognitive skills. Carefully consider each factor in the multiple response question, and determine relevant and irrelevant data before selecting your answer(s). You need to do exactly as the question asks, selecting *all* of the options that apply. No partial credit is given for some correct selections. Remember, *all* correct options must be selected for the answer to be correct. If you do not select all of the correct options or you include an incorrect option in your selections, then the test item is incorrect.

NCLEX® EXAM TIP

You should prepare to encounter several questions in the multiple response format on the NCLEX exam.

Test-Taking Strategies: Multiple Response

Always read the data carefully in the question.
Determine exactly what the question is asking (subject of the question).
Think about the cognitive skill(s) being measured.
Identify strategic words.
Note whether the question contains a positive or negative event query.
Use nursing knowledge and clinical learning experiences.
If a disorder is presented in the question, think about the pathophysiology associated with the disorder.
Visualize and form a mental image of the situation in the question, and think about what applies.
Read each option to yourself one at a time. If it applies to the situation, say "yes" to yourself and select the option. If it does not apply to the situation, say "no" to yourself and do not select the option.

SAMPLE QUESTION: Multiple Response

The nurse is caring for a client receiving intravenous (IV) therapy who is exhibiting manifestations of circulatory overload. What interventions would the nurse take? **Select all that apply.**

- ☐ Remove the IV.
- ☑ Monitor vital signs.
- ☑ Prepare to administer oxygen.
- ☑ Prepare to administer a diuretic.
- ☑ Place the client in an upright position.
- ☑ Notify the primary health care provider.

TEST-TAKING STRATEGY

This multiple response question requires that you select *all* interventions in the care of a client with circulatory overload, which is the subject of the question. Apply the cognitive skill, *take action*, and as you read each option and say "yes" or "no" to yourself, think about the pathophysiology associated with circulatory overload and recall that it results from excess fluid in the circulatory system. Visualize and form a mental image of the situation to help you determine that removing the IV is an incorrect action because IV access is needed to administer emergency medications.

▮▶ TIP FOR THE NURSING STUDENT

Circulatory overload means that there is an increased amount of fluid in the body, known as *increased blood volume* or *fluid overload*. This condition results in difficulty breathing and an elevation in the blood pressure. Circulatory overload is commonly caused by intravenous therapy and can result in complications, such as heart failure or pulmonary edema (fluid in the lungs). This is a critical situation requiring notification of the primary health care provider, and the goal of treatment is to rid the body of excess fluid. You will learn more about circulatory overload in your foundations and medical-surgical nursing courses when you focus on fluid and electrolyte imbalances.

What Test-Taking Strategies Are Helpful for Answering Ordered Response Questions?

In an ordered response question, you may be asked to use the computer mouse and to "drag and drop" the answers presented in order of priority. These questions usually ask you to prioritize nursing interventions or steps in a procedure. Information is presented in a question, and based on the data, you need to determine what you would do first, second, third, and so forth. Helpful test-taking strategies that are important for questions requiring prioritizing include the ABCs—airway, breathing, and circulation; Maslow's Hierarchy of Needs theory; and the steps of the nursing process. Applying the cognitive skill, *prioritize hypotheses* will be helpful in answering these question types. Refer to Chapter 8 for additional information on strategies for answering questions that require you to prioritize.

Test-Taking Strategies: Ordered Response

Use the ABCs—airway, breathing, and circulation.
Use Maslow's Hierarchy of Needs theory.
Use the steps of the nursing process.
Look for strategic words.
Determine whether the question identifies a positive or negative event query.
Think about the cognitive skill(s) being measured.
Visualize and form a mental image of the client or clinical event.
Use teaching and learning principles; remember, the client's readiness to learn is a first action.
Remember, hands are always washed first before any client contact.
Remember, treatments and procedures are always explained to the client before implementation.
Remember, the nurse checks for a signed informed consent before any invasive procedure.
Documenting a client's condition and response to treatment is done after care and implementation of treatments.

SAMPLE QUESTION: Ordered Response

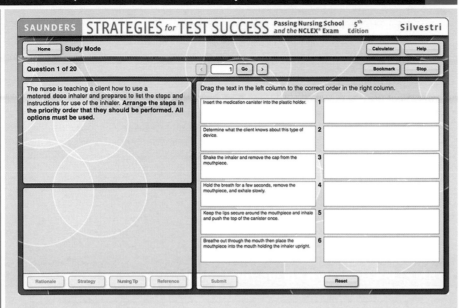

TEST-TAKING STRATEGY

Focus on the subject, an ordered response question that requires you to list in order of priority the steps and instructions in teaching a client how to use a metered-dose inhaler. Three strategies are important to consider when answering this question. First, use teaching and learning principles, recalling that it is important to first determine what the client knows about this medication administration system. Second, visualize the procedure and form a mental image as to how this medication system should be used; this will direct you to the correct order for its use. Third, apply the cognitive judgment skill *generate solutions*, and note that this is a procedural question, which asks you to determine steps in performing actions.

▌▌▶ TIP FOR THE NURSING STUDENT

A metered-dose inhaler is used to treat certain respiratory health problems, such as asthma or chronic obstructive pulmonary disease (COPD). The device provides a specified amount of the prescribed medication and disperses it into the lungs on inhalation. You will learn more about metered-dose inhalers in your pharmacology nursing course and fundamentals nursing course.

What Test-Taking Strategies Are Helpful for Answering Figure/Illustration Questions?

In a figure/illustration question, you are provided with a visual item, and you need to answer the question based on that item. Some examples of figures/illustrations that you may note on the NCLEX examination include rhythm strips, orthopedic or other assistive devices, anatomical areas of the body, or medication labels, to name a few. Some figure/illustration questions are in a multiple-choice or multiple response format. In other words, you are presented with a visual item and a question, and based on this information you need to answer by selecting the correct options. Other figure/illustration questions may require that you use the computer mouse to point and click on a part of the figure or may be in a fill-in-the-blank format. For example, you may be provided with a medication label and a question that requires you to calculate the dosage of a medication and type in the answer. The important concept to remember is that a figure/illustration question could be presented in any format, including multiple choice, fill-in-the-blank, multiple response, ordered response, or chart/exhibit. Any of the six cognitive skills could be measured in this question type, depending on the information presented.

Test-Taking Strategies: Figure/Illustration

Read all of the data in the question carefully, and focus on the figure/illustration.

Think about what the figure/illustration is representing.

Ask yourself, "What is the question asking?"

Focus on the subject of the question.

Look for strategic words.

Determine whether the question identifies a positive or negative event query.

Think about the cognitive skill(s) being measured.

Use nursing knowledge and clinical learning experiences.

Focus on the question format (fill-in-the-blank, multiple response, ordered response, chart/exhibit), and use the test-taking strategies for answering that type of question.

 SAMPLE QUESTION: Figure/Illustration

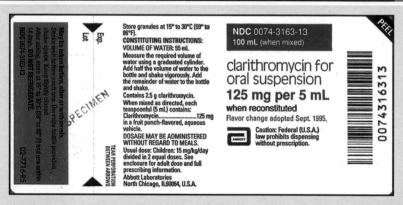

(From Kee J, Marshall S: *Clinical calculations: with applications to general and specialty areas*, ed 7, Philadelphia, 2012, Saunders.)

Clarithromycin oral suspension 250 mg twice daily has been prescribed for a client with pharyngitis. How many milliliters (mL) would the nurse prepare to administer one dose?

ANSWER:

[   ] mL

ANSWER: 10

TEST-TAKING STRATEGY

Focus on the subject, a figure/illustration question in a fill-in-the-blank format that requires you to perform a calculation. In other words, you are required to focus on the figure/illustration of the medication label, to perform a calculation to determine the amount of milliliters to administer in one dose, and to type in the answer. Use nursing knowledge of the formula for medication calculation doses, and apply the cognitive skill, *generate solutions.* On a pencil-and-paper test, perform the calculation on scrap paper and verify the amount using a calculator. On NCLEX, perform the calculation on the erasable noteboard, and verify the amount using the on-screen calculator. The formula and calculation are presented here.

Formula:

$$\frac{\text{Desired}}{\text{Available}} \times mL = mL \text{ per dose}$$

$$\frac{250mg}{125mg} \times 5mL = 10mL$$

TIP FOR THE NURSING STUDENT

Medication calculations are performed to determine the volume or amount of medication to be administered based on the dosage prescribed and the amount or volume that the nurse has available in the medication bottle. You will most likely be required to pass a medication calculation test before entering each clinical rotation, depending on the policy at your nursing school. You will learn more about medication calculations in your foundations course or related math courses before you enter the clinical setting.

What Test-Taking Strategies Are Helpful for Answering Chart/Exhibit Questions?

A chart/exhibit question will most likely provide you with data from a client's medical record and ask you a question about that data. These types of questions also may provide you with an exhibit of some type, such as a physician's prescription form with written orders or a laboratory form listing results from various laboratory tests. These questions will most likely be in the multiple choice format, but they also may be presented in other alternate item question formats. You may need to apply more than one of the six cognitive skills with these question types, as there will be much information to consider. You will need to determine relevant and irrelevant data, and potentially the appropriate nursing actions and evaluation for the scenario.

Test-Taking Strategies: Chart/Exhibit

Read all of the data in each tab in the chart or exhibit.
Avoid "skimming over" the information presented.
Focus on the subject of the question.
Determine relevant and irrelevant data.
Identify a relationship between the subject of the question and the data provided.
Look for strategic words.
Determine whether the question identifies a positive or negative event query.
Think about the cognitive skill(s) being measured.
Reread the data provided, and use nursing knowledge and clinical learning experiences to answer correctly.
Note the question format being presented, and use the test-taking strategies for that type of question.

SAMPLE QUESTION: Chart/Exhibit

Prednisone is prescribed for a hospitalized client with severe rheumatoid arthritis. Which laboratory result would the nurse monitor **most** closely?

CLIENT'S CHART

History	Medications	Diagnostic tests
Diabetes mellitus Gout Hypertension	Insulin glargine: 16 units subcutaneous daily at bedtime Allopurinol: 100 mg oral daily Atorvastatin: 10 mg oral daily Metoprolol tartrate: 50 mg oral daily Ramipril: 5 mg oral daily	Electrocardiogram: Normal sinus rhythm, rate 75 bpm Chest x-ray: Normal

1. Lipase level
2. Chloride level
3. Uric acid level
4. Blood glucose level

ANSWER: 4

TEST-TAKING STRATEGY

This chart/exhibit question provides you with a multiple choice question and data from a client's medical chart. Note all of the data in the question and the client's chart. Note the strategic word "most" and focus on the subject of the question: the laboratory test to monitor for the client taking prednisone. Apply the six cognitive skills as appropriate, and use nursing knowledge about the interactions and effects of prednisone to assist in answering. Recalling that this medication may increase the blood glucose level will direct you to the correct option.

TIP FOR THE NURSING STUDENT

Rheumatoid arthritis is a debilitating disease that has an autoimmune (self-attacking) component that causes inflammation and sometimes deformities of the joints. It is a disease that is marked by remission and exacerbation, with painful symptoms during exacerbation of the disease. You will learn more about rheumatoid arthritis in your medical-surgical nursing course.

What Test-Taking Strategies Are Helpful for Answering Graphic Item Option Questions?

A graphic item option question will provide you with a written question and images as the options. This type of question will most likely be in the multiple choice format. For example, a question may contain normal versus abnormal physical assessment findings, requiring you to discern between them. Depending on the information in the question, you will need to apply one or more of the six cognitive skills with these question types.

Test-Taking Strategies: Graphic Item Options

Look for strategic words.
Note the format of the question presented.
Think about the cognitive skill(s) being measured.
Use nursing knowledge, and relate clinical experiences to the subject of the question.
Once you have determined the subject and identified what the question is asking, examine each graphic option to choose the best answer.

SAMPLE QUESTION: Graphic Item Option

The nurse is told that an assigned client is in Buck's traction. Upon entering the client's room, the nurse would expect to see which device?

1.

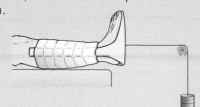

(Figure from Lewis S, Dirksen S, Heitkemper M, Bucher L, Camera I: *Medical-surgical nursing: assessment and management of clinical problems*, ed 8, St. Louis, 2011, Mosby.)

2.

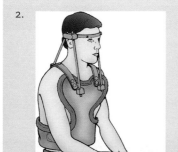

(Figure adapted from Urden LD: *Priorities in critical care nursing*, ed 5, St. Louis, 2007, Mosby.)

3.

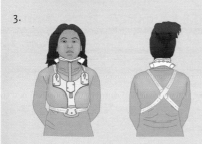

(Figure from Lewis S, Dirksen S, Heitkemper M, Bucher L, Camera I: *Medical-surgical nursing: assessment and management of clinical problems*, ed 8, St. Louis, 2011, Mosby.)

4.

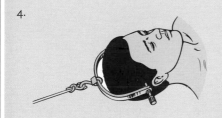

(Figure from Perry A, Potter P: *Clinical nursing skills and techniques*, ed 7, St. Louis, 2006, Mosby).

ANSWER: 1

TEST-TAKING STRATEGY

This question provides you with a graphic for each option and asks you to identify the option that illustrates Buck's traction. Therefore, the subject of the question is Buck's traction. Apply the cognitive skill, *recognize cues*, and use nursing knowledge to answer the question. Recall that Buck's traction is a type of skin traction, then look at each graphic in the options to answer correctly.

▐▶ TIP FOR THE NURSING STUDENT

Buck's traction is used to immobilize, position, or align a lower extremity. It is most commonly used when a person sustains a hip fracture and is awaiting surgery. It is also used to treat a contracture or disease of the hip or knee. It usually uses ropes, weights, and pulleys and a frame at the foot of the bed to apply the necessary weight. You will learn more about Buck's traction in your medical-surgical nursing course.

What Test-Taking Strategies Are Helpful for Answering Audio Questions?

An audio question requires you to wear a set of headphones. You are instructed to click on the icon to play the sound and listen to or watch the content. A question is presented based on the content. The format of the question will most likely be a multiple choice or multiple response type. An example of an audio question might be basic lung sounds, heart sounds, or bowel sounds, requiring you to identify the correct sound being heard to answer the question. Depending on the information in the question, you will need to apply one or more of the six cognitive skills. Audio practice questions can be located on the accompanying Evolve site.

Test-Taking Strategies: Audio Questions

Click on the icon to play the sound; you may replay the sound as many times as necessary.
Focus on the subject once you determine what the question is asking.
Note the format of the question you are answering.
Think about the cognitive skill(s) being measured.
Use nursing knowledge and relate clinical experiences to the subject of the question.

 SAMPLE QUESTION: Audio

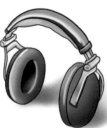

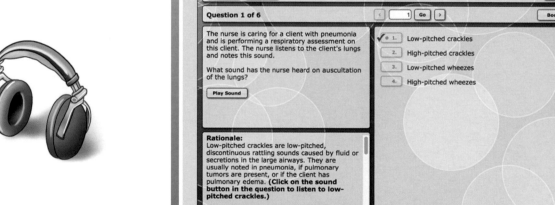

TEST-TAKING STRATEGY

This question type provides you with the question, an icon to listen to the sound the question is asking about, and your answer options. This type of question usually is in multiple choice format. Click on the icon to play the sound; you can replay the audio recording as many times as necessary. Use nursing knowledge and apply the cognitive skills, *recognize and analyze cues*, to relate to the subject of the question: the breath sound heard in a client with pneumonia. These types of questions commonly ask about physical assessment findings.

▐▌▶ TIP FOR THE NURSING STUDENT

Breath sounds are auscultated, or listened to, using a stethoscope. These sounds are assessed to determine the presence of alterations or complications in the lungs. You will learn more about the types of normal and abnormal breath sounds in your health and physical assessment nursing course.

Smart Study Tip

Scope of Practice
Audio questions ask about a subject or content area that is within the nursing scope of practice. Audio questions require you to listen to breath sounds, heart sounds, or bowel sounds representing a component of a nursing assessment.

What Test-Taking Strategies are Helpful for Answering NGN Items?

The NCJMM and the NGN item types that will be presented in the exam continue to develop as the NCSBN progresses in its research to determine the best ways to measure clinical judgment. The NCSBN plans to start to include these item types as scored test items in the spring of 2023. Currently, the major types of test items that will be used are highlight, drop-down, multiple response, multiple choice, and drag and drop. There are variations of some of these types. See Chapter 1 for information on the current variations for each type. The NCSBN research is still in progress, so additional variations may present. Also, see Table 1-2 for major item types and descriptions. Some sample NGN items are located below. Additionally, these types of questions can be located on the Evolve site accompanying this book.

NGN Items and Case Studies

The NGN test items will be accompanied by case studies—standalone case studies and unfolding case studies. An *NGN standalone case study* presents a client scenario *at one point in time* or *multiple points over time*. The client scenario will be followed by an NGN test item that measures some of the cognitive skills/processes. Currently, the NCSBN indicates that the item types that will accompany the standalone case study will be the bow-tie (presents a client scenario at one point in time) or a trend item (presents a client scenario at multiple points over time). These two innovative item types are still being researched.

An *NGN unfolding case study* presents a client scenario that *changes over time through multiple phases of care*. The unfolding case will begin with a one- to two-sentence introductory statement. Then, the client scenario data will be presented as part of the medical record for most items. The medical record presented for each item within an unfolding case will have one or more tabs that will be accessible for the test-taker. The data in this type of client scenario are more comprehensive than in the standalone case study as the "story" unfolds. All six of the cognitive skills will be measured in an unfolding case using the NGN test item formats.

Test-Taking Strategies: NGN Items

Read all of the data in the case scenario.
Avoid "skimming over" the data presented.
Note the question format being presented, and use the test-taking strategies for that type of question, if applicable. For NGN items, you will need to consider many aspects of the case scenario and think beyond what is presented in the case in order to correctly answer.
Review the client data presented for each question.
Apply the relevant clinical judgment skill(s) to assist in answering the question.
Use nursing knowledge, clinical judgment, and clinical learning experiences to answer correctly.

NCLEX EXAM TIP

NGN test items will include a case study. Be sure to read all of the data provided, determine relevant and irrelevant data, and use clinical judgment to make decisions regarding client care. The best way to become familiar with these item types is to practice as many of these test items as possible.

SAMPLE QUESTION: Multiple Response Select All That Apply

COGNITIVE SKILL: TAKE ACTION

The nurse is caring for a 62-year-old female who underwent elective repair of hiatal hernia. Client is postoperative and has been on the postoperative unit for 2 hours 45 minutes. She arrived on the nursing unit at 1215. The following data are documented.

Health History	Nurses' Notes	Vital Signs	Diagnostic Results
Client presented to acute care facility for an elective repair of hiatal hernia. Prior to the surgery, the client reports persistent nausea, vomiting, and heartburn for the last several months. She also reports having intermittent generalized abdominal pain with associated shortness of breath. Past medical history includes hypertension, hyperlipidemia, osteoarthritis, and obesity. Past surgical history includes cesarean section × 2 with tubal ligation and right total hip arthroplasty.	1215: Client received from postanesthesia care unit. Denies pain. Appears in no distress. Plan to continue to monitor, and initiate postoperative prescriptions. 1400: Ongoing monitoring of VS and physical assessment findings. Reports pain 2/10. Appears short of breath and noted to be grimacing. Chest x-ray ordered.	1215: T: 36.8° C (98.2° F) O_2: 95% 3L/NC BP: 132/76 mm Hg P: 90 bpm RR: 16 bpm 1230: T: 36.6° C (97.8° F) O_2: 95% 3L/NC BP: 128/76 mmHg P: 92 bpm RR: 16 bpm 1300: T: 36.8° C (98.2° F) O_2: 92% 3L/NC BP: 122/74 mm Hg P: 90 bpm RR: 20 bpm 1330: T: 37.3° C (99.2° F) O_2: 90% 4 L/NC BP: 126/72 mm Hg P: 102 bpm RR: 24 bpm 1400: T: 37.4° C (99.4° F) O_2: 90% 4 L/NC BP: 120/70 mm Hg P: 102 bpm RR: 24 bpm	Chest x-ray: Localized infiltrate in the right lower lobe of the lung. Diffuse opacity indicative of atelectasis. Postoperative changes noted. Previous study consistent with hiatal hernia and clear lungs.

Based on the data noted in the medical record and the current assessment findings, which actions would the nurse take? **Select all that apply.**

☐ 1. Increase oxygen.
☐ 2. Notify the surgeon.
☐ 3. Ambulate the client.
☐ 4. Call the rapid-response team.
☐ 5. Assist the client to an upright position.
☐ 6. Administer prescribed pain medications.

ANSWER:

1, 2, 3, 5, 6

TEST-TAKING STRATEGY

The client in this question is experiencing a complication related to surgery, specifically atelectasis. Actions to take include increasing the oxygen, notifying the surgeon, ambulating the client, assisting the client to an upright position, and administering prescribed pain medications. These actions will assist the client to relieve the atelectasis, which is likely the cause of the abnormal clinical manifestations and confirmation on chest x-ray. Administering pain medication will assist in easing discomfort associated with coughing and deep breathing. Calling the rapid-response team may not be necessary with the other interventions, unless the client's status continues to deteriorate.

This question type provides you with background data, current data, the question, and your options. This question type allows you to select one or more options at a time, and partial credit for correct answers is allowed. Use nursing knowledge to determine relevant and irrelevant data, to cluster important findings to create a clinical picture, and to relate to the subject of the question: nursing actions to take in managing a postoperative complication, specifically atelectasis. Apply the clinical judgment/cognitive skill, *take action*. These types of questions commonly ask about history, physical assessment findings including vital signs, laboratory and diagnostic test results, and important nursing actions to ensure client safety.

▐▶ TIP FOR THE NURSING STUDENT

A hiatal hernia occurs when the upper part of the stomach bulges through an opening in the diaphragm. It may be addressed with surgical intervention. A complication for any surgical client, but especially the client with a hiatal hernia, is atelectasis because of the location of the surgical procedure. You will learn more about hernias and other gastrointestinal problems, as well as more about aspiration pneumonia, in your medical-surgical nursing course.

SAMPLE QUESTION: Matrix Multiple Choice

COGNITIVE SKILL: ANALYZE CUES

The nurse is caring for a 19-year-old male client who presented to the emergency department with complaints of right lower abdominal pain.

Health History	Nurses' Notes	Vital Signs	Diagnostic Results
Client presented to emergency department (ED) with complaints of abdominal pain × 1 day. Pain is described as sharp and localized to the right lower quadrant of the abdomen, rated 8/10, worsened by movement, associated with nausea and vomiting. Past medical history and past surgical history are negative. The client arrived in the ED at 0700 and was seen and examined by the emergency physician at 0715.	0700: Client oriented to ED holding room, call light in reach. 0715: Seen by the physician; orders written. 0730: Received prescription for morphine 5 mg IV once for severe pain. 0745: Administered morphine 5 mg IV as prescribed. Prescription received for CBC and stat CT abdomen with contrast.	0710: T: 37.4° C (99.4° F) O$_2$: 96% RA BP: 144/86 mm Hg P: 112 bpm RR: 24 bpm 0815: T: 38.2° C (100.8° F) O$_2$: 97% RA BP: 128/78 mm Hg P: 98 bpm RR: 20 bpm	CBC: WBC: 16,000/mm³ (16 × 10⁹/L) Segmented neutrophils: 75% (8.3 × 10⁹/L) Band neutrophils: 9% (1 × 10⁹/L) Lymphocytes: 20% (0.1 × 10⁹/L) Monocytes: 2% (0.1 × 10⁹/L) Eosinophils: 3% (0.38 × 10⁹/L) Basophils: 1% (0.05 × 10⁹/L) RBC: 5.2 × 10¹²/L Platelets: 240,000/ mm³ (240 × 10⁹/L) Hemoglobin: 16 g/dL (160 g/L) Hematocrit: 45% (0.45 volume fraction) CT abdomen: Periappendiceal inflammation with fat stranding, thickening of the lateral conal fascia, ileocecal lymph node enlargement, and inflammatory thickening of the contiguous structures.

For each assessment finding, click to specify if the finding does not require immediate follow-up or if there is a need for immediate follow-up.

Assessment Findings	Does not require immediate follow-up	Requires immediate follow-up
Temperature changed from 37.4° C (99.4° F) to 38.2° C (100.8° F)	☐	☐
Blood pressure changed from 144/86 mm Hg to 128/78 mm Hg	☐	☐
Pulse changed from 112 bpm to 98 bpm	☐	☐
Respiratory rate changed from 24 bpm to 20 bpm	☐	☐
WBC: 16,000/mm³ (16 x 10⁹/L)	☐	☐
Segmented neutrophils: 75% (8.3 x 10⁹/L)	☐	☐
Platelets: 240,000/mm³ (240 x 10⁹/L)	☐	☐
CT abdomen findings	☐	☐

ANSWER:

Assessment Findings	Does not require immediate follow-up	Requires immediate follow-up
Temperature changed from 37.4° C (99.4° F) to 38.2° C (100.8° F)	☐	☑
Blood pressure changed from 144/86 mm Hg to 128/78 mm Hg	☑	☐
Pulse changed from 112 bpm to 98 bpm	☑	☐
Respiratory rate changed from 24 bpm to 20 bpm	☑	☐
WBC: 16,000/mm³ (16 x 10⁹/L)	☐	☑
Segmented neutrophils: 75% (8.3 x 10⁹/L)	☐	☑
Platelets: 240,000/mm³ (240 x 10⁹/L)	☑	☐
CT abdomen findings	☐	☑

TEST-TAKING STRATEGY

Assessment findings requiring immediate follow-up include the elevated temperature, elevated WBC count and segmented neutrophil result, as well as the CT abdomen findings. These results are concerning indicating an acute abdomen and require additional action. The other findings indicate an improvement in clinical status or are normal and therefore do not require follow-up at this time.

Apply the clinical judgment/cognitive skill, *analyze cues,* and make connections between the client's presentation and the laboratory and CT findings to determine what problem the client is experiencing. This question type provides you with background data, current data, the question, and your options. In this question type, each row can have 1 response selected. You will not be able to move on to the next item unless 1 response is selected in each row.

▐▶ TIP FOR THE NURSING STUDENT

Appendicitis is an inflammation of the appendix, which is a structure located on the colon on the right lower side of the abdomen. Symptoms may include anorexia, nausea, vomiting, and abdominal pain. The temperature may be elevated along with the WBC and segmented neutrophil count. You will learn more about appendicitis in your medical-surgical nursing course.

SAMPLE QUESTION: Drop-Down Cloze

COGNITIVE SKILL: PRIORITIZE HYPOTHESES

The nurse is caring for a 79-year-old female admitted to the medical unit with altered mental status.

Health History	Nurses' Notes	Vital Signs	Diagnostic Results
Client presented to emergency department (ED) accompanied by family member, who reports confusion in the client for the last 3 days. Family member reports client having decreased appetite and generalized malaise. The client arrived in the ED at 1900 and was seen and examined by the ED physician at 1915.	1900: Client and family member oriented to ED holding room, call light in reach. 1930: Received prescriptions for CBC, BMP, and UA.	1910: T: 37.8° C (100.0° F) O$_2$: 96% RA BP: 88/42 mm Hg P: 108 bpm RR: 18 bpm	CBC: WBC: 12,000/mm³ (12 x 10⁹/L) Neutrophils: 69% (7.6 x 10⁹/L) Band neutrophils: 15% (1.6 x 10⁹/L) Lymphocytes: 10% (0.05 x 10⁹/L) Monocytes: 2% (0.1 x 10⁹/L) Eosinophils: 3% (0.3 x 10⁹/L) Basophils: 1% (0.05 x 10⁹/L) RBC: 4.2 x 10¹²/L Platelets: 180,000/mm³ (180 x 10⁹/L) Hemoglobin: 11 g/dL (110 g/L) Hematocrit: 48% (0.48 volume fraction) BMP: Sodium: 145 mEq/L (145 mmol/L) Potassium: 3.8 mEq/L (3.8 mmol/L) Calcium: 9.8 mg/dL (2.5 mmol/L) Chloride: 102 mEq/L (102 mmol/L) Glucose: 110 mg/dL (6.1 mmol/L) Albumin: 4.0 g/dL (40 g/L) Blood urea nitrogen: 20 mg/dL (7.1 mmol/L) Creatinine: 2.0 mg/dL (176.4 mcmol/L) Urinalysis: pH 4.5 Bilirubin negative Glucose negative Protein moderate Specific gravity 1.038 Leukocytes positive Nitrites positive Bacteria positive

The nurse is initiating the client's plan of care. The nurse would **first** address the client's _____1_____ by administering prescribed _____2_____. The nurse determines that the clinical findings are probably related to _____3_____.

Options for 1	Options for 2	Options for 3
Blood pressure	Intravenous fluids	Urinary tract infection
Nausea	Ondansetron	Acute kidney injury
Temperature	Acetaminophen	Renal calculi
White blood cell count	Antibiotics	Acute abdominal condition
Heart rate	Antidysrhythmics	Hyperglycemia
Oxygen saturation	Supplemental oxygen	Dehydration

ANSWER: The nurse is initiating the client's plan of care. The nurse would first address the client's <u>blood pressure</u> by administering <u>intravenous fluids</u>. The nurse determines that the clinical findings are probably related to <u>urinary tract infection</u>.

TEST-TAKING STRATEGY

When looking at the data in the medical record, the nurse would determine that the blood pressure was a priority finding; therefore, the nurse would address this first. Intravenous fluids would be administered to assist in increasing the blood pressure. The clinical findings are probably due to a urinary tract infection, given that the urinalysis is positive for bacteria, leukocytes, and nitrites; the client may be experiencing urosepsis and impending septic shock.

This question type provides you with background data, current data, the question, and your options. This question type allows you to select one option from a drop-down list. There may be more than one drop-down list with this item type and the options may be words or phrases. Use nursing knowledge to determine relevant and irrelevant data, to cluster important findings and visualize a clinical picture, and to relate to the subject of the question: nursing actions to take in managing an older adult client presenting with altered mental status. Apply the clinical judgment/cognitive skill, *prioritize hypotheses,* to determine the client's priority and other needs. These types of questions commonly ask about history, physical assessment findings including vital signs, laboratory and diagnostic test results, and important nursing actions to ensure client safety.

▮▶ TIP FOR THE NURSING STUDENT

Urinary tract infection is an infection of any part of the urinary tract, including the urethra, bladder, ureters, or kidneys. Older adult clients are at risk for urinary tract infections and may present with atypical clinical signs and symptoms due to factors related to aging. You will learn more about urinary tract infection in your medical-surgical nursing course, and you will learn more about changes related to aging in your gerontological nursing course.

SAMPLE QUESTION: Highlight Text

COGNITIVE SKILL: RECOGNIZE CUES

A 22-year-old male client arrives via ambulance to the emergency department (ED) with complaints of palpitations and weakness. He reports he was on a ladder while working in his garage when he suddenly started to feel shaky and dizzy. He reports that he drinks energy drinks on a daily basis as well as fitness supplements before going to the gym. The emergency physician prescribes a stat electrocardiogram (ECG) and D-dimer and cardiac markers to be drawn. The nurse documents the following findings as part of the assessment:
- Continued reports of palpitations and weakness
- Heart rate = 140 beats per minute and irregular
- Respirations = 22 breaths per minute
- Blood pressure = 110/78 mm Hg
- Creatinine kinase isoenzyme = 4 ng/mL (4 mcg/L)
- Troponin T (cTnT): <0.1 ng/mL (0.1 mcg/L)
- D-dimer <50 ng/mL (3.0 mmol/L)
- ECG shows atrial fibrillation with rapid ventricular response

Highlight the findings that require follow-up by the nurse.

ANSWER:
- <mark>Continued reports of palpitations and weakness</mark>
- <mark>Heart rate = 140 beats per minute (bpm) and irregular</mark>
- Respirations = 22 breaths per minute
- Blood pressure = 110/78 mm Hg
- Creatinine kinase isoenzyme = 4 ng/mL (4 mcg/L)
- Troponin T (cTnT): <0.1 ng/mL (0.1 mcg/L)
- D-dimer <50 ng/mL (3.0 mmol/L)
- <mark>ECG shows atrial fibrillation with rapid ventricular response</mark>

TEST-TAKING STRATEGY

Findings requiring follow-up by the nurse include continued reports of palpitations and weakness, heart rate 140 bpm and irregular, and ECG showing atrial fibrillation with rapid ventricular response. This is a life-threatening dysrhythmia and can result in significant reductions in cardiac output. The respirations, blood pressure, and laboratory results are reassuring and do not require follow-up at this time.

This question type provides you with background data, current data, the question, and your options. This question type allows you to select your answer by highlighting words or phrases. You can select and deselect highlighted words or phrases after reading a portion of the client's medical record. Apply the clinical judgment/cognitive skill, *recognize cues.* Use nursing knowledge to determine relevant and irrelevant data, to cluster important findings to visualize a clinical picture, and to relate to the subject of the question: clinical assessment findings requiring follow-up by the nurse. These types of questions commonly focus on determining normal and abnormal clinical assessment and diagnostic findings.

⫸ TIP FOR THE NURSING STUDENT

Atrial fibrillation is an irregular heart rate or dysrhythmia that is associated with inadequate blood flow, or perfusion, to vital organs and extremities. Atrial fibrillation with rapid ventricular response is a life threatening dysrhythmia because of the resulting decrease in cardiac output. You will learn more about atrial fibrillation and other cardiac dysrhythmias in your medical-surgical nursing course.

SAMPLE QUESTION: Matrix Multiple Choice

COGNITIVE SKILL: GENERATE SOLUTIONS

The nurse is caring for an 87-year-old male admitted 1 day ago for exacerbation of chronic obstructive pulmonary disease (COPD).

Health History	Nurses' Notes	Vital Signs	Diagnostic Results
Client presented to emergency department (ED) complaining of shortness of breath for the last 3 days. Client is on continuous home oxygen at 1.5 L/min NC. Reports associated weakness and increased use of inhalers. The client arrived in the ED at 0800 and was seen and examined by the emergency physician at 0815.	0800: Client oriented to ED holding room, call light in reach. Focused respiratory assessment shows increased work of breathing and wheezing in bilateral lower lobes of the lungs. 0830: Received prescriptions for albuterol/ipratropium breathing treatment, 1 view chest x-ray. 0845: Albuterol/ipratropium treatment administered, tolerated well. Work of breathing improved and lung sounds clear bilaterally.	0800: T: 36.6° C (97.8° F) O_2: 84% 1.5L NC BP: 158/84 mm Hg P: 104 bpm RR: 25 bpm 0900: T: 36.8° C (98.2° F) O_2: 90% 1.5L NC BP: 150/78 mm Hg P: 112 bpm RR: 20 bpm	Chest x-ray: Bilateral lungs enlarged, with flattened diaphragm, bullae, and hyperinflation of the alveoli.

What actions would the nurse take to address the COPD exacerbation?

For each action below, click to specify whether the action would be:

Anticipated: an action that the nurse would anticipate taking to resolve the problem

Nonessential: an action that the nurse could take without harming the client, but the action would be unlikely to address the problem

Contraindicated: an action that could harm the client and that should not be taken

Action	Anticipated	Nonessential	Contraindicated
Monitor oxygenation status	☐	☐	☐
Administer methylprednisolone	☐	☐	☐
Increase oxygen	☐	☐	☐
Request a prescription for an electrocardiogram	☐	☐	☐
Encourage use of incentive spirometer	☐	☐	☐
Use humidified oxygen	☐	☐	☐
Request a prescription for coagulation factors	☐	☐	☐
Administer as-needed blood pressure medications	☐	☐	☐

ANSWER:

What actions would the nurse take to address the COPD exacerbation?

For each action below, click to specify whether the action would be:

Anticipated: an action that the nurse would anticipate taking to resolve the problem

Nonessential: an action that the nurse could take without harming the client, but the action would be unlikely to address the problem

Contraindicated: an action that could harm the client and that should not be taken

Action	Anticipated	Nonessential	Contraindicated
Monitor oxygenation status	☒	☐	☐
Administer methylprednisolone	☒	☐	☐
Increase oxygen	☐	☐	☒
Request a prescription for an electrocardiogram	☐	☒	☐
Encourage use of incentive spirometer	☒	☐	☐
Use humidified oxygen	☒	☐	☐
Request a prescription for coagulation factors	☐	☒	☐
Administer as-needed blood pressure medications	☐	☒	☐

Anticipated actions include the following as indicated treatment for COPD exacerbation: monitoring oxygenation status, administering methylprednisolone, encouraging the use of an incentive spirometer to assist in inflating alveoli, and using humidified oxygen for comfort during oxygen therapy. Nonessential actions include the following: requesting a prescription for an ECG since the client is displaying no symptoms of cardiac issues; requesting a prescription for coagulation factors as bleeding risk is not a concern at this time; and administering as-needed blood pressure medications. The blood pressure is elevated but not critical, and this intervention will not specifically address the COPD exacerbation. Increasing oxygen would not be done for COPD exacerbation because of the risk for diminishing the drive to breathe. In COPD, the drive to breathe comes from a low oxygen level rather than a high carbon dioxide level, and when oxygen is supplemented too much, it is possible that this drive can be affected.

TEST-TAKING STRATEGY

This question type provides you with background data, current data, the question, and your options. In this question type, each row can have 1 response selected. You will not be able to move on to the next item unless 1 response is selected in each row. Use nursing knowledge to determine relevant and irrelevant data, to cluster important findings to visualize a clinical picture, and to relate to the subject of the question: nursing actions in the management of the client with COPD exacerbation. Apply the clinical judgment skill *generating solutions* to plan anticipated actions. These types of questions commonly focus on determining normal and abnormal clinical assessment and diagnostic findings, developing a plan of care, and nursing actions to ensure client safety.

▐▌▶ TIP FOR THE NURSING STUDENT

COPD is a disease of the lung causing chronic inflammatory changes and resulting in obstructed airflow in the lungs. The disease is progressive, and management is targeted at improving the symptoms and slowing disease progression. You will learn more about COPD in your medical-surgical nursing course.

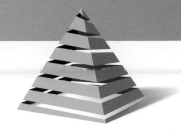

CHAPTER **6**

How to Avoid "Reading Into the Question"

One of the pitfalls that can cause a problem when trying to answer a question correctly is "reading into the question." This means you are considering issues beyond the information presented in the question. Except for NGN items, avoid thinking beyond what is presented in the question. Some strategies you can use to prevent this include the following:

- Identifying the ingredients of a question
- Reading the question carefully and looking for strategic words or phrases
- Thinking about the clinical judgment/cognitive skill to apply in answering the question
- Focusing on the data in the question
- Recognizing cues in the data to determine if an abnormality exists
- Analyzing cues by connecting data to the client's clinical presentation and determining if the data is expected or unexpected
- Prioritizing hypotheses by ranking client needs and concern
- Generating solutions by using hypotheses to determine interventions for an expected outcome
- Taking action by implementing the generated solutions addressing the highest priorities or hypotheses
- Evaluating outcomes by comparing observed outcomes with expected ones
- Focusing on the client of the question and ensuring client safety
- Identifying the subject of the question and what the question is asking
- Considering all available resources
- Avoiding the "What if?" syndrome
- Using the process of elimination

Clinical Judgment and Clinical Decision-Making

Clinical judgment is a process employed when the nurse considers the details of a clinical situation and is able to identify relevant factors and make sound clinical decisions in the disposition of client care. As a nurse, it is important to understand the client's baseline data and background to effectively apply clinical judgment to client care. This is a skill that is built and refined over time. Also, use clinical judgment when answering test questions. When applying this skill to test questions, it will help if you can determine the significant factors in the information presented in the question. Refer to chapters 1 and 5 for specific information about applying the Clinical Judgment Measurement Model developed by the National Council of State Boards of Nursing (NCSBN).

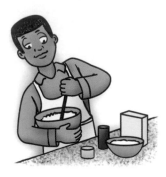

Ingredients of a Question

What Are the Ingredients of a Question?

Test questions contain a case event, a question query, and options. It is important to identify the ingredients of a question as you read it because this will help you sort out the facts and determine what the question is asking.

What Is the Case Event?

The case event is the "heart" of the question. It provides both relevant and irrelevant information that you need to think about to answer the question.

What Is the Question Query?

The question query is a statement that generally follows the case event and asks you something specific about it.

What Are the Options?

The options are all the answers presented with the question.

Examples of some types of questions that may appear in your nursing exams or on the NCLEX exam and the specific ingredients of the questions are provided in this section. The answers to these example questions and the test-taking strategy also are provided. Additionally, Chapter 5 provides information about the various question types that will be in your nursing exams and the NCLEX exam.

 INGREDIENTS OF A QUESTION: Multiple Choice

Case Event: The nurse is reviewing the laboratory results of a client who is receiving magnesium sulfate by IV infusion and notes that the magnesium level is 3.5 mg/dL (1.44 mmol/L).
Question Query: Based on this laboratory result, the nurse would **most likely** expect to note which finding in the client?
Options:
1. Tremors
2. Hyperactive reflexes
3. Respiratory depression
4. No specific findings because this value is a normal level

ANSWER: 3

TEST-TAKING STRATEGY

Apply the clinical judgment/cognitive skill, *analyze cues*, and note the **strategic words**, *most likely*. Knowing that the level identified in the question is elevated will assist in eliminating option 4. Next, eliminate options 1 and 2 because they are **comparable or alike**. Remember to use nursing knowledge, **focus on the information** in the case event, identify what the question is asking (the **subject**), make connections between the data and what is expected, note the **strategic words**, read carefully, and use the process of elimination.

⯈ TIP FOR THE NURSING STUDENT:

You need to know that the normal magnesium level is 1.8 - 2.6 mEq/L (0.74 to 1.07 mmol/L); therefore, the magnesium level presented in the question is elevated. Next you need to know the signs and symptoms indicative of an elevated magnesium level. You will learn normal laboratory values in your foundations of nursing course. Learn the normal magnesium level and the signs and symptoms of a magnesium imbalance.

INGREDIENTS OF A QUESTION: Fill in the Blank

Case Event: The primary health care provider prescribes an intravenous (IV) antibiotic to be administered in 50 mL 0.9% normal saline and to infuse in 30 minutes. The drop factor for the IV tubing is 15 gtt/mL.

Question Query: The nurse would plan to set the flow rate of the infusion at how many drops per minute? **Fill in the blank.**

ANSWER: 25

TEST-TAKING STRATEGY:

Apply the clinical judgment/cognitive skill, *generate solutions,* and note the words *set the flow rate* in the query. Read the question carefully, focusing on the **subject,** drops per minute. Note that 50 mL fluid is to infuse in 30 minutes and the drop factor is 15. Use the formula for calculating an IV infusion to answer the question. Always double-check the calculation, make sure that the answer makes sense, and verify your answer using a calculator. Remember to use nursing knowledge, **focus on the information** in the case event, identify what the question is asking (the **subject**), and note the words in the query.

▪▪▶ TIP FOR THE NURSING STUDENT

In this question, you need to know the formula for calculating an IV flow rate. You will most likely learn about medication calculations and IV flow rates in your foundations of nursing course. The formula and the calculation for this question are as follows:

$$\frac{\text{Total volume to be infused} \times \text{Drop factor}}{\text{Time in minutes}} = \text{Drops per minute}$$

$$\frac{50 \times 15}{30} = 25$$

NCLEX® EXAM TIP

Use the formula for calculating an IV infusion. Perform the calculation on the noteboard provided to you, and use the computer's on-screen calculator to verify your answer. Read carefully because in calculation questions you may be asked to round the answer to the nearest whole number or to one decimal place. If rounding is necessary, perform at the end of the calculation.

INGREDIENTS OF A QUESTION: Multiple Response

Case Event: The nurse enters a hospitalized client's room and discovers that the client is having a tonic-clonic seizure.

Question Query: Which actions would the nurse implement? **Select all that apply.**

Options:
- ☐ **1.** Call a code.
- ☐ **2.** Check airway patency.
- ☐ **3.** Establish an IV access.
- ☐ **4.** Protect the client from injury.
- ☐ **5.** Restrain the client's extremities loosely.
- ☐ **6.** Document the characteristics of the seizure that the client exhibits.

ANSWER: 2, 3, 4, 6

TEST-TAKING STRATEGY:

Apply the clinical judgment/cognitive skill, *take action.* Read each option carefully and note the **subject,** the nursing actions in the event of a seizure. In this type of question, it is helpful to visualize the event to assist in determining the nurse's actions. Remember that a patent airway and client safety are your priority. Use nursing knowledge, **focus on the information** in the case event, identify what the question is asking (the **subject**), read carefully, and use the process of elimination.

▪▪▶ TIP FOR THE NURSING STUDENT

You need to know that a seizure is an abnormal sudden excessive discharge of electrical activity within the brain. You also need to know what you would do if a client has a seizure. What you need to remember is that a patent airway and client safety are your priorities. You will learn about seizures when you study neurological problems.

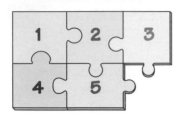

INGREDIENTS OF A QUESTION: Prioritizing (Ordered Response)

Case Event: The nurse is preparing to change an abdominal dressing using sterile technique.
Question Query: What is the order of **priority** that the nurse would take to perform this procedure? **Arrange the actions in the order of priority that they would be performed. All options must be used.**

Unordered Options	Ordered Responses
Wash hands.	Explain the procedure to the client.
Set up a sterile field.	Wash hands.
Explain the procedure to the client.	Set up a sterile field.
Document the characteristics of the wound.	Don clean gloves and remove the old dressing.
Don sterile gloves, clean the site as prescribed, and apply a new dressing.	Don sterile gloves, clean the site as prescribed, and apply a new dressing.
Don clean gloves and remove the old dressing.	Document the characteristics of the wound.

TEST-TAKING STRATEGY

Apply the clinical judgment/cognitive skill, *take action*. Read each option carefully and note the strategic word, *priority*. In this type of question, it is helpful to visualize the event to assist in determining the nurse's order of actions. Remember to use nursing knowledge, read carefully, focus on the information in the case event, identify what the question is asking (the subject), and note the strategic word.

◗◗▶ TIP FOR THE NURSING STUDENT

You need to know the principles that are related to asepsis and the technique for changing a sterile dressing, which you will learn in your fundamentals of nursing class. Learn these principles and techniques because they are critical in preventing infection in the client.

NCLEX® EXAM TIP

For a prioritizing (ordered-response) question on the NCLEX exam, you will need to use the computer mouse to drag and drop the unordered options in order of priority (ordered responses).

INGREDIENTS OF A QUESTION: Figure or Illustration

Case Event: The nurse is checking the arterial pulses on an adult client.
Question Query: Select the area where the nurse would palpate the carotid pulse. **Refer to figure.**

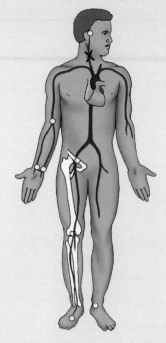

(Figure from Ignatavicius D, et al.: *Medical surgical nursing: Concepts for interprofessional collaborative care*, ed 10, Elsevier, 2021, p. 624.)

ANSWER: The answer is indicated by the circle marked with the X.

TEST-TAKING STRATEGY

Apply the clinical judgment/cognitive skill, *take action*. Note the subject, the location of the carotid pulse. In this type of question, it is helpful to visualize the pulse points for assessment of arterial pulses to identify the correct answer. Remember to use nursing knowledge, read carefully, focus on the information in the case event, and identify what the question is asking (the subject).

▯▶ TIP FOR THE NURSING STUDENT

You need to know where the arterial pulse points are located. Use what you learned in anatomy class to assist in answering this question. You will also learn these pulse points in your foundations of nursing class and in your physical assessment class. Be sure to learn these pulse points for assessment of arterial pulses.

 ## Strategic Words or Strategic Phrases

Always read every word in the question carefully. As you read, look for strategic words or strategic phrases in the case event and query of the question. Strategic words or strategic phrases focus your attention on specific or critical points that you need to consider when answering the question.

Some strategic words or strategic phrases may indicate that all the options are correct, in which case you will need to prioritize to select the correct option. Remember, as you read the question, look for the strategic words or strategic phrases; they will make a difference with regard to how you will answer the question.

What Are the Commonly Used Strategic Words or Strategic Phrases to Look For?

Common Strategic Words or Strategic Phrases

Best
Early
Late
Effective
Essential
First
Highest priority
Immediate
Initial
Next
Most
Most appropriate
Most important
Most likely
Need for follow-up
Need for further teaching *or* need for further education
Primary
Priority
Increased
Decreased

Use of Strategic Words or Strategic Phrases in a Question

You may be asking yourself: "How are these strategic words or strategic phrases used in a question?" Following are some examples of question queries that contain strategic words:

What is the *best* nursing action?
Which is an *early* sign of hypoxia?
Which is a *late* sign of shock?
The nurse determines that the treatment is *effective* if which is noted?
Which item is *essential* in the care of the client?
Which is the *immediate* nursing action?
What is the *initial* nursing action?
The nurse would take which action *first*?
Which client need is the *highest priority*?
Which action would the nurse take *next*?
The client is *most* at risk for which complication?
Which response to the client is *most appropriate*?
Which nursing action is *most important*?
The client is *most likely* at risk for which disorder?
Which assessment finding indicates the *need for follow-up*?
Which client statement indicates the *need for further teaching*?
What is the *primary* clinical manifestation of diabetes mellitus?
Which nursing action is the *priority*?
The nurse would expect which laboratory value to be *increased*?
The nurse would expect which vital sign to be *decreased*?

The Subject of the Question

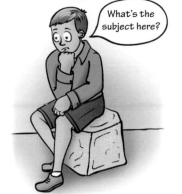

What Is the Subject of the Question?

The subject of the question is the specific content that the question is asking about. It is important to read every word in the question. As you read and note the strategic words or strategic phrases, determine what the question is asking. Identifying and focusing on the subject of the question will help you eliminate the incorrect options and direct you to the correct option.

SMART STUDY TIP

Student-to-Student

The questions on nursing exams cover subjects that you have learned in your nursing course. Focus on these subject areas when preparing for a nursing exam. If your instructor gives you a study guide for the exam, review all subject areas on the study guide.

NCLEX® EXAM TIP

There are hundreds of subjects that you could be asked about when you take the NCLEX exam. This is understandable, especially when you think about all the information that you needed to learn in nursing school. A test question may ask about any Client Needs area of the NCLEX Test Plan, any content area of nursing, or anything that has to do with the role and responsibilities of the nurse. Therefore, the list of subjects that could be tested is never-ending. It is extremely helpful to obtain a copy of the detailed NCLEX Test Plan, which is published by the National Council of State Boards of Nursing (NCSBN). This Test Plan, which identifies some of the content and activities that will be tested on the NCLEX exam, can be obtained at no fee at the NCSBN website (www.ncsbn.org). Be sure to download the detailed Test Plan.

 SAMPLE QUESTION: The Subject of the Question

Case Event: A hospitalized client with metastatic cancer is receiving a continuous intravenous (IV) infusion of morphine sulfate to alleviate pain.

Question Query: The nurse would monitor the client for which adverse effect of the medication?

Subject: In this question, note that the client is receiving morphine sulfate and that the question asks about an adverse effect of the medication. Therefore, the subject of this question is an adverse effect of morphine sulfate.

Options:
1. Nausea
2. Sedation
3. Dizziness
4. Skeletal muscle flaccidity

ANSWER: 4

TEST-TAKING STRATEGY

Apply the clinical judgment/cognitive skill, *recognize cues.* Read every word in the question, and specifically determine what the question is asking. The subject of the question is the adverse effect of morphine sulfate. Nausea, sedation, and dizziness are side effects of morphine sulfate that the client may experience, but they are not adverse effects. Remember to focus on the subject and on the information in the question and what the question is asking!

NCLEX® EXAM TIP

On the NCLEX exam, do not be surprised if you are given questions that contain content with which you are totally unfamiliar or are only vaguely familiar. This happens to many who take this examination. When it does happen, read the question carefully and focus on the subject.

Sometimes you do not even need to know much about the content to answer the question. In addition, with some of these unfamiliar questions, you may be able to use nursing knowledge from a different content area to answer the question. Do not become alarmed and anxious if you receive a question with unfamiliar content. Sit back, take a deep breath, read carefully, focus on the subject, and use nursing knowledge from a different content area and test-taking strategies to answer the question.

SMART STUDY TIP

Lifestyle Planning

Be sure to plan daily study times in your schedule. Reviewing class notes and highlighted text book notes daily will help to reinforce knowledge.

▐▶ TIP FOR THE NURSING STUDENT

You need to know that morphine sulfate is an opioid analgesic and that it causes depression of the central nervous system. Next, noting that the question is asking about an adverse or toxic effect will assist in answering correctly. You will learn about morphine sulfate in your nursing courses, and it is important that you are very familiar with the side effects and adverse and toxic effects of the medication. In addition to skeletal muscle flaccidity, a major concern is that the medication causes respiratory depression. Learn the side effects and adverse effects of this medication.

Using Nursing Knowledge and the Process of Elimination

Why Is Nursing Knowledge So Important?

Nursing knowledge is needed to assist in answering test questions because the knowledge provides information that you need to think about critically to make clinical judgments to answer the question. If you can use your nursing knowledge to answer the question, then by all means do so!

What Does It Mean to Use the Process of Elimination?

The process of elimination involves reading each option for a question and removing the options that are incorrect and do not address the subject of the question. Using the process of elimination is extremely important when you are reading the options to a question and trying to determine the correct answer. Do not hastily select an option because it sounds good. Always read every option carefully before selecting an answer.

Some students read a question, and before looking at the options they determine a correct answer. This is a helpful strategy for answering a test question, because you are using nursing knowledge to help answer the question correctly. The problem with this strategy is that you may have an answer to the question in mind, but when you look at the options, your answer is not there. This can be very frustrating and anxiety provoking. Let's look at an example.

❓ SAMPLE QUESTION: The Process of Elimination

Case Event: A client who has type 1 diabetes mellitus describes shakiness and hunger 2 hours after receiving a dose of regular insulin.
Question Query: The nurse determines that the client is having a hypoglycemic reaction and prepares to give the client which **best** item to treat the reaction?
  After you read this question, you may immediately think, "Orange juice! Yes, orange juice is the best item! I know the answer to this question." Then you look at the options and find the following:
Options:
1. Milk
2. Diet soda
3. Sugar-free gelatin
4. Sugar-free cookies

ANSWER: 1

TEST-TAKING STRATEGY

Your answer, orange juice, is not there! So now what do you do? Apply the clinical judgment/cognitive skill, *generate solutions*. You need to use your nursing knowledge and think about what thought processes led you to identify orange juice as the answer to the question. Note the **strategic word**, *best*. Remember that a food item that contains 10 to

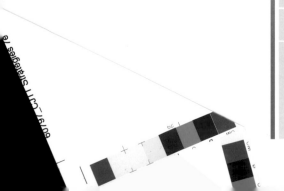

15 g carbohydrate is used to treat a hypoglycemic reaction. Now look at your options and use the process of elimination. In this question you can eliminate options 2, 3, and 4 because these items are comparable or alike and do not contain carbohydrates.

⏩ TIP FOR THE NURSING STUDENT

You need to know that diabetes mellitus is a chronic disorder of impaired carbohydrate, protein, and lipid metabolism that is caused by a deficiency of effective insulin. You also need to know that hypoglycemia is a complication of diabetes mellitus, and you need to know the signs of hypoglycemia. You will learn a great deal about diabetes mellitus during your nursing courses because it is a prevalent health problem. In this question you can use medical terminology skills to determine that *hypoglycemic* means a low blood glucose level. When the blood glucose is low, glucose needs to be provided to the client. The only item in the options that will provide a form of glucose is milk. Learn about diabetes mellitus, the signs of hypoglycemia, and its treatment.

Determining If an Abnormality Exists

Determine if an abnormality exists. Look at data in the question and in the responses and decide what is abnormal. Pay closer attention to this information as you answer the question.

❓ SAMPLE QUESTION: Determining If an Abnormality Exists

Case Event: The nurse is caring for a client who is taking digoxin and is monitoring routine laboratory values.

Question Query: Which laboratory value requires the **need for follow-up** by the nurse?

Options:

1. Sodium 138 mEq/L (138 mmol/L)
2. Potassium 3.4 mEq/L (3.4 mmol/L)
3. Phosphorus 3.0 mg/dL (0.97 mmol/L)
4. Magnesium 1.8 mEq/L (0.74 mmol/L)

ANSWER: 2

TEST-TAKING STRATEGY

Apply the clinical judgment/cognitive skill, *analyze cues.* Note the strategic words, *need for follow-up.* The first step in approaching the answer to this question is to determine if an abnormality exists.

The client is taking digoxin. The laboratory values noted in the options are all normal except potassium. Make connections between the data in the question and the options. Recall that the potassium level must stay consistent while the client is taking digoxin in order to prevent adverse effects from occurring. Remember to determine if an abnormality exists in the event before choosing the correct option.

⏩ TIP FOR THE NURSING STUDENT

Digoxin is a medication that has positive inotropic actions, which means that it helps the heart pump more effectively. Digoxin has a very narrow therapeutic index, which puts the client at risk for digoxin toxicity. Therefore, serum digoxin levels are monitored routinely. In addition to this, a consistent electrolyte balance (particularly potassium) is needed in order for the digoxin to be effective in management of the health problem it is prescribed for. You will learn about digoxin, its adverse effects, and nursing implications when you study heart problems and pharmacological interventions.

Focusing on the Data in the Question and Ensuring Client Safety

Focus only on the data in the question, read every word, and make a decision about what the question is asking. Reread the question more than one time; ask yourself, "What is this question asking?" and "What content is this question testing?"

 SAMPLE QUESTION: Focusing on the Data in the Question and Ensuring Client Safety

Case Event: The nurse is providing discharge instructions to a client with diabetes mellitus. The client's HgbA1C level is 10%.
Question Query: How would the nurse inform the client?
Options:
1. "Increase the amount of vegetables and water intake in your diet regimen."
2. "Change the time of day you exercise because it may cause hypoglycemia."
3. "Continue with the same diet and exercise regimen you are currently using."
4. "Utilize a high-intensity exercise regimen and decrease carbohydrate consumption."

ANSWER: 1

TEST-TAKING STRATEGY

Apply the clinical judgment/cognitive skill, *generate solutions*. Focus on the data in the question, an HgbA1C level of 10%. This is above the recommended range for a client with diabetes mellitus and indicates poor glycemic control. Choose the option that addresses the data in the question and ensures client safety.

Option 1 is a safe recommendation to make to a diabetic client and will help reduce the HgbA1C level. Changing the time of day for exercise and continuing with the same diet and exercise regimen will not address the problem in the question. Utilizing a high-intensity exercise regimen and decreasing carbohydrate consumption could potentially result in a hypoglycemic reaction and does not ensure client safety.

 TIP FOR THE NURSING STUDENT

Diabetes mellitus is a condition where carbohydrate metabolism is affected, and it can result in high blood glucose or low blood glucose levels. There are two types of diabetes mellitus and various contributing factors to this health problem. One method of monitoring diabetes mellitus is to measure the HgbA1C level, which is a blood test that provides information about glycemic control over the past 2 to 3 months and provides information that is helpful in tailoring the client's treatment regimen. You will learn about the laboratory tests used to monitor diabetes mellitus when you study endocrine problems.

 Focusing on the Client of the Question

Focus on the client in the question. At times, other people are discussed in the question that also affect how the question should be answered. Remember the concepts of client-centered and family-centered care.

 SAMPLE QUESTION: Focusing on the Client

Case Event: The nurse is caring for a terminally ill client. The client's wife, who has served as the caregiver, is at the bedside. She states, "I really hope my husband can just get better so we can go home."
Question Query: What statement would the nurse make to the client's wife?
Options:
1. "Has the doctor spoken with you about your husband's plan of care?"
2. "It sounds like this is difficult for you. What do you know about your husband's condition?"

3. "I hope your husband gets better too. It would be wonderful for you to be able to take him home."
4. "I know this is a difficult situation. I've seen this many times before. The spouse always has a hard time."

ANSWER: 2

TEST-TAKING STRATEGY

Apply the clinical judgment/cognitive skill, *take action*. Focus on the **client of the question**, which in this case is the client's spouse. Also, use **therapeutic communication techniques.**

The correct option acknowledges the spouse's feelings and asks for further information to determine her understanding of the situation. Option 1 does not acknowledge her feelings. Option 3 may offer false reassurance and false hope. Option 4 does not address the spouse's feelings and may cause further emotional distress.

TIP FOR THE NURSING STUDENT

When a client is terminally ill, oftentimes nurses need to consider the care of the client as well as care of the family members. Family members may be active in providing care to terminally ill clients and are at risk for caregiver strain and burnout. Respite care is one option that would be offered, if possible, for caregivers and family members of a terminally ill client. You will learn about therapeutic communication techniques and care to a terminally ill client in your foundations of nursing course.

Considering All Available Resources

Consider available resources as you answer the question. When you answer a test question, remember that you have all available supplies and equipment needed to care for the client at the bedside. You do not need to leave the client to obtain supplies from a treatment or supply room. Remember that you will have all resources you need to provide quality client care.

SAMPLE QUESTION: Consider All Available Resources

Case Event: The nurse is called to the room to assist a client with a chest tube. The client states it felt like the tube pulled out. The nurse assesses the client and finds that the tube has dislodged and is lying on the floor.

Question Query: What action would the nurse take **next**?

Options:

1. Obtain a pair of sterile gloves.
2. Contact the charge nurse for help.
3. Submerge the dislodged tube into sterile water.
4. Cover the insertion site with an occlusive dressing.

ANSWER: 4

TEST-TAKING STRATEGY

Apply the clinical judgment/cognitive skill, *take action.* Note the **strategic word,** *next.* When providing care to a client, particularly in emergency situations, **consider available resources** and keep in mind that all of the resources needed to provide client care will be readily available. Most students would eliminate options 1 and 3 first, knowing these actions are not necessary in this scenario. From the remaining options, you may think, "I don't have an occlusive dressing with me in this situation, so let me call for help first." Remember, you have everything you need wherever and whenever you need it!

> **▮▮▶ TIP FOR THE NURSING STUDENT**
>
> A chest tube may be needed if the client has fluid buildup in the lung (pleural effusion) or has a collapsed lung (pneumothorax). These complications can occur as a result of injury or various health problems. As the nurse managing care of the client with a chest tube, it is necessary to anticipate the possible complications and monitor the client closely. You will learn about chest tubes and the care involved when you study respiratory problems.

 ## What Do You Do If You Eliminate Two Options and Are Unsure of the Final Two?

As you use the process of elimination to rule out the incorrect options, it is likely that you will be able to easily eliminate two of the four options in a multiple-choice question. Now what do you do with the last two options, and how do you proceed to select the correct one? Follow these helpful steps when you are trying to decide which of the last two options is correct.

1. Read the question again.
2. Identify the case event from the query of the question.
3. Look for the strategic words or strategic phrases.
4. Identify the subject of the question.
5. Ask yourself, "What is the question asking?"
6. Think about the clinical judgment/cognitive skill that you need to apply.
7. Read the options again.
8. Eliminate the options that do not apply or relate to the situation.
9. Make your final choice by focusing on what the question is asking, using nursing knowledge, and implementing test-taking strategies.

What Is the "What If?" Syndrome?

The "What if?" syndrome occurs when you read a test question and instead of simply focusing on the information in the question, you start asking yourself, "Well, what if?" You need to avoid asking yourself this question because this leads you right into the dreaded pitfall of "reading into the question." Read the question carefully, identify strategic words or strategic phrases, focus on the subject of the question, and think about the clinical judgment/cognitive skill that you need to apply. You may need to think critically to answer the question, but stay on track! Asking yourself "What if?" moves you off track with regard to what the question is asking. Let's look at two questions and then examine the ways to avoid reading into them.

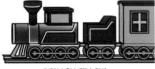

STAY ON TRACK!

> **❓ SAMPLE QUESTION 1**
>
> *Case Event:* The nurse is changing the tapes on a newly inserted tracheostomy tube. The client coughs, and the tube is dislodged.
> *Question Query:* What is the **initial** nursing action?
> 1. Grasp the retention sutures to spread the opening.
> 2. Call the primary health care provider to reinsert the tube.
> 3. Call the respiratory therapy department to reinsert the tube.
> 4. Cover the tracheostomy site with a sterile dressing to prevent infection.
> Now you may immediately think, "The tube is dislodged, and I need the primary health care provider!" Read the question carefully. Note the strategic word, *initial*, and focus on the information in the question—the client's tube is dislodged. The question is asking you for an *initial* nursing action, so that is what you need to look for. This will direct you to option 1. Use nursing knowledge and test-taking strategies to assist in answering the question.
>
> **ANSWER: 1**

TEST-TAKING STRATEGY

Apply the clinical judgment/cognitive skill, *take action*. Note the **strategic word**, initial, and focus on the **information in the question**. Eliminate options 2 and 3 first because they are **comparable or alike** and will delay the immediate intervention needed. Eliminate option 4 because this action will block the airway. If the tube is accidentally dislodged, the initial nursing action is to grasp the retention sutures and spread the opening. In addition, use of the **ABCs—airway, breathing, and circulation**—will direct you to the correct option.

➡ TIP FOR THE NURSING STUDENT

A tracheostomy is an opening into the trachea that is created surgically for the purpose of establishing an airway. You will learn about the care of a client with a tracheostomy tube when you learn about nursing care for a client with a respiratory problem, but the important thing to remember for any client is that maintaining a patent airway is the nurse's priority. In this question the only nursing action that will open the airway is the action identified in option 1. You will learn about tracheostomy care and the nurse's responsibilities in the care of the client when you study respiratory problems.

SAMPLE QUESTION 2

Case Event: The nurse is caring for a hospitalized client with a diagnosis of heart failure who suddenly reports shortness of breath and dyspnea.
Question Query: The nurse would take which **immediate** action?
1. Get an order for oxygen.
2. Prepare to administer furosemide.
3. Elevate the head of the client's bed.
4. Call the primary health care provider.
Now you may immediately think that the client has developed pulmonary edema, a complication of heart failure, and needs a diuretic. Although pulmonary edema is a complication of heart failure, there is no information in the question indicating the presence of pulmonary edema. The question simply states that the client suddenly reports shortness of breath and dyspnea. Read the question carefully. Note the **strategic word**, *immediate*, and **focus on the subject**—the client's symptoms. The question is asking you for a nursing action, so that is what you need to look for. This will direct you to option 3. Use nursing knowledge and test-taking strategies to assist in answering the question.

ANSWER: 3

TEST-TAKING STRATEGY

Apply the clinical judgment/cognitive skill, *take action* and focus on the **information in the question**. Note the **strategic word**, *immediate*. Think about the client's symptoms and look for the *immediate* nursing action. Although the primary health care provider may need to be notified, this is not the immediate action. Although oxygen may need to be administered, taking the time to get an order delays immediate intervention. Furosemide is a diuretic and may or may not be prescribed for the client. Because no data in the question indicate the presence of pulmonary edema, option 3 is correct.

➡ TIP FOR THE NURSING STUDENT

Heart failure is an inability of the heart to maintain adequate circulation to meet the metabolic needs of the body because of an impaired pumping ability. Pulmonary edema is a serious complication of heart failure in which fluid accumulates in the pulmonary system as a result of the impaired pumping ability of the heart. You will learn about heart failure and pulmonary edema when you learn about cardiac problems. One thing to remember is that with all clients, airway is the priority, and that as the nurse, you need to take an immediate action that will assist the client to breathe easily. In many questions that ask for an immediate action, the action that identifies a client position is usually the immediate action, as long as the position is a correct one. For clients with respiratory or cardiac problems, elevation of the client's head will assist with breathing. Learn about heart failure and pulmonary edema, the signs and symptoms, and immediate nursing actions to take.

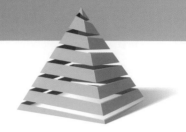

CHAPTER 7

Positive and Negative Event Queries

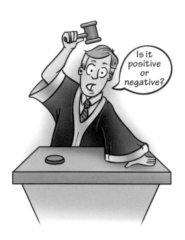

The questions presented on the National Council Licensure Examination (NCLEX®) are written to include either a positive or a negative event query. Primarily, the questions are written as positive event queries; however, you need to be prepared for either type.

SMART STUDY TIP

Student-to-Student

One of the first things you should do when reading a test question is identify whether the query is positive or negative. If you do this, you will look at the scenario in the appropriate context, and this will increase the likelihood of answering the question correctly.

Positive Event Queries

 ### What Is a Positive Event Query?

> **Positive event query: Select an option that is positive or correct!**

A positive event query asks you to make a decision and select the option that is accurate or correct with regard to the data presented in the question. How will you know that the question includes a positive event query? Read the question carefully and focus on the query of the question. The query contains words or phrases that indicate the question includes a positive event query.

What Words and Phrases Are Commonly Used in Positive Event Queries?

Remember to read the question carefully and focus on the query of the question because the query contains words or phrases that indicate the question includes a positive event query. Several examples of queries and sample questions that indicate the question includes a positive event query are listed next.

Positive Event Queries: Examples of Words and Phrases		
Early	Initial	Select all that apply
Late	First	Understands
Most likely	Immediately	Has been achieved
Greatest	Most appropriate	Adequately tolerating
Highest	Priority	Most important
Best	Effective	Essential

Positive Event Queries: Examples of Queries

What is the **earliest** sign of a change in level of consciousness?
Which is a **late** sign of shock?

The nurse **most likely** expects to note which finding?

Which individual is at the **greatest** risk for committing suicide?

Which intervention is of **highest priority** in the preoperative teaching plan?

What **best** action would the nurse implement?

What is the **initial** nursing action?

Which action would the nurse take **first?**

Based on these findings, the nurse would **immediately** take which action?

Which nursing action is **most appropriate?**

The nurse would make which **most appropriate** response to the client?

List in order of **priority** the actions that the nurse would take.

Which assessment finding indicates that the medication was **effective?**

Select all that apply.

Which statement made by the client indicates the **best** understanding of how to prevent transmission of the disease?

Which outcome would indicate that the **most important** goal has been achieved for this client?

The nurse determines that the client is **adequately tolerating** the procedure if which observation is made?

Which item is **essential** to have at the bedside?

Positive Event Queries: Sample Questions

SAMPLE QUESTION 1

Case Event: A client with suspected active lung tuberculosis is being scheduled for diagnostic tests.

Positive Event Query: The nurse anticipates that which diagnostic test will **most likely** be prescribed to confirm the diagnosis?

1. Chest x-ray
2. Skin testing
3. Sputum culture
4. White blood cell count

ANSWER: 3

TEST-TAKING STRATEGY:

This question identifies an example of a positive event query. Apply the clinical judgment/cognitive skill, *generate solutions.* Note the strategic words, *most likely.* Additional noteworthy words are *active* (noted in the question) and *confirm* (noted in the query). Focus on the diagnosis presented in the question and the associated pathophysiology to assist in directing you to option 3. Remember that tuberculosis is an infectious disease caused by *Mycobacterium tuberculosis,* and the demonstration of tubercle bacilli using bacteriology is essential for establishing a diagnosis. It is not possible to make a diagnosis solely on the basis of a chest x-ray, and a positive reaction to a skin test indicates the presence of tuberculosis infection but does not show whether the infection is active or dormant. A white blood cell count may be increased, but it is not specifically related to the presence of tuberculosis. Remember to note the wording in the query and focus on the strategic words!

▮▶ TIP FOR THE NURSING STUDENT

Tuberculosis is an infectious disease of the lung caused by the acid-fast bacillus *Mycobacterium tuberculosis.* It is generally transmitted by the inhalation of infected droplets and usually affects the lungs, although infection of multiple organ systems can occur. It is a major public health concern because of its infectious nature. Because of the presence of the acid-fast bacillus in the lung, the way that the infection is confirmed is by its presence in the sputum. You may have already learned about this disease during your microbiology course, but will learn more about it when you study the respiratory system and infectious diseases. Be sure to learn about this infectious disease.

SMART STUDY TIP

Scope of Practice

As the nurse, you will not be prescribing diagnostic tests, but you must understand preprocedure preparation and postprocedure care and the associated client teaching points. Nurses play an active role in the treatment process of assigned clients and are integral in the management and delivery of quality care.

SMART STUDY TIP

Preparing for Clinical

As a nursing student, you will be expected to deliver safe care to your assigned clients. Be sure to know if your clients are on any type of transmission-based precautions, and institute these precautions in the care of your clients. This is important because it relates to infection control. Your clinical instructor will be observing to ensure that you follow these precautions!

SAMPLE QUESTION 2

Case Event: The nurse is preparing to administer digoxin 0.25 mg orally. The label on the medication bottle reads "digoxin 0.125 mg per tablet."

Positive Event Query: How many tablet(s) will the nurse plan to administer to the client?

ANSWER: 2 tablets

TEST-TAKING STRATEGY:

Apply the clinical judgment/cognitive skill, *generate solutions*. Focus on the subject, calculating a medication dose. Note the words *plan to administer*. Focus on the information in the question and that a dose of 0.25 mg is prescribed. Use the formula for calculating a medication dose to answer the question. Always double-check the calculation and verify your answer using a calculator. Remember to use nursing knowledge, focus on the information in the question, and identify what the question is asking (the subject).

▐▶ TIP FOR THE NURSING STUDENT

In this question you need to know the formula for calculating a medication dose. You will learn about medication calculations in your foundations of nursing course. The formula and the calculation for this question are as follows:

$$\frac{Desired}{Available} \times Quantity = number\ of\ tablet(s)$$

$$\frac{0.25\,mg}{0.125\,mg} \times 1\,tablet = 2\,tablets$$

SAMPLE QUESTION 3

Case Event: The nurse is caring for an infant in the post-operative period.

Positive Event Query: Which nursing interventions apply in the care of an infant after a cleft lip repair (cheiloplasty)? **Select all that apply.**

- ☐ 1. Position the child on the abdomen.
- ☐ 2. Observe for bleeding at the operative site.
- ☐ 3. Keep elbow restraints on the infant at all times.
- ☐ 4. Cleanse the suture line gently after feeding the infant.
- ☐ 5. Institute measures that will prevent vigorous and sustained crying.
- ☐ 6. Assist the mother with breastfeeding if this is the feeding method of choice.

ANSWER: 2, 4, 5, 6

TEST-TAKING STRATEGY:

Apply the clinical judgment/cognitive skill, *generate solutions*. Focus on the subject, nursing interventions after a cleft lip repair. Eliminate option 3 first because of the closed-ended word, *all*. Next, visualize each intervention and think about its effect on the surgical repair to assist in selecting the correct interventions. Remember to focus on the subject and the surgical procedure!

▐▶ TIP FOR THE NURSING STUDENT

A cleft lip is a craniofacial malformation that results from the incomplete fusion of the embryonic structures surrounding the primitive oral cavity. It may be unilateral or bilateral. Closure of the lip defect is usually done between 6 and 12 weeks of age as long as the infant is free of any oral, respiratory, or systemic infection. Interventions in the postoperative period are directed toward protecting the operative site, preventing infection, and maintaining nutrition. Keeping these goals of care in mind will assist in answering the question correctly. You will learn about disorders of the newborn and infant in your newborn care and pediatric nursing courses. Learn about cleft lip repair and the important nursing interventions.

SAMPLE QUESTION 4

Case Event: The nurse is performing cardiopulmonary resuscitation on a 6-month-old infant.

Positive Event Query: Which anatomical area would the nurse palpate to assess circulation?

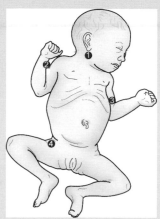

(Figure from Lowdermilk D, Perry A: *Maternity & women's health care*, ed 8, St Louis, 2004, Mosby.)

ANSWER: 3

TEST-TAKING STRATEGY:

Apply the clinical judgment/cognitive skill, *take action*. Focus on the subject, assessing circulation in a 6-month-old infant. Visualize the body structure of a 6-month-old infant and recall that the very short and fat neck of the infant makes the carotid pulse difficult to palpate. In an infant younger than 12 months, the brachial pulse is used to assess circulation. Remember to focus on the subject!

➡ TIP FOR THE BEGINNING NURSING STUDENT

You need to know where the arterial pulse points are located, but you also need to note that this question focuses on the 6-month-old infant. Use what you learned in anatomy class, foundations of nursing class, and physical assessment class. You will also learn more about the infant in your newborn care and pediatric nursing courses. Think about the anatomical structure of the 6-month-old infant, and remember that in an infant younger than 12 months, the brachial pulse is used to assess circulation.

SAMPLE QUESTION 5

Case Event: The nurse is caring for a client who suddenly develops pulmonary edema.

Positive Event Query: Arrange the nursing interventions in the **priority** order that they would be performed. **All options must be used.**

Unordered Options	Ordered Responses
Check lung sounds.	Place the client in high Fowler's position.
Place oxygen on the client.	Place oxygen on the client.
Place the client in high Fowler's position.	Place the client on a cardiac monitor and pulse oximetry.
Place the client on a cardiac monitor and pulse oximetry.	Check lung sounds.
Prepare to insert a urinary catheter and to administer furosemide.	Prepare to insert a urinary catheter and to administer furosemide.
Prepare the client for endotracheal intubation and mechanical ventilation.	Prepare the client for endotracheal intubation and mechanical ventilation.

TEST-TAKING STRATEGY:

Apply the clinical judgment/cognitive skill, *take action*. Focus on the subject, care for the client with pulmonary edema. Think about the pathophysiology associated with pulmonary edema. This will assist in determining that positioning the client in high Fowler's position would be the first action so that breathing will be easier for the client. Next, use the ABCs—airway, breathing, and circulation—to guide your selections. This will assist in determining that administering oxygen to the client would be the next action, followed by placing the client on a cardiac monitor and pulse oximetry to determine a baseline. Next check the lung sounds, because this is an assessment or data collection procedure, and you would want to evaluate the status of lung sounds so that you will be able to determine the response to furosemide when it is administered. The urinary catheter is also inserted so the urine output can be assessed as a response to the furosemide. If there is no response to the treatment, then finally the client may need intubation and mechanical ventilation. Remember to focus on the subject!

⫸ TIP FOR THE NURSING STUDENT

Pulmonary edema is a life-threatening event that can result from severe heart failure. In pulmonary edema, the left ventricle of the heart fails to eject sufficient blood, and pressure increases in the lungs because of the accumulated fluid. The client has severe dyspnea and struggles for air. Therefore, interventions are aimed at alleviating this severe dyspnea and removing the excess fluid from the body. You will learn about pulmonary edema in your medical-surgical nursing course when you study cardiovascular problems. Be sure to learn the signs and symptoms of heart failure and pulmonary edema and the associated interventions.

Negative Event Queries

What Is a Negative Event Query?

A negative event query asks you to make a decision and select the option that is inaccurate or incorrect with regard to the data presented in the question. How will you know that the question includes a negative event query? Read the question carefully and focus on the query of the question. The query contains words or phrases that indicate the question includes a negative event query. Generally, negative event queries are used in evaluation-type questions and evaluate the effectiveness of a treatment, procedure, medication, or teaching.

What Words and Phrases Are Commonly Used in Negative Event Queries?

Remember to read the question carefully and focus on the query of the question because the query contains words or phrases that indicate the question includes a negative event query. Examples of words and phrases are listed in the following box. In addition, examples of negative event queries and sample questions that indicate the question includes a negative event query are listed next.

Negative Event Queries: Examples of Words and Phrases

Least likely	Needs additional instructions
Least priority	Have not yet been met
Least helpful	Indicates the need for follow-up
Ineffective	Has not met the outcome criteria

Negative Event Queries: Examples of Queries

Which individual is **least likely** to develop coronary artery disease?

Which client problem is of **least priority?**

Which approach by the nurse would be **least helpful** in assisting this client?

The nurse determines that the medication is **ineffective** if the client continues to experience which symptom?

The nurse determines that the family **needs additional instructions** if the nurse observed which action being done by the family?

Which outcome indicates to the nurse that the goals **have not yet been met?**

Which assessment finding indicates the **need for follow-up?**

The nurse determines that the client **has not met the outcome criteria** by discharge if which observation is made?

SMART STUDY TIP

Scope of Practice

Negative event query type questions may ask about what you, as a nurse, need to follow up on in the care of your assigned clients. In other words, the question asks about what nursing actions need to be further implemented to ensure delivery of quality client care.

Negative Event Queries: Sample Questions

SAMPLE QUESTION 1

Case Event: The nurse is reviewing the nursing care plan of a hospitalized client with sickle cell crisis.

Negative Event Query: Which client problem is the **least priority?**

1. Generalized pain
2. Signs of dehydration
3. Inability to cope with the disease
4. Lack of perfusion to peripheral tissues

ANSWER: 3

TEST-TAKING STRATEGY:

Apply the clinical judgment/cognitive skill, *prioritize hypotheses*. Focus on the words *least priority*. According to Maslow's Hierarchy of Needs theory, physiological needs are the priority, followed by safety needs, and then psychosocial needs. Using Maslow's theory will direct you to option 3 because this is the only option that addresses a psychosocial need. Remember to focus on the words *least priority*. These words indicate a negative event query.

⏩ TIP FOR THE NURSING STUDENT

Sickle cell disease is a genetic disorder that results in chronic anemia, pain, organ damage, and disability. The client also has an increased risk for infection. In sickle cell disease, the hemoglobin contains an abnormal beta chain known as *hemoglobin S*. The hemoglobin S is sensitive to oxygen changes occurring on the red blood cells; when decreased oxygen states occur, the abnormal cells pile together, distorting its shape, and these cells form a sickle shape, become rigid, and block blood flow. The client with sickle cell disease can have episodes of crises that occur in response to conditions that cause hypoxemia. This causes acute pain. The primary treatment for crisis consists of hydration, comfort measures with analgesics, and oxygen administration. You will learn about sickle cell disease when you study hematological problems. Be sure to learn about the causes of crisis and its treatment measures.

SAMPLE QUESTION 2

Case Event: The nurse has collected data from four clients examined in the health care clinic.
Negative Event Query: Which client is **least likely** to develop coronary artery disease?
1. A client who is obese, is inactive, and has a stressful lifestyle
2. A client with a blood cholesterol level of 289 mg/dL (7.47 mmol/L)
3. A client who has been smoking 2 packs of cigarettes daily for the past 20 years
4. A client with hypertension whose blood pressure has been maintained at 118/78 mm Hg

ANSWER: 4

TEST-TAKING STRATEGY:

Apply the clinical judgment/cognitive skill, *analyze cues.* Focus on the data in the question and note the words *least likely.* Recalling the risk factors associated with coronary artery disease will direct you to option 4. Option 4 is the only option that identifies a risk factor (hypertension) that has been modified and controlled. Remember to focus on the words *least likely.* These words indicate a negative event query.

❚❚▶ TIP FOR THE NURSING STUDENT

Coronary artery disease affects the arteries that supply blood to the myocardium. When blood flow to the myocardium is partially or completely blocked, ischemia or infarction of the myocardium can occur and the client suffers a heart attack. Coronary artery disease is a major concern because it is a life-threatening health problem; this is why great emphasis is placed on reducing or eliminating the modifiable risk factors such as obesity, high blood pressure, stress, smoking, and high cholesterol. You will learn about coronary artery disease when you study the cardiovascular system in medical-surgical nursing. Be sure to learn the associated risk factors and measures to reduce or eliminate them.

 SAMPLE QUESTION 3

Case Event: The nurse is caring for a client with aphasia.
Negative Event Query: Which nursing action will be **ineffective** when communicating with the client?
1. Increasing environmental stimuli
2. Speaking with a normal volume or tone
3. Presenting one thought or idea at a time
4. Asking questions that can be answered "yes" or "no"

ANSWER: 1

TEST-TAKING STRATEGY:

Apply the clinical judgment/cognitive skill, *generate solutions.* Focus on the data in the question and the client's diagnosis and note the word *ineffective.* Recalling that the client with aphasia may need extra time to comprehend and respond to communication will direct you to option 1. Increased environmental stimuli may be distracting and disrupting to communication efforts. Remember to focus on the word *ineffective*! This word indicates a negative event query.

❚❚▶ TIP FOR THE NURSING STUDENT

Aphasia is an abnormal neurological condition in which language function is disordered or absent because of injury to certain areas of the cerebral cortex. This condition is most often seen in a client with a stroke (brain attack). The aphasic client needs repetitive directions to understand and complete a task, and each task needs to be broken down into parts, with directions given one step at a time. The client needs time to process the information. This is why increased environmental stimuli can be disruptive to the communication process. You will learn about aphasia when you study the neurological system in your medical-surgical nursing course. Be sure to learn about the nursing interventions for a client with aphasia.

SMART STUDY TIP

Student-to-Student

Negative event queries are one of the hardest types of questions to answer correctly. Be on the lookout for the words or phrases that indicate the question contains a negative event query, and be sure to reread the question before submitting your answer!

SAMPLE QUESTION 4

Case Event: The nurse is collecting data from a client who has been taking omeprazole as prescribed.

Negative Event Query: The nurse determines that the medication is **ineffective** if the client continues to experience which symptom?

1. Dizziness
2. Heartburn
3. Headaches
4. Muscle pains

ANSWER: 2

TEST-TAKING STRATEGY:

Apply the clinical judgment/cognitive skill, *evaluate outcomes*. Focus on the data in the question and note the name of the medication and the word *ineffective*. Recalling that omeprazole is a gastric acid pump inhibitor (most medication names that end with the letters -*zole* are gastric acid pump inhibitors) will direct you to option 2. Remember to focus on the word *ineffective*! This word indicates a negative event query.

⦿ TIP FOR THE NURSING STUDENT

Omeprazole is a gastric acid pump inhibitor that is most often used to treat gastrointestinal disorders, such as esophagitis, gastroesophageal reflux disease, and certain stomach ulcers. Therefore, this medication will assist in relieving heartburn. You will learn about this medication when you study pharmacology and when you study gastrointestinal problems in your medical-surgical nursing course. Be sure to learn the action, intended effect, contraindications, and client teaching points for this medication.

SAMPLE QUESTION 5

Case Event: A client treated for an episode of hyperthermia is being discharged to home from the emergency department, and the nurse provides discharge instructions.

Negative Event Query: The nurse determines that the client **needs additional instructions** if the client states intentions to implement which measure?

1. Resume full activity level immediately
2. Increase fluid intake for the next 24 hours
3. Stay in a cool environment when possible
4. Monitor voiding for adequacy of urine output

ANSWER: 1

TEST-TAKING STRATEGY:

Apply the clinical judgment/cognitive skill, *evaluate outcomes*. Focus on the strategic words, *needs additional instructions*. Select the client statement that indicates that the nurse needs to provide further instructions. Resumption of full activity immediately is not helpful; rather, rest periods are indicated. Remember to focus on the strategic words, *needs additional instructions*. These words indicate a negative event query.

⦿ TIP FOR THE NURSING STUDENT

Hyperthermia is a condition in which the client's body temperature is elevated above his or her normal range. It can be caused by various factors, such as a hot environment, vigorous activity, medications or anesthesia, increased metabolic rate, illness or trauma, dehydration, or the inability to perspire. Treatment involves lowering the body temperature and treating and eliminating its cause. You will learn about hyperthermia during your nursing program in many of your courses. Be sure to focus on the causes of the hyperthermia and its treatment.

SAMPLE QUESTION 6

Case Event: Malnutrition has been diagnosed for an unconscious client.

Negative Event Query: Which outcome indicates to the nurse that the goals for this client **have not yet been met?**

1. Stable weight
2. Intake equaling output
3. Total protein 4.5 g/dL (45 g/L)
4. Blood urea nitrogen (BUN) 12 mg/dL (4.28 mmol/L)

ANSWER: 3

TEST-TAKING STRATEGY:

Apply the clinical judgment/cognitive skill, *evaluate outcomes*. Focus on the subject, *goals have not yet been met*. Because stable weight and equal intake and output are satisfactory indicators and the BUN is a normal value, option 3 is the answer to the question. Also recall that the total protein reference range is 6.4 to 8.3 g/dL (64 to 83 g/L). Remember to focus on the subject, *goals have not yet been met!* These words indicate a negative event query.

▐▶ TIP FOR THE NURSING STUDENT

Malnutrition indicates that the client's intake of nutrients is insufficient to meet the client's metabolic needs. This can be due to various causes such as, but not limited to, disease, injury, malabsorption, social factors, or cultural factors. Nursing interventions focus on addressing the nutritional deficits. You will learn about malnutrition in your nutrition or foundations of nursing course.

CHAPTER 8

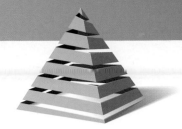

Questions Requiring Prioritization

Many test questions in the National Council Licensure Examination (NCLEX®) require you to use the skill of prioritizing nursing actions. Most prioritizing questions are presented in the multiple-choice format; however, you may also be presented with a question in the prioritizing (ordered-response) format or other formats. Prioritizing questions address content in any nursing area. These types of questions can be difficult because when a question requires prioritization, all options may be correct, but you need to determine the correct order of action or highest priority. Some test-taking strategies that you can use to assist in answering these questions correctly include noting the strategic words or strategic phrases that indicate the need to prioritize; the ABCs—airway, breathing, and circulation; Maslow's Hierarchy of Needs theory; the steps of the nursing process, and applying clinical judgment and cognitive skills. The cognitive skills most useful for prioritizing questions will be *prioritize hypotheses*, *generate solutions*, and *take action*. Let's review the definition of prioritizing and these test taking strategies.

 ## Prioritizing

What Does Prioritizing Mean?

Prioritizing means that you need to rank the client's problems in order of importance. It is important to read a question carefully and focus on the information in the question because the order of importance may vary depending on the subject of the question, the clinical setting, the client's condition, and the client's needs. It also is important to consider what the client deems a priority, which may be quite different from what the nurse thinks is most important. Remember to always consider what the client believes is the priority when planning care.

When you prioritize, you are deciding which client needs or problems require immediate action and which ones could be delayed until a later time because they are not urgent. As you read a question and are trying to determine which option identifies the nurse's priority, use the priority classification system to rank nursing actions as a high, intermediate (middle), or low priority. The description of these three types of classifications is listed next. An additional guideline to use when prioritizing is to think about whether the nursing action is indicated (appropriate or necessary), non-essential (makes no difference or not necessary), or contraindicated (could be harmful).

 ## Priority Classification System

High Priority: a client need that is life-threatening or, if untreated, could result in harm to the client

Intermediate (Middle) Priority: a nonemergency and non–life-threatening client need that does not require immediate attention

Low Priority: a client need that is not directly related to the client's illness or prognosis, is not urgent, and does not require immediate attention

Guides for Prioritizing

Strategic words or phrases
The ABCs
Maslow's Hierarchy of Needs theory
The steps of the nursing process (clinical problem-solving process)
Clinical judgment

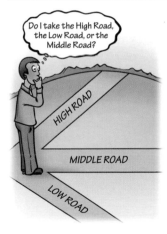

Do I take the High Road, the Low Road, or the Middle Road?

HIGH ROAD
MIDDLE ROAD
LOW ROAD

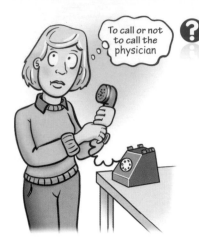

To call or not to call the physician

When Is It a Priority to Select the Option "Call the Physician"?

An important point to remember is that the NCLEX exam tests your competence and ability to care for a client and to implement necessary measures in a particular situation. It is critically important to read the question carefully, note the information in the question, and read all available options. One other point to remember is that if an option identities an intervention that requires a physician's order, then answer the question as if there is already an actual order for the intervention. If the question describes a client situation that is not life-threatening and there is an option that directly relates to a nursing action relevant to the situation, then it is best to select that option and not the option that indicates to "call the physician." Remember that there is usually an action that the nurse would take in a non–life-threatening situation before calling the physician. *Note:* For those nursing students who are studying to become licensed practical/vocational nurses rather than registered nurses, it is very important to report immediately any changes in a client's condition to the registered nurse.

If the question presents a client situation that is life-threatening, then the correct option *may* be to call the physician. Unfortunately, this is not always clear-cut and can present a dilemma in your efforts to answer a question correctly. That is why it is so important to carefully read the question and all the options. Let us review some sample questions that illustrate when to and when not to select the option "call the physician."

SAMPLE QUESTION: When TO Select the Option "Call the Physician" as the Priority Action

Case Event: The nurse is caring for a client who just returned from the recovery room after a tonsillectomy and adenoidectomy. The client is restless, and the pulse rate is increased. The nurse continues to assess the client, but the client begins to vomit large amounts of bright red blood.
Question Query: What is the **immediate** nursing action?
1. Call the surgeon.
2. Continue to assess the client.
3. Obtain a flashlight and gauze.
4. Check the client's blood pressure.

ANSWER: 1

TEST-TAKING STRATEGY
Read the question carefully, noting the strategic word, *immediate* and apply the clinical judgment/cognitive skill, *take action.* Several other noteworthy words in this question include *restless, pulse rate is increased, large amounts,* and *bright red blood.* The subject of the question is that the client is actively bleeding and is exhibiting signs of shock (restlessness and increased pulse rate), indicating a life-threatening situation. Remember to always read each option carefully. In this situation and from the options provided, the nurse would contact the physician and in this question, it is the surgeon. Options 2, 3, and 4 would delay necessary interventions needed in this life-threatening situation.

⏩ TIP FOR THE NURSING STUDENT
Whenever you note that a client is bleeding and the amount is large and bright red, you would become concerned because this indicates active bleeding. Active bleeding is a concern after any type of surgery, including a tonsillectomy and adenoidectomy, and indicates a potential life-threatening situation. You will learn about postoperative complications in your foundations of nursing course, and you will learn specifically about tonsillectomy and adenoidectomy in your pediatrics nursing course. Be sure to learn the postoperative complications and the immediate nursing interventions.

SMART STUDY TIP

Preparing for Clinical

When caring for a pediatric client, family-centered care is always a focus. Although the child is your primary client, the child's family is an additional client whose needs you must be sensitive to and address while caring for the child.

SAMPLE QUESTION: When NOT TO Select the Option "Call the Physician" as the Priority Action

Case Event: The nurse enters a client's room and finds the client slumped over in bed. The nurse quickly assesses the client and discovers that the client is not breathing and there is no pulse.

Question Query: The nurse would take which **immediate** action?

1. Sit the client upright in bed.
2. Call the physician.
3. Begin cardiopulmonary resuscitation (CPR).
4. Place oxygen via a nasal cannula on the client.

ANSWER: 3

TEST-TAKING STRATEGY

Read the question carefully, note the strategic word, *immediate*, and focus on the subject—the client is not breathing and there is no pulse. Apply the clinical judgment/cognitive skill, *take action*. Although the information in the question indicates a life-threatening situation, you need to read all options carefully. In this situation and based on the options provided, the nurse needs to intervene *immediately*. Although the physician needs to be called, the *immediate* nursing action would be to begin CPR. Options 1 and 4 are incorrect because neither of these options will provide immediate assistance to this client.

➤ TIP FOR THE NURSING STUDENT

It is important to read all the information in the question and focus on every word. Note that the client is not breathing and there is no pulse. Therefore, you need to begin CPR. You were most likely required to obtain health care certification in basic life support and CPR before entering nursing school. Be sure to review these procedures, especially because you will be caring for clients during your clinical experiences in your nursing program.

SAMPLE QUESTION: When NOT TO Select the Option "Call the Physician" as the Priority Action

Case Event: A nurse is caring for a postoperative client who suddenly becomes restless.

Question Query: The nurse would take which **most appropriate** action?

1. Notify the surgeon.
2. Medicate the client for pain.
3. Check the client's vital signs.
4. Talk to the client in a calm voice.

ANSWER: 3

TEST-TAKING STRATEGY

Read the question carefully, note the strategic words, *most appropriate*, and focus on the subject—a postoperative client who becomes restless. Additionally, focus on the data in the question. No data in the question indicate that the client has pain; therefore, eliminate option 2. Apply the clinical judgment/cognitive skill, *take action*. Because option 4 is a psychosocial action rather than a physiological one (physiological needs are the priority), eliminate that option using Maslow's Hierarchy of Needs theory.

Recall that restlessness can be an early sign of shock. However, no data in the question indicate a life-threatening condition. Therefore, the nurse would gather more data about the client's condition and would *most appropriately* check the client's vital signs.

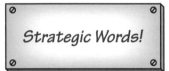

SMART STUDY TIP

Scope of Practice

As a nurse, it is your responsibility to determine when a nursing action needs to be taken before calling the physician. Remember that most often, a nursing action is usually taken before notifying the physician.

TIP FOR THE NURSING STUDENT

One complication after surgery is the development of shock, which is usually due to bleeding or an excessive loss of blood during the surgical procedure. The nurse monitors the postoperative client for signs of shock. One of the earliest signs of shock is restlessness. If restlessness is noted, the nurse would check the client's vital signs next. In shock, the nurse would note that the blood pressure decreases and the pulse rate increases. You will learn about shock as a postoperative complication in your foundations of nursing course. Be sure to focus on the signs of shock and the immediate nursing interventions.

 ## Strategic Words or Strategic Phrases

What Strategic Words or Strategic Phrases Indicate the Need to Prioritize Nursing Actions?

Remember that when a question requires prioritization, all options may be correct; therefore, you need to determine the correct order of nursing action(s). Read the question carefully, and look for the strategic words or strategic phrases in the question that indicate the need to prioritize. Some common strategic words or strategic phrases that indicate the need to prioritize are listed next and are followed by sample questions to illustrate how some of these words or phrases are used in a question.

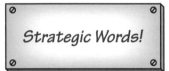
Strategic Words!

NCLEX® EXAM TIP

Remember that many, if not most, questions on the NCLEX exam will require you to prioritize. This means that you can expect the options presented for the question will all be correct options and you will need to use prioritizing skills to answer correctly. Remember to look for the strategic words in the event query to assist in answering correctly!

Common Strategic Words and Phrases That Indicate the Need to Prioritize		
Best	Initial	Next
Essential	Most	Order of priority
First	Most appropriate	Primary
Highest priority	Most important	Priority
Immediately	Most likely	Vital

 ### SAMPLE QUESTION: Prioritizing and Strategic Words

Case Event: The nurse is caring for a hospitalized client with angina pectoris (coronary artery disease) who begins to experience chest pain. The nurse administers a sublingual nitroglycerin tablet as prescribed, but the pain is unrelieved. The nurse checks the client's blood pressure and notes that it is stable.

Question Query: Which action would the nurse take **next**?

1. Reposition the client.
2. Call the client's family.
3. Administer another nitroglycerin tablet.
4. Contact the client's consulting cardiologist.

ANSWER: 3

TEST-TAKING STRATEGY

Note the strategic word, *next*, and focus on the subject—the client is experiencing chest pain. Apply the clinical judgment/cognitive skill, *take action*. Recalling that for a hospitalized client the nurse would administer 3 nitroglycerin tablets 5 minutes apart from each other to relieve chest pain will assist in directing you to option 3. Repositioning the client will not alleviate pain associated with coronary artery disease. The nurse would call the physician or cardiologist if 3 nitroglycerin tablets administered 5 minutes apart from each other did not alleviate the pain. There is no useful reason to call the client's family at this time.

TIP FOR THE NURSING STUDENT

Angina pectoris refers to chest pain that is most often caused by a lack of oxygen to myocardial tissue and occurs as a result of atherosclerosis (clogged blood vessels) or spasm of the coronary arteries. The pain may be relieved by rest and vasodilation of the coronary arteries by medication such as nitroglycerin. The usual protocol for administering nitroglycerin to a hospitalized client is to administer a total of 3 tablets, 5 minutes apart each, to relieve the chest pain. In other words, a nitroglycerin tablet is administered, and if the pain is not relieved in 5 minutes, another is administered. This is repeated in 5 minutes, 1 more time, if the pain is not relieved by the second nitroglycerin tablet. After administering 3 nitroglycerin tablets, if the pain is still unrelieved, the physician or cardiologist is called. It is also important for the nurse to monitor the client's blood pressure because nitroglycerin causes a drop in blood pressure. You will learn about angina pectoris, coronary artery disease, and nitroglycerin during your medical-surgical nursing course. Because this is a major, life-threatening disorder, it is critical that you learn about its signs and symptoms and immediate treatment.

SMART STUDY TIP

Lifestyle Planning

Allowing time for yourself and fun time with family and friends is a priority in your success in nursing school. Don't forget to include this important aspect of your life in your schedule on a regular basis! Planning ahead and setting realistic daily goals for yourself will ensure you are able to build this into your busy schedule.

SAMPLE QUESTION: Prioritizing and Strategic Words

Case Event: An infant with tetralogy of Fallot experiences a hypercyanotic spell during a blood draw.

Question Query: The nurse would take which action **first?**

1. Place the infant in a knee–chest position.
2. Administer intravenous (IV) fluids as prescribed.
3. Administer 100% oxygen by face mask as prescribed.
4. Administer morphine sulfate subcutaneously as prescribed.

ANSWER: 1

TEST-TAKING STRATEGY

Note the **strategic word**, *first,* and focus on the **subject** of the question—a hypercyanotic spell. Apply the clinical judgment/cognitive skill, *take action.* In questions that require you to determine the first nursing action, if one of the options indicates client positioning, that option may be the correct one. Positioning a client can relieve a symptom and is an intervention that takes only seconds to implement. Placing the infant in the knee–chest position reduces the venous return from the legs (which is desaturated) and increases systemic vascular resistance, which diverts more blood flow into the pulmonary artery. Your next action would be to administer oxygen to the infant. Remembering that morphine sulfate reduces spasm that occurs with these spells and that IV fluids are not always needed to treat these spells will assist in determining the order of priority for the remaining two interventions.

TIP FOR THE NURSING STUDENT

Tetralogy of Fallot is a congenital cardiac anomaly that consists of 4 defects in the heart: pulmonary stenosis, ventricular septal defect, malposition of the aorta so that it arises from the septal defect or the right ventricle, and right ventricular hypertrophy. The treatment consists primarily of supportive measures and palliative surgical procedures until the child is old enough to tolerate total corrective surgery. It would be helpful to review the anatomy and physiology of the heart. In addition, you will learn about tetralogy of Fallot when you take your pediatrics nursing course.

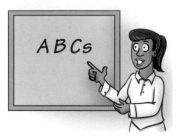

ABCs

Use the ABCs to prioritize!

The ABCs

What Are the ABCs, and How Will They Help Answer a Prioritizing Question?

The ABCs—airway, breathing, and circulation—direct the order of priority of nursing actions. Airway is always the first priority in caring for any client. When a question requires prioritization, use the ABCs to help determine the correct option. If an option addresses maintenance of a patent airway, that will be the correct option. If none of the options address the airway, move to B (breathing), followed by C (circulation). One exception is if the question asks about cardiopulmonary resuscitation. In these questions, remember to follow CAB—circulation (compressions), airway, and breathing—to prioritize. Some sample questions of how the ABC—airway, breathing, and circulation—strategy works are provided next.

SAMPLE QUESTION: The ABCs

Case Event: A client with a diagnosis of cancer is receiving morphine sulfate for pain.
Question Query: When preparing the plan of care for the client, the nurse would include which **priority** action?
1. Monitor stools.
2. Monitor urine output.
3. Encourage fluid intake.
4. Encourage the client to cough and deep breathe.

ANSWER: 4

TEST-TAKING STRATEGY

Note the strategic word, *priority*, and focus on the subject—morphine sulfate. Apply the clinical judgment/cognitive skill, *generate solutions*. Use the ABCs—airway, breathing, and circulation—as a guide to direct you to the correct option. Recall that morphine sulfate suppresses the cough reflex and the respiratory reflex. Although options 1, 2, and 3 are components of the plan of care, the correct option addresses airway. Remember to use the ABCs to prioritize.

▮▶ TIP FOR THE NURSING STUDENT

Morphine sulfate is an opioid analgesic that is used to alleviate pain. One of the primary concerns when a client receives morphine sulfate is that the medication depresses the respiratory and cough reflex. Therefore, the nurse focuses primarily on the client's respiratory status when administering morphine sulfate. You will learn about morphine sulfate in your medical-surgical nursing courses and in your pharmacology course.

SAMPLE QUESTION: The ABCs

Case Event: The nurse is assessing the client's condition after cardioversion.
Question Query: Which observation would be of **highest priority**?
1. Blood pressure
2. Status of airway
3. Oxygen flow rate
4. Level of consciousness

ANSWER: 2

TEST-TAKING STRATEGY

Note the strategic words, *highest priority*, and focus on the subject—monitoring a client after cardioversion. Apply the clinical judgment/cognitive skill, *prioritize hypotheses*. Nursing responsibilities after cardioversion include maintenance of a patent airway, oxygen administration, assessment of vital signs and level of consciousness, and dysrhythmia detection. Airway, however, is always the highest priority. Use the ABCs—airway, breathing, and circulation to direct you to option 2.

TIP FOR THE NURSING STUDENT

Cardioversion is a procedure in which an electrical shock is delivered to the heart with the use of a defibrillator. Cardioversion is used to slow the heart or to restore the heart to a normal sinus rhythm when medication therapy is ineffective. You will learn about cardioversion when you study cardiac disorders and dysrhythmias in your medical-surgical nursing course.

SAMPLE QUESTION: The ABCs

Case Event: The nurse is providing preoperative teaching to a client scheduled for a cholecystectomy.

Question Query: Which intervention would be of **highest priority** in the preoperative teaching plan?

1. Teaching leg exercises
2. Providing instructions regarding fluid intake
3. Teaching coughing and deep-breathing exercises
4. Assessing the client's understanding of the surgical procedure

ANSWER: 3

TEST-TAKING STRATEGY

Note the strategic words, *highest priority*, and note the subject—preoperative plan of care. Apply the clinical judgment/cognitive skill, *prioritize hypotheses*. Use the ABCs—airway, breathing, and circulation—to answer the question. Option 3 relates to airway. After cholecystectomy, breathing tends to be shallow because deep breathing is painful as a result of the location of the surgical procedure. Although all options are a component of the preoperative teaching plan, teaching the importance of performing coughing and deep-breathing exercises is the priority in the preoperative plan of care.

TIP FOR THE NURSING STUDENT

A cholecystectomy is the removal of the gallbladder, usually performed via laparoscopic procedure. You can use medical terminology skills to determine what cholecystectomy refers to: *cholecyst-* means gallbladder, and *-ectomy* means removal of. Next, using your knowledge of anatomy, think about the anatomical location of the gallbladder. Because of its close anatomical location to the diaphragm, it makes sense that the client would have difficulty coughing and deep breathing after surgery. You will learn about coughing and deep breathing exercises for the post-operative client in your foundations of nursing course.

Maslow's Hierarchy of Needs Theory

What Is Maslow's Hierarchy of Needs Theory, and How Will It Help Answer Prioritizing Questions?

Abraham Maslow theorized that human needs are satisfied in a particular order, and he arranged human needs in a pyramid or hierarchy. According to Maslow, basic physiological needs, such as airway, breathing, circulation, water, food, and elimination, are the priority. These basic physiological needs are followed by safety and then the psychosocial needs, including security, love and belonging, self-esteem, and self-actualization, in that order.

Maslow's Hierarchy of Needs theory is a helpful guide when prioritizing client needs. When you are answering a question that requires you to prioritize, select an option that relates to a physiological need, remembering that physiological needs are the first priority.

If a physiological need is not addressed in the question or noted in one of the options, then continue to use Maslow's Hierarchy of Needs theory as a guide and look for the option that addresses safety. If neither physiological nor safety needs are addressed, look for the option that addresses the client's psychosocial need. See the illustration of Maslow's Hierarchy of Needs theory for a full list of needs. The sample questions that follow point out how Maslow's theory can be used as a guide when answering questions that require prioritizing.

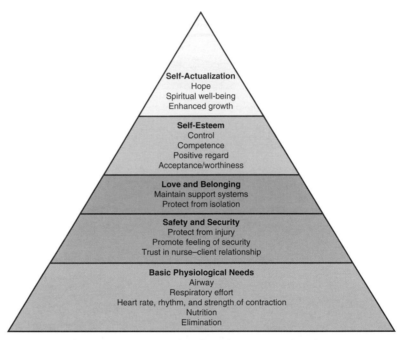

Nursing priorities from Maslow's Hierarchy of Needs. (From Harkreader H, Hogan MA, Thobaben M: *Fundamentals of nursing: caring and clinical judgment*, ed 3, Philadelphia, 2007, Saunders.)

 SAMPLE QUESTION: Maslow's Hierarchy of Needs

Case Event: The nurse is admitting a client with a diagnosis of posttraumatic stress disorder to the mental health unit. The client is confused and disoriented.

Question Query: During the assessment, what is the nurse's **primary** goal for this client?

1. Explain the unit rules.
2. Orient the client to the unit.
3. Stabilize the client's psychiatric needs.
4. Accept the client and make the client feel safe.

ANSWER: 4

TEST-TAKING STRATEGY

Note the strategic word, *primary,* and focus on the subject—a client being admitted to the mental health unit. Apply the clinical judgment/cognitive skill, *generate solutions.* Using Maslow's Hierarchy of Needs theory, remember that when a physiological need does not exist, safety needs take precedence. It is important to accept a client and make a confused and disoriented client feel safe. Orientation and explaining the unit rules are part of any admission process and this goal is not helpful to a confused and disoriented client. Stabilizing psychiatric needs is a long-term goal.

⚑ TIP FOR THE NURSING STUDENT

Posttraumatic stress disorder is a mental health disorder characterized by an acute emotional response to a traumatic event that involved severe environmental stress. This event could include situations such as a natural disaster, a terrorist attack, military combat, physical torture, rape, experiencing or witnessing an automobile crash or other type of accident, or witnessing a shooting or murder. You will learn about posttraumatic stress disorder in your psychiatric/mental health nursing course.

❓ SAMPLE QUESTION: Maslow's Hierarchy of Needs

Case Event: The nurse has developed a plan of care for a client diagnosed with anorexia nervosa.
Question Query: Which client problem would the nurse select as the **priority** in the plan of care?
1. Malnutrition
2. Inability to cope
3. Concern about body appearance
4. Lack of knowledge about nutrition

ANSWER: 1

TEST-TAKING STRATEGY

Note the strategic word *priority,* and focus on the subject—the priority problem for a client with anorexia nervosa. Apply the clinical judgment/cognitive skill, *prioritize hypotheses.* Use Maslow's Hierarchy of Needs theory to recall that physiological needs are the priority. This will assist in directing you to option 1. Options 2, 3, and 4 are psychosocial needs and are of a lesser priority.

⚑ TIP FOR THE NURSING STUDENT

Anorexia nervosa is a disorder characterized by a prolonged refusal to eat. The client believes that he or she is obese, although the body weight is well below the individual's normal expected weight. It results in emaciation, amenorrhea, an emotional disturbance concerning body image, and the fear of becoming obese. The condition is primarily seen in adolescent girls and is usually associated with emotional stress or conflict such as anger, fear, or anxiety. Treatment includes measures to improve nutritional status and therapy to overcome the emotional conflicts associated with the disorder. You will learn about anorexia nervosa in your psychiatric/mental health nursing course.

❓ SAMPLE QUESTION: Maslow's Hierarchy of Needs

Case Event: The nurse is preparing to teach a client how to use crutches. Before initiating the lesson, the nurse performs an assessment on the client.
Question Query: The **priority** nursing assessment would include which focus?
1. The client's feelings about the restricted mobility
2. The client's fear related to the use of the crutches
3. The client's muscle strength and previous activity level
4. The client's understanding of the need for increased mobility

ANSWER: 3

TEST-TAKING STRATEGY

Note the strategic word *priority,* and focus on the subject—teaching a client how to use crutches. Apply the clinical judgment/cognitive skill, *prioritize hypotheses.* Using Maslow's Hierarchy of Needs theory, remember that physiological needs take precedence over psychosocial needs. This should direct you to option 3. Assessing muscle strength will help determine whether the client has enough strength for crutch walking and if muscle-strengthening exercises are necessary. Previous activity level will provide information related to the tolerance of activity. Options 1, 2, and 4 are also components of the assessment but relate to psychosocial needs.

�ᴵ TIP FOR THE NURSING STUDENT

Crutches are devices that are usually made of wood or metal and that aid a person in walking. Crutches require the use of some upper and lower body muscle strength; otherwise injury, such as a fall, can occur. It is also important for the nurse to determine the client's previous activity level to determine if crutches would be an appropriate assistive device. If the client's previous activity level was minimal and muscle strength is poor, crutches would not be an appropriate ambulatory device, and the client would be at risk for injury with their use. It is also important for the crutches to be fitted properly and for the individual to be taught how to safely walk using them to achieve a stable gait. You will learn about the use of crutches and other assistive devices for ambulation in your foundations of nursing course.

❓ Nursing Process (Clinical Problem-Solving Process)

How Will the Nursing Process (Clinical Problem-Solving Process) Help Answer Prioritizing Questions?

The Test Plan for the NCLEX exam identifies the nursing process (clinical problem-solving process) as an Integrated Process. The nursing process provides a systematic method for providing care to a client. For the student studying to become a registered nurse, these steps include assessment, analysis, planning, implementation, and evaluation. For the student studying to become a licensed practical/vocational nurse, these steps include data collection, planning, implementation, and evaluation. These steps are usually followed in sequence, with assessment/data collection being the first step and evaluation being the last step. However, once the nursing process begins, it becomes a cyclical process. The steps of the nursing process can be used as a guide to help you when answering questions that require prioritization. Remember that it is always important to read the question carefully to determine what the question is asking. When a question asks for the first or initial nursing action, use these steps and look for an assessment/data collection action in one of the options. If an assessment/data collection action is not addressed in one of the options, then continue to use the nursing process in a systematic order. See the accompanying illustration of the steps of the nursing process for the student studying to become a registered nurse, and the illustration of the steps of the nursing process (clinical problem-solving process) for the student studying to become a licensed practical/vocational nurse. A de-

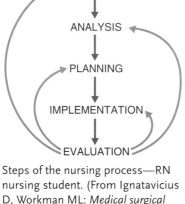

Steps of the nursing process—RN nursing student. (From Ignatavicius D, Workman ML: *Medical surgical nursing: patient-centered collaborative care*, ed 6, Philadelphia, 2006, Saunders.)

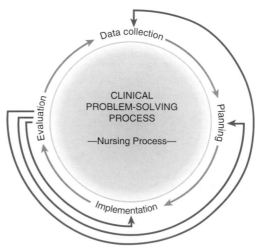

Steps of the nursing process—PN nursing student.

cription for each step follows. The cognitive skills of the NCSBN's Clinical Judgment Measurement Model (NCJMM) can be applied to practice and test-taking similarly as the steps of the nursing process, and can be seen as somewhat parallel. The assessment/data collection step is similar to *recognize cues*. Analysis is similar to *analyze cues* and *prioritize hypotheses*. Planning is similar to *generate solutions* and implementation is similar to *take action*. Finally, evaluation is similar to *evaluate outcomes*.

Cognitive Skills	Step of the Nursing Process
Recognize Cues	Assessment
Analyze Cues	Analysis
Prioritize Hypotheses	Analysis
Generate Solutions	Planning
Take Action	Implementation
Evaluate Outcomes	Evaluation

Assessment/Data Collection

Assessment/data collection questions address the process of gathering subjective and objective data relative to the client, confirming that data, and communicating and documenting the data. Assessment/data collection is similar to the cognitive skill, *recognize cues*. Applying the cognitive skill, *recognize cues* requires you to identify relevant assessment data.

Remember that assessment/data collection is the first step in the nursing process. When you are asked to select your first or initial nursing action, look for an option that addresses assessment/data collection. If an option contains the concept of assessment or the collection of client data, it is best to select that option. Some strategic words to look for in the options that indicate an assessment/data collection action are listed in the box to the right. A sample question follows.

If an assessment/data collection action is not noted in one of the options, follow the steps of the nursing process (clinical problem-solving process) as your guide in selecting your initial or first action. *Possible exception to this guideline for prioritizing:* If the question presents an emergency situation, read carefully; in an emergency situation, an intervention may be the priority!

> **Use the steps of the nursing process (clinical problem-solving process) to prioritize!**

Strategic Words in Options That Indicate Assessment/ Data Collection

Ascertain
Assess
Check
Collect
Determine
Find out
Identify
Monitor
Observe
Obtain information
Recognize

? SAMPLE QUESTION: Assessment/Data Collection

Case Event: A nurse is teaching a client with coronary artery disease about dietary measures that need to be followed.

Question Query: During the session the client expresses frustration in learning the dietary regimen. The nurse would take which **initial** action?

1. Notify the cardiologist.
2. Continue with the dietary teaching.
3. Identify the cause of the frustration.
4. Tell the client that the diet needs to be followed.

ANSWER: 3

TEST-TAKING STRATEGY

Note the strategic word, *initial*, and focus on the subject—a nursing action. Use the steps of the nursing process and apply the clinical judgment/cognitive skill, *take action*. In this question, the nurse needs to take an action and collect data in order to recognize cues that are relevant.

Of the options presented, the only assessment/data collection action is option 3. Options 1, 2, and 4 identify the implementation step of the nursing process. The initial action is to identify the cause of the frustration. Remember that assessment/data collection is the first step of the nursing process.

▪▶ TIP FOR THE NURSING STUDENT

Coronary artery disease affects the arteries that supply blood to the myocardium. When blood flow to the myocardium is partially or completely blocked, ischemia or infarction of the myocardium can occur, and the client experiences a heart attack. Because coronary artery disease is life-threatening, great emphasis is placed on reducing or eliminating the modifiable risk factors, such as obesity, high blood pressure, stress, smoking, and high cholesterol. Dietary measures include limiting foods high in cholesterol. High-fat foods, such as fried foods, are high in cholesterol. Because cholesterol is also found in foods of animal origin, meats such as organ meats, beef, bacon, and sausage are high in cholesterol. You will learn about coronary artery disease when you study the cardiovascular system in medical-surgical nursing, and you will learn about the foods high in cholesterol when you study nutrition related to cardiovascular disorders. Be sure to learn about these foods that are high in cholesterol because you will need to teach your client with cardiovascular disease about limiting them in the diet.

SMART STUDY TIP

Student-to-Student

Analysis questions are higher-level questions and require analysis and application of learned knowledge, as well as determining the priority nursing action. In addition to basic knowledge, these questions require practice to perfect your ability to answer them correctly.

Analysis

Beware! Analysis questions are the most difficult because they require understanding of the principles of physiological responses and require interpretation of the data on the basis of assessment. Analysis is similar to the cognitive skill, *analyze cues* and requires you to connect data to the client's presentation and determine if the data is expected or unexpected. Analysis questions also require critical thinking and determining the rationale for therapeutic interventions that may be addressed in the question; therefore, many questions on the NCLEX exam are analysis-type questions. Questions that address this step of the nursing process also may require determining client needs or problems and prioritizing hypotheses. *Prioritizing hypotheses* is a cognitive skill that requires analysis and ranking client needs or problems in order of priority. Remember to read the question carefully, identify the strategic words and the subject, and use the process of elimination to select the correct option. An example of an analysis-type question is provided next.

 SAMPLE QUESTION: Analysis

Case Event: The nurse is reviewing the laboratory results of an infant suspected of having pyloric stenosis.

Question Query: Which laboratory finding would the nurse **most likely** expect to note in this infant?

1. A blood pH of 7.50
2. A blood pH of 7.30
3. A blood bicarbonate of 21 mEq/L
4. A blood bicarbonate of 28 mEq/L

ANSWER: 1

TEST-TAKING STRATEGY

Note the strategic words, *most likely*, and focus on the subject—laboratory results. Apply the clinical judgment/cognitive skill, *analyze cues*. Make a connection between the data, that the infant has pyloric stenosis, and the expected finding. It is necessary to understand the physiology associated with pyloric stenosis and that metabolic alkalosis is likely to occur as a result of vomiting. Next, it is necessary to know which laboratory findings would be noted in this acid–base condition. The normal pH ranges from 7.35 to 7.45. In an alkalotic condition the pH is elevated. In an acidotic condition the pH is lower than normal. Options 3 and 4 identify normal bicarbonate levels. Analysis of these data will direct you to the correct option.

▌▶ TIP FOR THE NURSING STUDENT

Pyloric stenosis is a condition in which a narrowing of the pyloric sphincter at the outlet of the stomach occurs. This results in an obstruction that blocks the flow of food into the small intestine. The condition primarily occurs as a congenital defect in newborns. The infant experiences forceful projectile vomiting, causing the loss of hydrochloric acid, which results in metabolic alkalosis in the infant. The condition is treated by surgical correction. You will learn about acid–base disorders in your foundations of nursing course and in your medical-surgical nursing course. You will also learn about pyloric stenosis in your maternity and newborn course and in your pediatrics nursing course.

Planning

Planning questions frequently address creating a client plan of care. These questions require using hypotheses in determining goals and outcome criteria for goals of care, planning interventions, and communicating and documenting the plan of care. With regard to questions that address the planning step of the nursing process, keep two important points in mind. First, remember that this is a nursing examination, and the answer to the question most likely involves something related to the nursing plan rather than to the medical plan, unless the question asks what you anticipate the physician or specialist will prescribe. The second point to remember relates to questions that contain options listing client problems or hypotheses and require you to generate solutions. In these questions, it is important to remember that actual client problems rather than potential or at-risk client problems will most likely be the priority when generating solutions and planning care. Read the information in the question carefully; this information will guide you to select the correct option in this type of question. An example of a planning type of question is provided next.

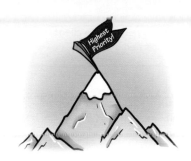

❓ SAMPLE QUESTION: Planning

Case Event: The nurse is reviewing the plan of care for a client with a diagnosis of sickle cell anemia.

Question Query: Which client problem would the nurse select as receiving the **highest priority** when planning care?

1. Dehydration
2. Nervousness about the disease
3. Embarrassment about appearance
4. Inability to cope with lifestyle limitations imposed as a result of the disease

ANSWER: 1

TEST-TAKING STRATEGY

Note the strategic words, *highest priority*, and focus on the subject—a client problem in the plan of care. Apply the clinical judgment/cognitive skill, *generate solutions* to plan care. To correctly answer this question, use Maslow's Hierarchy of Needs theory, remembering that physiological needs come first. Using this guideline will direct you to option 1. *Dehydration* is a physiological need and is the priority client problem when planning care. Options 2, 3, and 4 are psychosocial needs and may or may not be a concern for the client, but remember that physiological needs are the priority.

❚❚➤ TIP FOR THE NURSING STUDENT

Sickle cell anemia is a severe and chronic incurable anemic condition in which the abnormal hemoglobin called *hemoglobin S* (Hb S) results in distortion and fragility of the erythrocytes. It is characterized by crises in which the sickled cells clump and cause obstruction of the blood vessels. Joint pain, thrombosis, fever, lethargy, weakness, and splenomegaly occur. You may have learned about sickle cell anemia in your anatomy and physiology course. You will also learn more about this type of anemia in your medical-surgical nursing course and pediatrics course. Sickle cell anemia also may be discussed in your maternity nursing course because this type of anemia in a pregnant client places the client at risk for complications during the pregnancy.

Implementation

Implementation questions address the process of organizing and managing care, counseling and teaching, providing care to achieve established goals, supervising and coordinating care, and communicating and documenting nursing interventions. These questions also address the cognitive skill, *take action*, in which the nurse implements the generated solutions addressing the highest priorities or hypotheses. Because the NCLEX exam tests your competence and ability to function as a professional nurse, many questions on the examination are implementation or take action-type questions.

> You have only one client to be concerned about!

> Answer the question from an ideal and textbook perspective!

> Answer the question as if the nurse had all the time available to care for the client and all the resources needed at the client's bedside!

When you are presented with a question on NCLEX that requires you to determine what the nurse will do, there are two important points to keep in mind. The first point is that the only client that you need to be concerned about is the client in the question; remember that the client in the question is your only assigned client. This is an important point to bear in mind as you are trying to select the correct option.

The second important point to keep in mind when you are answering NCLEX questions is that you need to answer the question from a textbook perspective; you also need to answer the question as if the nurse has all the time available to care for the client and all the needed resources available at the client's bedside.

To illustrate these important points, let us look at the following sample questions.

SAMPLE QUESTION: Implementation

Case Event: The nurse is caring for a preoperative client who verbalizes a great deal of anxiety about the surgical procedure scheduled in 2 hours.

Question Query: Which action by the nurse would **best** alleviate the client's anxiety?

1. Stay with the client until he is brought to the operating room.
2. Call the client's wife, and ask her to visit the client before surgery.
3. Talk to the client for 15 minutes, and return shortly thereafter to check on the client.
4. Tell the client that you will spend some time answering his questions as soon as you get your other tasks completed.

ANSWER: 1

TEST-TAKING STRATEGY

Note the strategic word, *best,* and focus on the subject—alleviating the client's anxiety. Apply the clinical judgment/cognitive skill, *take action.* As you are reading the options, you may hesitate to select option 1 and may say to yourself, "I could never stay with a client for 2 hours. I would never get any of my other clients taken care of." Stop right there and remember that on the NCLEX exam, the only client you are caring for is the client in the question. Therefore, option 1 is the *best* option.

▌▶ TIP FOR THE NURSING STUDENT

A preoperative client is a client who is either preparing for surgery or is waiting to be transferred to the operating room. Often these clients are anxious about the surgery, and the nurse is responsible for alleviating the anxiety. You will learn about the many ways to alleviate a client's anxiety, but one way is to be present and available for the client to answer questions if necessary and to provide comfort. Many times just the nurse's presence provides comfort to a client. You will learn about caring for the client having surgery in your foundations of nursing course, and you will also learn about the many measures that you can implement to alleviate a client's anxiety.

SAMPLE QUESTION: Implementation

Case Event: The nurse is caring for a client after a cardiac catheterization. The client suddenly reports a feeling of wetness in the groin at the catheter insertion site.

Question Query: The nurse checks the site, notes that the client is actively bleeding, and would take which **best** action?

1. Contact the cardiologist.
2. Check the client's peripheral pulse in the affected extremity.
3. Don a sterile glove and place pressure on the insertion site using sterile gauze.
4. Don a clean glove and place pressure on the insertion site with the gloved hand.

ANSWER: 3

TEST-TAKING STRATEGY

Note the **strategic word**, *best,* and focus on the **subject**—a nursing action for a client who is bleeding. Apply the clinical judgment/cognitive skill, *take action*. Active bleeding indicates the need for intervention and the application of pressure at the site of bleeding. This directs you to options 3 and 4 as the possible correct options. You may hesitate to select option 3 because you may say to yourself, "I would not use the sterile gloves or gauze, because by the time I went to the supply room, obtained these sterile items, and returned to the room, the client would have lost a critically large amount of blood." Stop right there, and remember that on the NCLEX exam, you have all the resources needed and readily available at the client's bedside. Because the catheter insertion site is an open area, the best option is to don a sterile glove and place pressure on the insertion site using sterile gauze.

TIP FOR THE NURSING STUDENT

A cardiac catheterization is a diagnostic procedure in which a catheter is introduced into a large blood vessel and a contrast dye is injected through the circulatory system of the heart. This procedure is primarily done to assess the status of the coronary arteries in the heart and to determine if any blockage is present and, if so, the extent of the blockage. After the procedure the client is at risk for bleeding, infection, thrombophlebitis, and dysrhythmias (irregular heartbeat patterns). You will learn about this important cardiac diagnostic procedure when you study cardiovascular disorders in your medical-surgical nursing course.

Evaluation

Evaluation questions focus on comparing the actual outcomes of care with the expected outcomes and on how the nurse would monitor or make a judgment concerning a client's response to therapy or to a nursing action. The cognitive skill tested in these questions is *evaluate outcomes*. These questions also address evaluating the client's ability to implement self-care, health care team members' ability to implement care, and the process of communicating and documenting evaluation findings.

In an evaluation question, it is important to note if the question includes a negative event query. Look for the words or phrases that indicate a negative event query because they may be used in evaluation-type questions and ask for inaccurate information related to the subject of the question. (Words or phrases used in a negative event query are listed in Chapter 7.) Following is an example of an evaluation-type question.

SMART STUDY TIP

Scope of Practice

Evaluation is performed by both registered nurses (RNs) and licensed practical nurses (LPNs) or licensed vocational nurses (LVNs). These types of questions ask about outcomes for care administered and teaching. In addition, when answering questions that differentiate between the role of RNs and LPNs/LVNs, remember that LPNs/LVNs do not assess or analyze data (they collect data and report the data to the RN). They also reinforce teaching initiated by the RN.

SAMPLE QUESTION: Evaluation

Case Event: A client recovering from an exacerbation of left-sided heart failure has a problem with tolerating activity.

Question Query: The nurse determines that the client **best** tolerates mild exercise if the client exhibits which change in vital signs during activity?

1. Pulse rate increased from 80 to 104 beats/min
2. Oxygen saturation decreased from 96% to 91%
3. Respiratory rate increased from 16 to 19 breaths/min
4. Blood pressure decreased from 140/86 to 110/68 mm Hg

ANSWER: 3

TEST-TAKING STRATEGY

Note the strategic word, *best,* and focus on the subject—the client's ability to tolerate exercise. Apply the clinical judgment/cognitive skill, *evaluate outcomes.* Use the process of elimination and nursing knowledge regarding normal vital sign values. Options 1 and 2 are incorrect because they represent changes from normal to abnormal values. A decrease in blood pressure of more than 10 mm Hg could indicate an orthostatic hypotensive change and that the client is not tolerating the exercise. The only option that identifies values that remain within the normal range is option 3.

▶ TIP FOR THE NURSING STUDENT

Heart failure is an inability of the heart to maintain adequate circulation to meet the metabolic needs of the body because of an impaired pumping ability. Because of the imbalance of the oxygen supply and demand that occurs in this disorder, activity intolerance can be a problem for the client. In the case of a client with heart failure, activity intolerance refers to an insufficient amount of physiological energy necessary to tolerate or complete the desired activity or exercise. You will learn about heart failure in your medical-surgical nursing course when you learn about cardiac disorders. One important thing to remember is that with all clients, airway is the priority.

CHAPTER 9

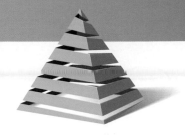

Leading and Managing, Delegating, and Assignment-Making Questions

The nurse is both a leader and a manager. As a leader and a manager, the nurse needs to assume many roles and responsibilities. Some of these roles include managing, organizing, and prioritizing care; making client care or related task assignments and delegating care; supervising care delivered by other health care providers; and managing time efficiently. The National Council Licensure Examination (NCLEX®) Test Plan identifies the content related to these roles and responsibilities in the Safe and Effective Care Environment Client Needs category. The Test Plan can be obtained at www.ncsbn.org. It is important to review the information related to this content area to ensure that you are well prepared for questions regarding the roles and responsibilities of the nurse as a leader and a manager. In addition, new graduates are more commonly being transitioned to supervisory or management roles early on in their career. This chapter reviews these roles and responsibilities of the nurse and other health care providers, including the licensed practical or vocational nurse and the assistive personnel. This chapter also reviews the guidelines and principles related to delegating and assignment-making, which are two important roles of the nurse. In addition, this chapter identifies guidelines for time management, because managing time efficiently is a key factor for completing activities and tasks within a defined time period and is a necessary skill as a nurse.

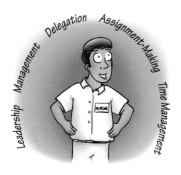

 ## Delegation and Assignment-Making

What Is Delegation?

Delegation is the process of transferring a selected nursing task in a client situation to an individual who is competent to perform that specific task. It involves sharing activities and achieving outcomes with other individuals who have the competency to accomplish the task. The nurse practice act and any other practice limitations, such as agency policies and procedures, define the aspects of care that can be delegated and the tasks and activities that need to be performed by the registered nurse, those that can be performed by the licensed practical nurse or licensed vocational nurse, and those that can be performed by assistive personnel. When delegating an activity, the nurse needs to determine the degree of supervision that the delegatee may require and provide supervision as appropriate.

> **Delegation:** Transferring a nursing task to an individual who is competent to perform the task.

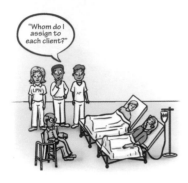

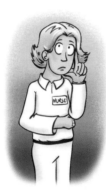

Assignment-Making: Planning care activities for a client or a group of clients and determining who will provide the care or perform certain activities.

What Is Assignment-Making?

Assignment-making is a specific activity that involves planning care activities for a client or a group of clients and determining specifically who will provide the care or perform certain activities. As with delegating, the nurse practice act and any other practice limitations, such as agency policies and procedures, which define the aspects of care, need to be used as a guide when planning assignments for activities and client care. Supervision of performance of the activity as appropriate also is important.

What Are the Important Points to Keep in Mind When Delegating or Making Assignments?

When you are answering questions related to either delegating or assignment-making, keep two important points in mind. First, even though a task or activity may be delegated to someone, the nurse who delegates the task or activity maintains accountability for the overall nursing care of the client. Remember that only the task, not the ultimate accountability, may be delegated to another.

The second point to keep in mind is that the NCLEX exam is a national examination. Therefore, use general guidelines regarding what a health care provider can competently and legally perform to answer the question correctly. On NCLEX, avoid using agency policies and procedures and agency position descriptions to answer the question, unless the question provides information to do so, because they are specific to the agency.

Let us review two sample questions: one that illustrates the use of general guidelines related to delegating and assignment-making and one that relates to specific agency policies and procedures.

❓ SAMPLE QUESTION: General Guidelines

Case Event: The nurse is planning client assignments for the day and has a licensed practical nurse (LPN) and an assistive personnel (AP) on the nursing team.

Question Query: The nurse **most appropriately** assigns which client to the LPN?

1. A client with a tracheostomy who requires frequent suctioning
2. A client who requires the collection of urine for a 24-hour period
3. A client recovering from pneumonia who requires ambulation every 3 hours
4. A client who requires turning and repositioning every 2 hours and range-of-motion exercises every 4 hours

ANSWER: 1

TEST-TAKING STRATEGY

Note the strategic words, *most appropriately*. Apply the clinical judgment/cognitive skill, *generate solutions*, for this question. This question requires that you determine which client would most appropriately be assigned to the LPN. No information in the question indicates the need to use agency policies, procedures, or position descriptions to determine the most appropriate assignment; therefore, use general guidelines. As you read each option, think about and visualize the client's needs. The client described in option 1 has needs that cannot be met by the AP. Remember that the health care provider needs to be competent and skilled to perform the assigned task or client activity.

❚❚▶ TIP FOR THE NURSING STUDENT

You will learn about the specific roles and responsibilities of various health care providers in your foundations of nursing course. You will also learn more specific content about these roles and responsibilities when you discuss leadership and management roles of the nurse. The important thing to remember is that the registered nurse is educationally prepared to assume the highest level of responsibility. The licensed practical or vocational nurse can assume some responsibilities that are invasive, and the assistive personnel can assume responsibilities that are noninvasive. A tracheostomy is a surgically created opening into the neck that provides an airway for a client who is unable to breathe through the upper airway. A client with a tracheostomy requires suctioning, which involves, as needed, the insertion of a tube that provides suction to remove secretions to maintain a clear airway. This is an invasive procedure, and thus a licensed nurse needs to be assigned to this client. The collection of urine, ambulating a client, and turning and repositioning and range-of-motion exercises are noninvasive procedures and thus can be assigned to assistive personnel.

SAMPLE QUESTION: Specific Agency Policies and Procedures

Case Event: The licensed nurse employed in a hospital is assigning client care activities to an assistive personnel (AP). The AP is a senior nursing student and works at the hospital as an AP part-time on weekends. The hospital position description for a nursing student who is employed as an AP indicates that he or she may perform basic procedures learned in nursing school if supervised by a licensed nurse.

Question Query: Based on the hospital's position description, the licensed nurse assigns which **most appropriate** activity to this AP?

1. Change a sterile abdominal dressing
2. Hang a unit of red blood cells on a client
3. Insert an intravenous catheter into an infant
4. Administer digoxin by intravenous (IV) push

ANSWER: 1

TEST-TAKING STRATEGY

Apply the clinical judgment/cognitive skill, *generate solutions,* to this question. In this question, information is provided that directs you to use the hospital's position description to determine the most appropriate activity to assign to the AP. The strategic words in the question are *most appropriate.* Based on the data in the question and in the options, it is best to select the least invasive activity. Also, recall that blood administration and medication administration must be performed by a licensed health care provider. Inserting an IV catheter into an infant is an invasive procedure that needs to be performed by a health care provider specially trained to perform it. Remember that the health care provider needs to be competent and skilled to perform the assigned task or client activity.

⏩ TIP FOR THE NURSING STUDENT

When answering assignment-making questions, remember to focus on who the task is being assigned to and remember to select the least invasive task if the health care provider is not licensed. Hanging red blood cells means that the client will receive blood by the IV route, and this is a highly invasive procedure. Inserting an IV catheter and administering digoxin (a cardiac medication) intravenously are also highly invasive procedures that need to be performed by licensed personnel. Changing a sterile dressing is also invasive to some degree and requires education in its performance to maintain sterility. You will learn about the specific roles and responsibilities of various health care providers in your foundations of nursing course. You will also learn more specific content about these roles and responsibilities when you discuss leadership and management roles of the nurse.

SMART STUDY TIP

Lifestyle Planning

Many nursing students choose to do nursing internships or externships while in nursing school. This is an excellent opportunity and provides valuable experience for nursing students and for graduates. If your schedule permits, you should explore the availability of these positions!

🔺 What Principles and Guidelines Can Be Used to Delegate and Make Assignments?

If you are presented with a question on an examination that requires you to delegate or plan assignments for a group of clients, certain principles and guidelines can be used to assist in answering the question correctly. As you are using the process of elimination to determine the correct option, keep these principles and guidelines in mind. Also, read each option carefully. Think about and visualize the client's needs to

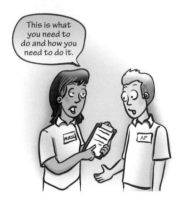

determine which health care provider could best meet the client's needs. Following is a review of these principles and guidelines for delegating and assignment-making.

Principles and Guidelines for Delegating and Assignment-Making

1. Always ensure client safety—never select an option that could potentially harm the client.
2. Focus on the subject of the question and what the question is asking; for example, is the question asking you to delegate to a registered nurse, a licensed practical or vocational nurse, or assistive personnel?
3. Determine which tasks or client care activities can be delegated and to whom, and match the task to the delegatee on the basis of agency policies and procedures, or position descriptions as appropriate; that is, think about the activities that the delegatee can safely and legally perform. Always remember that on NCLEX, state- and agency-specific guidelines will not be addressed.
4. Think about individual variations in work abilities, and determine the degree of supervision that may be required; for example, if the question asks you to delegate or assign a client care activity to a new graduate, you must think about the need for providing adequate supervision and the need to teach the new graduate about the assigned activity.
5. Always provide directions to the delegatee that are clear, concise, accurate, and complete and that validate the person's understanding of the directions and expectations; that is, ask the delegatee to verbalize the procedure for performing the task or activity that was delegated.
6. Communicate a feeling of confidence to the delegatee, and provide feedback promptly after the task or activity is performed regarding his or her performance; ensure that the delegatee completed the task, and evaluate the outcome of the care provided.
7. Provide the delegatee with a timeline for completion of the task or activity; for example, if a client is scheduled for a diagnostic test and an activity or task needs to be completed before the test, it is important to identify this timeline to the delegatee.
8. Maintain continuity of care as much as possible when assigning client care; for example, it is best for the client to be cared for by the nurse with whom the client has developed a therapeutic relationship. However, it is also important to remember that in some client situations, maintaining continuity of care would be unfavorable with regard to ensuring a safe environment for a health care provider, such as with the client with an infectious disease or the client with a radiation implant.

 SAMPLE QUESTION: Assignment-Making

Case Event: The nurse is planning the client assignments for the day and is reviewing client data and the needs of the clients on the nursing team.

Question Query: To maintain continuity of care, the nurse would ensure that which client is cared for by the nurse who cared for the client on the previous day?

1. A client with active tuberculosis
2. A client with herpes zoster (chickenpox)
3. A client with a cervical radiation implant
4. A client recently diagnosed with inoperable cancer

ANSWER: 4

TEST-TAKING STRATEGY

Focus on the subject of the question—to maintain continuity of care. Apply the clinical judgment/cognitive skill, *generate solutions*, to this question. Read each option carefully, keeping two points in mind: the client's needs and ensuring a safe environment for the health care provider. The clients described in options 1, 2, and 3 can potentially present a risk to the health care provider. The client in option 4 will likely have psychosocial needs that can best be met if the client is cared for by a health care provider with whom the client has developed a therapeutic relationship.

TIP FOR THE NURSING STUDENT

Tuberculosis is an infection caused by an acid-fast bacillus known as *Mycobacterium tuberculosis* and usually affects the lungs, although infection of multiple organ systems can occur. In its active stage it is highly contagious and is transmitted by the inhalation of infected droplets. Herpes zoster (chickenpox) is an acute and highly contagious viral disease caused by the varicella zoster virus. This disease is transmitted by close contact with an infected person. A radiation implant is a device that is placed internally into a client to treat cancer. This type of therapy is also known as *brachytherapy*. When a radiation implant is in place, the client is strictly isolated because the implant emits radiation and can affect and be harmful to other individuals. Cancer, also known as a *neoplasm*, is an abnormal growth. It is characterized by the uncontrolled growth of cells that invades surrounding tissue and spreads (metastasizes) to other parts of the body. Cancer is not a contagious disorder. You will learn about the spread of infectious diseases in your foundations of nursing course. You will also learn about tuberculosis and radiation implants in your medical-surgical nursing course and about herpes zoster (chickenpox) in your pediatrics course.

Who Can Do What?

There are some general guidelines to follow when answering a question that requires determining what tasks and client care activities should be assigned to which health care provider. Remember that these are general guidelines, and the general guidelines are the ones that you need to follow when taking a national examination. These guidelines (listed next) are followed by sample questions in both multiple response and multiple choice formats.

Assistive Personnel (AP)

Generally, noninvasive tasks and basic client care activities can be assigned to an assistive personnel. Some of these tasks and activities may include:
Ambulation
Basic skin care
Bathing
Client transport
Grooming
Hygiene measures
Positioning
Range-of-motion exercises
Some specimen collections, such as urine or stool

Licensed Practical or Vocational Nurse

In addition to the tasks that the AP can perform, a licensed practical or vocational nurse can perform certain invasive tasks and client care activities. Some of these additional tasks may include:
Administering oral medications
Administering intramuscular injections
Administering subcutaneous injections
Administering intradermal medications
Administering medications by the rectal, vaginal, eye, ear, nose, or topical routes
Administering medications by a gastrointestinal tube
Administering some selected IV piggyback medications
Changing dressings
Irrigating wounds
Monitoring an IV flow rate
Suctioning

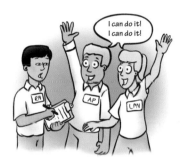

SMART STUDY TIP

Preparing for Clinical

As a student in clinical, other health care providers on the nursing unit can be very valuable resources to you during your rotations. Ask questions and ask them to assist with tasks, and you will learn a lot about client care.

Teaching about basic hygienic and nutritional measures

Urinary catheterization

Using the nursing process (clinical problem-solving process): data collection, planning, implementing, and evaluating

Registered Nurse

The registered nurse is competent to perform many tasks and client care activities. In addition to the tasks and client care activities that a licensed practical or vocational nurse can perform, the registered nurse can perform numerous other procedures. To assist you in differentiating the role of the registered nurse and the licensed practical or vocational nurse, some tasks and client care activities that only the registered nurse can perform are:

Administering IV medications by continuous IV, by piggyback, and by IV push

Initiating client teaching

Using the nursing process: assessment, analyzing data, planning, implementing, and evaluating

SAMPLE QUESTION: Multiple Response

Case Event: The nurse is planning the client assignments for the day and has a registered nurse, a licensed practical nurse, and assistive personnel on the nursing team.

Question Query: Which clients can be safely assigned to the licensed practical nurse? **Select all that apply.**

☐ **1.** A client scheduled for an ultrasound of the heart

☐ **2.** A client with an open abdominal wound who requires wound irrigations every 3 hours

☐ **3.** A client with a spinal cord injury who requires intermittent urinary catheterization every 4 hours

☐ **4.** A client newly diagnosed with diabetes mellitus who requires teaching about insulin administration

☐ **5.** A client with pulmonary edema who was admitted to the hospital 2 hours ago and requires frequent respiratory assessments

☐ **6.** A client with a central IV line who is receiving parenteral nutrition and lipids and has a prescription to receive 2 units of packed red blood cells

ANSWER: 1, 2, 3

TEST-TAKING STRATEGY

Focus on the **subject** of the question—a client assignment to a licensed practical nurse. Apply the clinical judgment/cognitive skill, *generate solutions*, to this question. Use general principles and guidelines to assist in answering the question correctly. Think about and visualize the client's needs, and determine whether the licensed practical nurse can competently and legally perform activities to meet these needs. Initial teaching about insulin administration needs to be done by a registered nurse. Client assessment is done by the registered nurse; however, the licensed practical nurse can collect data. A client with a central IV line who needs to receive blood transfusions needs to be cared for initially by a registered nurse. In addition, this client has complex needs with regard to the central IV line because the client is also receiving parenteral nutrition and lipids and has a prescription to receive a blood transfusion. Remember that the health care provider needs to be competent and skilled to perform the assigned task or client activity.

⏩ TIP FOR THE NURSING STUDENT

An ultrasound of the heart is a noninvasive procedure in which the heart chambers and valves are visualized and examined for abnormalities. There is no client preparation for the procedure, and the procedure is painless for the client. Wound irrigations may be prescribed for certain clients who have wound infections or are at risk for a wound infection. This procedure requires sterile technique and cleansing of the wound with a sterile solution, such as normal saline, or another type of solution as prescribed by the primary health care provider. A spinal cord injury occurs as a result of a traumatic disruption of the spinal cord, such as from a car or other type of accident or from some sort of violent impact. Such trauma can cause varying degrees of paralysis; depending on the level of injury in the spinal cord, some individuals lose the ability to urinate on their own. As a result, these individuals require urinary catheterization (insertion of a tube to drain the bladder), an invasive procedure. Diabetes mellitus is a disorder of carbohydrate, fat, and protein metabolism that occurs primarily as a result of a deficiency or complete lack of insulin secretion by the beta cells of the pancreas or resistance to insulin. Many clients with diabetes mellitus require insulin (although some may be controlled with oral medications). Insulin needs to be administered by subcutaneous injection, and these clients need to learn how to properly administer it. In addition to insulin, diet and exercise are important components of management of the disease. Heart failure is an inability of the heart to maintain adequate circulation to meet the metabolic needs of the body because of an impaired pumping ability. Pulmonary edema is a serious complication of heart failure in which fluid accumulates in the pulmonary system as a result of the impaired pumping ability of the heart. A client with pulmonary edema requires frequent respiratory assessments. The registered nurse is the health care provider who is responsible for client assessment. A central IV line is one that is inserted into a central vein, usually the subclavian vein. Clients with this type of IV line can receive solutions such as parenteral nutrition (a solution containing a high concentration of nutrients and glucose) and lipids (fat emulsion to prevent fatty acid deficiency) through the line. Red blood cells, usually administered to a client with anemia, can also be administered through a central IV line, and a registered nurse is responsible for administering the blood transfusion. You will learn about these client conditions in your foundations of nursing course and in your medical-surgical nursing course.

SAMPLE QUESTION: Multiple Choice

Case Event: The nurse is planning client assignments for the day and needs to assign 4 clients. There is a registered nurse, a licensed practical nurse, and 2 assistive personnel on the nursing team.

Question Query: Which client would the nurse **most appropriately** assign to the registered nurse?

1. A client requiring a bed bath
2. A client who requires frequent ambulation
3. A client with a right above-the-knee amputation who requires a dressing change
4. A client who was admitted to the hospital during the night after experiencing an acute asthma attack

ANSWER: 4

TEST-TAKING STRATEGY

Note the strategic words, *most appropriately,* and focus on the subject of the question—a client assignment to a registered nurse. Apply the clinical judgment/cognitive skill, *generate solutions,* to this question. Use general principles and guidelines to assist in answering the question correctly. Think about and visualize the client's needs. The client who was admitted to the hospital during the night after experiencing an acute asthma attack would most appropriately be assigned to the registered nurse because this client would require frequent respiratory assessments. The assistive personnel can most appropriately give a bed bath and ambulate a client. The licensed practical nurse can perform dressing changes. Remember that the health care provider needs to be competent and skilled to perform the assigned task or client activity.

▐▶ TIP FOR THE NURSING STUDENT

Asthma is a respiratory disorder that is characterized by recurring episodes of difficulty breathing (dyspnea), wheezing lung sounds, constriction of the bronchi, coughing, and the production of mucoid bronchial secretions. Acute attacks can occur that require aggressive treatment to maintain a patent airway. These clients require frequent respiratory assessment that needs to be done by a registered nurse. You will learn about asthma in your medical-surgical nursing course when you study respiratory problems. You will also learn about asthma in your pediatrics nursing course. You will learn about the procedure for giving a client a bed bath (bathing a client while the client is in bed) and will learn about the safe procedure for ambulating a client during your foundations of nursing course. These are noninvasive procedures and can therefore be assigned to assistive personnel because these health care providers are trained to perform these procedures safely. A right above-the-knee amputation means that the client underwent a surgical procedure in which the right limb to the level above the knee was surgically removed. This client requires dressing changes, which are an invasive procedure that requires sterile technique. The licensed practical or vocational nurse is trained to perform sterile dressing changes. You will also learn about the procedure for changing sterile dressings in your foundations of nursing course and in your medical-surgical nursing course.

 SAMPLE QUESTION: Multiple Choice

Case Event: The nurse is planning the client assignments for the day.
Question Query: Which assignment is **most appropriate** for the assistive personnel?
1. A client requiring colostomy irrigation
2. A client receiving continuous tube feedings
3. A client who requires stool specimen collections
4. A client with difficulty swallowing food and fluids

ANSWER: 3

TEST-TAKING STRATEGY

Note the strategic words, *most appropriate,* and focus on the subject of the question—a client assignment to an assistive personnel. Apply the clinical judgment/cognitive skill, *generate solutions,* to this question. Use general principles and guidelines to assist in answering the question correctly. Think about and visualize the client's needs, and determine whether the assistive personnel can competently and legally perform activities to meet these needs. In this situation the most appropriate assignment for an assistive personnel would be to care for the client who requires stool specimen collections. Colostomy irrigations and tube feedings are not performed by assistive personnel. The client with difficulty swallowing food and fluids is at risk for aspiration. Remember that the health care provider needs to be competent and skilled to perform the assigned task or client activity.

▮▶ TIP FOR THE NURSING STUDENT

A colostomy is the surgical creation of a stoma (an artificial anus) on the abdominal wall that allows for the elimination of feces (bowel contents). This is created for the client with a bowel tumor who is experiencing bowel obstruction or for the client with a tumor or other disorder who requires removal of part of the colon. The colostomy may require irrigations to empty the content of the colon. This is an invasive procedure that can be performed by the licensed practical or vocational nurse or the registered nurse. Tube feedings involve the administration of liquid food to a client through a tube placed in the client's stomach or other area of the client's gastrointestinal tract. Because this procedure places the client at risk for aspiration (breathing in fluid or food into the lungs, resulting in a blocked airway), a licensed nurse needs to perform this procedure. Likewise, a client having difficulty swallowing food and fluids is at risk for aspiration and requires care from a licensed nurse. The collection of stool specimens is a noninvasive procedure, and therefore assistive personnel can perform this procedure. You will learn about caring for these types of clients in your foundations of nursing course and in your medical-surgical nursing course.

Time Management

What Is Time Management, and Why Is It Important?

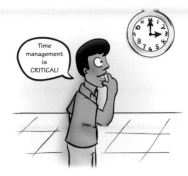

Time management is a technique used by the nurse to assist in completing tasks within a defined period. It involves learning how, when, and where to use one's time and involves establishing personal goals and time frames. Time management requires an ability to anticipate the day's activities, to combine activities when possible, and to avoid being interrupted by nonessential activities. It also involves efficiency in completing tasks quickly and thoroughly and effectiveness in deciding on the most important task to do and doing it correctly. The ability to manage time efficiently is important to complete tasks and client care activities within a reasonable time frame. In many client care situations, time management requires prioritizing. The nurse needs to be skilled in planning time resourcefully and needs to assist other health care providers with time management. Some principles and guidelines to use to assist in managing time efficiently are listed next.

 Principles and Guidelines of Time Management

Following is a list of the principles and guidelines of time management:
1. Identify tasks, obligations, and client care activities and write them down.
2. Organize the workday; identify which tasks and client care activities must be completed in specified time frames.
3. Prioritize client needs.
4. Anticipate the needs of the day and provide time for unexpected and unplanned tasks or client care activities that may arise.
5. Focus on beginning the daily tasks by working on the most important first, while keeping goals in mind; look at the final goal for the day, which will help break down tasks into manageable parts.
6. Begin client rounds at the beginning of the shift, assessing/collecting data on each assigned client.
7. Delegate tasks when appropriate.
8. Keep a daily hour-by-hour log to assist in providing structure to the tasks that must be accomplished, and cross tasks off the list as they are accomplished.
9. Use hospital and agency resources efficiently, anticipating resource needs and gathering the necessary supplies before beginning the task.
10. Organize paperwork and continuously document task completion and necessary client data throughout the day.
11. At the end of the day, evaluate the effectiveness of time management.

❓ SAMPLE QUESTION: Prioritizing and Time Management

Case Event: The nurse on the day shift is assigned to care for 4 clients.
Question Query: After the report from the night shift, which client would the nurse plan to assess/collect data from **first?**
1. Client scheduled for a cardiac catheterization at 10:00 AM
2. Client scheduled to have an electrocardiogram (ECG) at 11:00 AM
3. Client with pulmonary edema who was treated with furosemide at 5:00 AM
4. Client newly diagnosed with diabetes mellitus who is scheduled for discharge to home

ANSWER: 3

TEST-TAKING STRATEGY

Note the strategic word, *first*, and focus on the subject—which client the nurse plans to assess/collect data from first. Apply the clinical judgment/cognitive skill, *prioritize hypotheses*, to this question. This question describes a situation in which the nurse needs to prioritize and manage his or her time with regard to the assigned clients. Use the ABCs—airway, breathing, and circulation—to answer the question. Airway is always a high priority; therefore, the nurse would assess and collect data from the client with pulmonary edema who was treated with furosemide at 5:00 AM first. The nurse would next assess/collect data from the client scheduled for the cardiac catheterization because this client will require preprocedural preparation. The client scheduled for discharge would be attended to next because there may be discharge needs that require attention. The client scheduled for an ECG can be checked last.

▌▶ TIP FOR THE NURSING STUDENT

Heart failure is an inability of the heart to maintain adequate circulation to meet the metabolic needs of the body because of an impaired pumping ability. Pulmonary edema is a serious complication of heart failure in which fluid accumulates in the pulmonary system as a result of the impaired pumping ability of the heart. The client is treated with a diuretic, which is a medication that will result in an increased urine output, thus ridding the body of the excess fluid that accumulated in the pulmonary system. Furosemide is a diuretic. A major concern for the client with pulmonary edema is airway and breathing, so this is the reason why assessing/collecting data from this client is the priority. A cardiac catheterization is a diagnostic procedure in which a catheter is introduced into a large blood vessel and threaded through the circulatory system of the heart. This procedure is primarily done to assess the status of the coronary arteries in the heart and to determine if any blockage is present and if so, the extent of the blockage. The client requires some preprocedural preparation, such as ensuring informed consent has been obtained, checking for client allergies, obtaining height and weight and vital signs and noting the quality and presence of peripheral pulses, ensuring that an IV line is inserted, client teaching, and administering prescribed medications. Because this procedure is scheduled for 10:00 AM, this client can be assessed second. Diabetes mellitus is a disorder of carbohydrate, fat, and protein metabolism that occurs primarily as a result of a deficiency or complete lack of insulin secretion by the beta cells of the pancreas or resistance to insulin. Insulin therapy or oral medications, diet therapy, and an exercise regimen are important components for management of the disease to prevent complications, and the nurse needs to ensure that the client has been taught about management and understands the treatment prescribed for the disorder. Because the client is scheduled for discharge, it is important that the nurse ensure that the client's needs are met and that the client understands the prescribed treatment. Therefore, in this situation, this client is the nurse's third priority. An ECG is a diagnostic test that is performed using a device that records the electrical activity of the myocardium (heart) and detects the transmission of the cardiac impulse through the tissues of the heart muscle. This test can diagnose specific abnormalities of the heart. It is a noninvasive test that requires no specific preparation except for explaining the procedure to the client. Therefore, in this situation, this client would be the nurse's last priority. You will learn about time management in your foundations of nursing course and about caring for these types of clients in your medical-surgical nursing course.

CHAPTER 10

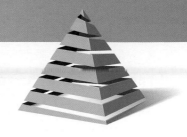

Communication Questions

Communication is a process in which information is exchanged, either verbally or nonverbally, between two or more individuals. According to the National Council of State Boards of Nursing (NCSBN), an Integrated Process of the Test Plan is a process that is foundational to the practice of nursing and is incorporated throughout the Client Needs categories of the Test Plan. In the National Council Licensure Examination (NCLEX®) Test Plan, the NCSBN identifies the concept of communication as a component of one of the Integrated Processes. In addition, in the Psychosocial Integrity category of Client Needs, therapeutic communication and cultural awareness/cultural influences on health are listed as content that is tested on the NCLEX exam. Therefore, it is likely that you will be presented with questions related to the communication process. Many of these questions require you to apply the clinical judgment/cognitive skill, *generate solutions*. This chapter reviews the guidelines to follow when answering communication questions and points out the importance of cultural and spiritual aspects when communicating and caring for clients. Several sample questions are included to illustrate how communication guidelines are used.

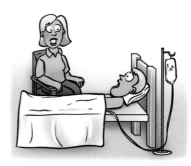

SMART STUDY TIP

Preparing for Clinical

As a nursing student, one thing your instructor will expect is that you have the ability to communicate with your assigned clients. Become very familiar with therapeutic and nontherapeutic communication techniques before your first clinical experience!

How Are Communication Concepts Tested in a Question?

Communication is an important characteristic of the nurse–client relationship. Therefore, test questions that refer to the concept of communication may address a client situation in any clinical setting and any nursing care area.

When we think about communication concepts and the nurse–client relationship, we usually visualize an interaction between the nurse and the client. Although this is an accurate visualization, it is important to broaden our thinking with regard to the communication process and the concepts that are tested on the examination. Test questions address not only the communication process between the nurse and the client but also the process between the nurse and a client's family member or significant other, or the nurse and another member of the health care team, such as another nurse, assistive personnel, or health care provider. For example, you may be asked about how you would respond to a staff member who makes an inappropriate statement or how you would respond to a primary health care provider who is demanding. Therefore, most questions that test the concept of communication relate to how the nurse should respond to the person with whom he or she is communicating.

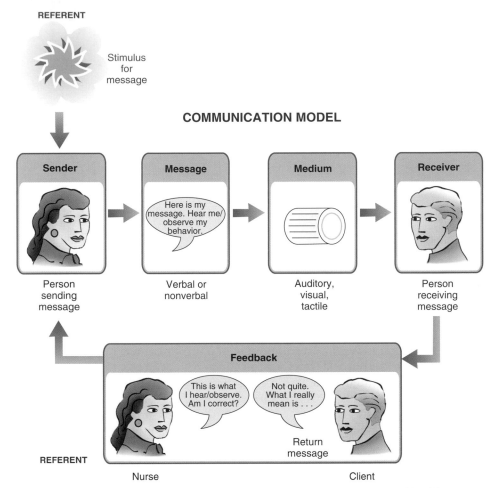

Communication model. (From Varcarolis EM: *Foundations of psychiatric mental health nursing,* ed 4, Philadelphia, 2002, Saunders.)

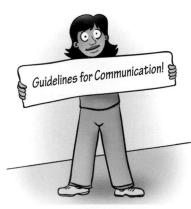

What Guidelines Can Be Used to Answer Communication Questions?

The five primary guidelines to use when answering communication questions are as follows:

1. Use therapeutic communication techniques to answer communication questions because of their effectiveness in the communication process. As you read the question and each option, find the option that is client focused and indicates the use of a therapeutic communication technique.

2. Nontherapeutic communication techniques are ineffective and should be avoided when responding to a client, a client's family member or significant other, or another member of the interprofessional health care team. As you read the question and each option, eliminate the options that indicate the use of a nontherapeutic communication technique.

3. Note the client of the question. The client could be the person with the health care problem, a client's family member or significant other, or another member of the interprofessional health care team. Look for the client-focused option because this will reflect a therapeutic technique.

4. Focus on feelings, concerns, anxieties, or fears. As you read the question and each option, look for the option that indicates the use of a therapeutic communication technique and focuses on the feelings, concerns, anxieties, or fears of the client of the question.

5. Consider cultural and spiritual differences and client preferences as you answer the question. If you note that a question contains information that identifies a specific cultural group, think about specific cultural and spiritual characteristics to answer the question correctly. Remember that some cultures may be unique with regard to characteristics related to the process of communication.

Guidelines for Communication

Note the client of the question.
Use therapeutic communication techniques.
Avoid nontherapeutic communication techniques.
Focus on the client's feelings, concerns, anxieties, or fears.
Select a client-focused option.
Consider cultural and spiritual differences and client preferences.

 ## Communication Techniques

What Are the Therapeutic Communication Techniques?

Using therapeutic communication techniques encourages the client, or other individual with whom the nurse is communicating, to express his or her thoughts and feelings. Many therapeutic communication techniques can be used to promote verbalization. The following table provides a brief review of these techniques.

Therapeutic Communication Techniques

Technique	Description
Active listening	Carefully noting what the client is saying and observing the client's nonverbal behavior
Broad openings	Encouraging the client to select topics for discussion
Clarifying	Providing a means for making the message clearer, correcting any misunderstandings, and promoting mutual understanding
Focusing	Directing the conversation on the topic being discussed
Informing	Giving information to the client
Offering self to help	Includes staying with the client, talking to the client, and offering to help the client
Open-ended questions	Encouraging conversation because these questions require more than one-word answers
Paraphrasing	Restating in different words what the client said
Reflecting	Directing the client's question or statement back to the client for consideration
Restating	Repeating what the client has said and directing the statement back to the client to provide the client the opportunity to clarify the message further if necessary
Silence	Allowing time for formulating thoughts
Summarizing	Stating briefly what was discussed during the conversation
Validating	Verifying that both the nurse and the client are interpreting the topic or message in the same way

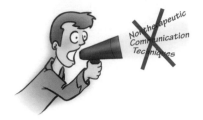

What Are the Nontherapeutic Communication Techniques?

Nontherapeutic communication techniques impair or block the flow of a conversation. They are also known as the barriers to an effective communication process. The nontherapeutic communication techniques need to be avoided when communicating because of their ineffectiveness. The following table briefly reviews some nontherapeutic communication techniques.

Nontherapeutic Communication Techniques	
Technique	**Description**
Approval	Implying that the client is thinking or doing the right thing and is not thinking or doing what is wrong; this may direct the client to focus on thinking or behavior that pleases the nurse
Asking excessive questions	Directly seeking information from the client without respect for the client's willingness or readiness to respond
Changing the subject	Avoiding addressing the client's thoughts, feelings, or concerns; implying that the client's statement is not important
Closed-ended questions	Questions that ask for specific information such as a "yes" or "no" answer and therefore inhibit communication
Disagreeing	Opposing the client's thinking or opinions, implying that the client is wrong
Disapproving	Indicating a negative value judgment about the client's behavior or thoughts
False reassurance	Making a statement that implies that the client has no reason to be worried or concerned; belittling a client's concerns
Giving advice	Assuming that the client cannot think for himself or herself, which inhibits problem-solving and fosters dependence
Minimizing the client's feelings	Making a statement that implies that the client's feelings are not important
Parroting	Repeating the client's words before determining what the client has said
Placing the client's feelings on hold	Avoiding addressing the client's thoughts, feelings, or concerns; making a statement that places the responsibility of addressing the client's thoughts, feelings, or concerns elsewhere or on another person
Value judgments	Making a comment that addresses the client's morals; this can make the client feel angry or guilty or as though he or she is not being supported or respected
"Why?" questions	Cause the client to feel defensive because many times he or she does not know the reason "why"; these types of questions also often imply criticism

SMART STUDY TIP

Scope of Practice

It is within the scope of nursing practice and is also the responsibility of the nurse to communicate with clients in a way that makes them feel comfortable and in a caring environment. Therapeutic communication is also very important for the client with a mental health problem.

Why Are Cultural Considerations Important?

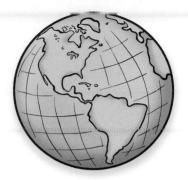

Communication involves three cultural characteristics: communication style, use of eye contact, and the meaning of touch. The nurse needs to be aware of certain cultural characteristics that relate to the communication process and other aspects of care that may differ from his or her own cultural uniqueness. Questions on the NCLEX exam may address the concept of communication with a client from a specific cultural group. If you note that a question contains information identifying a specific cultural group, think about specific cultural and spiritual characteristics to answer the question correctly.

 ## Other Cultural Considerations

Dietary Preferences

Being knowledgeable of ethnic dietary preferences is an important nursing responsibility. The nurse needs to incorporate the client's dietary preferences into the plan of care; otherwise, the client may not comply with health care recommendations. In addition, the nurse needs to ensure that the client receives an adequate nutritional intake to prevent nutritional deficiencies.

Food may have a symbolic meaning in some groups, and these beliefs need to be acknowledged by the nurse when planning care. Awareness and recognition of the value and importance of these beliefs will prevent imposition and guide the nurse's actions and decision-making to ensure culturally competent care.

End-of-Life Care Practices

End-of-life care practices may vary among groups, and it is important for the nurse to understand and incorporate these practices in the plan of care. For the dying client, maintaining the integrity of religious and spiritual rituals promotes a peaceful death. For the family members or significant others, maintaining religious and spiritual practices helps provide a sense of fulfilling obligations and helps promote acceptance of their loved one's death. Ask the client and/or family what religious and spiritual practices they want included in the plan of care.

Sample Communication Questions

Following are sample communication questions that illustrate the use of therapeutic and nontherapeutic communication techniques. Remember to use therapeutic communication techniques; focus on the client of the question; focus on the client's feelings, concerns, anxieties, and fears; and select the client-focused option.

SMART STUDY TIP

Lifestyle Planning

When caring for clients from a culture different from your own, consider their lifestyle choices when planning care. Never impose your lifestyle choices or cultural beliefs on a client. Ask the client and/or family what cultural preferences they want included in the plan of care.

Cultural Communication Points to Consider!

Communication style
Use of eye contact
Meaning of touch

? SAMPLE QUESTION 1

Case Event: A mother says to the nurse in the pediatrician's office, "I am afraid that my child might have another seizure."
Question Query: Which response by the nurse is therapeutic?
1. "Tell me what frightens you the most about seizures."
2. "Why worry about something that you cannot control?"
3. "Most children will never experience a second seizure."
4. "Phenytoin can prevent another seizure from occurring."

ANSWER: 1

TEST-TAKING STRATEGY

Use therapeutic communication techniques. Apply the clinical judgment/cognitive skill, *generate solutions*, to this question. Note that the client of the question is the mother. Option 1 is the only option that addresses the client's fears. Option 2 is a nontherapeutic response because it states that the mother should not worry. Options 3 and 4 are incorrect because the nurse is giving false reassurance to the mother that a seizure will not recur or can be prevented in this child. Remember to focus on the client's feelings, concerns, and fears and select the client-focused option.

▮▶ TIP FOR THE NURSING STUDENT

A seizure is a hyperexcitation of the neurons in the brain leading to a sudden, violent involuntary series of contractions of a group of muscles. There are different types of seizures. The most important nursing measures when a client experiences a seizure are to maintain a patent airway and to ensure safety for the client. You will learn about caring for a client with seizures when you study neurological disorders in your medical-surgical nursing course.

 SAMPLE QUESTION 2

Case Event: A client examined in the health care clinic has been diagnosed with hypertension and has been taking a prescribed antihypertensive medication. On a follow-up visit, the client says to the nurse, "I don't understand why I have to take this medication. It makes me feel awful."

Question Query: What is the **most appropriate** nursing response?

1. "You will need to ask your doctor about that."
2. "Everyone who takes that medication says the same thing."
3. "You have to take this medication if you want to prevent a stroke."
4. "Describe what you mean when you say that the medication makes you feel awful."

ANSWER: 4

TEST-TAKING STRATEGY

Note the strategic words, *most appropriate*. Apply the clinical judgment/cognitive skill, *generate solutions*, to this question. Focus on the client's feelings, concerns, and fears and select the client-focused option. Option 1 avoids the client's concern and places the client's feelings on hold. Option 2 minimizes the client's feelings and implies that the client's complaint is not important. In option 3 the nurse gives advice and also provides false reassurance that the medication will prevent a stroke. In this option, the nurse also avoids the client's complaint, is somewhat threatening, and may induce fear in the client. In option 4 the nurse uses the therapeutic communication technique of restating. In this technique, the nurse explores by repeating what the client has said and directing the statement back to the client to provide the client the opportunity to clarify the message further.

▮▶ TIP FOR THE NURSING STUDENT

Hypertension is a condition characterized by an elevated blood pressure above the normal value and is a known cardiovascular risk factor. Many times clients with hypertension do not even know that they are experiencing the disorder and are without signs and symptoms. This is why the disorder is sometimes called a *silent disease* and may not be discovered until a routine physical exam is performed. Antihypertensive medications are prescribed to lower the blood pressure, but unpleasant side effects of the medication can occur. This is why noncompliance can be a concern for clients with hypertension taking antihypertensive medications. You will learn about hypertension in your medical-surgical nursing course.

SAMPLE QUESTION 3

Case Event: A client with a history of cardiac disease is brought to the emergency department because of an episode of chest pain while mowing the lawn. During the assessment, the client tells the nurse that he stopped taking his cardiac medication.

Question Query: What is the **most appropriate** nursing response?

1. "Why did you stop taking your medication?"
2. "Tell me some of the reasons that led you to stop taking your medication."
3. "Everything is going to be just fine. We will get you started on those medications right away."
4. "You stopped the medication! Don't you know that you are never supposed to do that with cardiac medications?"

ANSWER: 2

TEST-TAKING STRATEGY

Note the strategic words, *most appropriate,* and use therapeutic communication techniques. Apply the clinical judgment/cognitive skill, *generate solutions,* to this question. Remember to focus on the client's feelings, concerns, and fears and select the client-focused option. Option 2 is an open-ended and broad opening question that will promote and encourage the client to communicate. The statement in option 1 uses the word *why.* Use of this word implies criticism and often makes the client feel defensive; in addition, many times the client does not know why he or she stopped the medication. In option 3 the nurse provides false reassurance by telling the client that everything is going to be fine. Also, the nurse avoids exploring the reason(s) that led the client to stop the medication. In option 4 the nurse demoralizes, belittles, and lectures the client, which is nontherapeutic.

▮▶ TIP FOR THE NURSING STUDENT

Cardiac disease can result from a variety of causes, including, but not limited to, angina pectoris (chest pain), myocardial infarction (heart attack), heart failure, or valvular disorders. If a client experiences chest pain, this could result from a lack of oxygen to the myocardial tissue and needs to be attended to immediately to prevent myocardial tissue death. You will learn about cardiac disease during your medical-surgical nursing course; because heart disease is a major health concern, focus on the ways to teach a client to prevent it.

SAMPLE QUESTION 4

Case Event: A client recently diagnosed with ovarian cancer says to the nurse, "I cannot believe this has happened to me. I wish that I were dead!"

Question Query: Which nursing response is therapeutic?

1. "Every client diagnosed with this type of cancer says the same thing."
2. "You must be feeling very upset. Are you thinking of hurting yourself?"
3. "I know what you mean, but there are a lot of treatments available for ovarian cancer."
4. "Why are you talking that way? Your children would not want to hear you say that, would they?"

ANSWER: 2

TEST-TAKING STRATEGY

Use therapeutic communication techniques. Apply the clinical judgment/cognitive skill, *generate solutions,* to this question. Remember to focus on the client's feelings, concerns, and fears and select the client-focused option. In option 2 the nurse focuses on the client's statement and addresses the client's feelings in the response. In options 1 and 3 the nurse minimizes the client's feelings. In addition, option 3 provides false reassurances. In option 4 the nurse uses the word *why*, which implies criticism and often makes the client feel defensive. In addition, option 4 focuses on the client's children and their feelings rather than on the client's feelings.

▌▶ TIP FOR THE NURSING STUDENT

Ovarian cancer is a malignant tumor of the ovary or ovaries. It is rarely detected in its early stages and is usually far advanced when diagnosed. Regularly scheduled pelvic examinations contribute significantly to early diagnosis; thus, it is important to teach clients about the importance of these pelvic examinations. You will learn about ovarian cancer and other types of cancer in your medical-surgical nursing course.

SAMPLE QUESTION 5

Case Event: Which nursing responses indicate the use of therapeutic communication techniques?

Question Query: **Select all that apply.**

1. "I know how you feel."
2. "You will do just fine, just wait and see."
3. "Don't worry about anything. You are in good hands!"
4. "Why do you still smoke when you know that you have cancer?"
5. "Let's talk more about the reasons you are not following your diet."
6. "You are feeling anxious because of the conversation that you had with your boss yesterday."

ANSWER: 5, 6

TEST-TAKING STRATEGY

Focus on the subject, the use of therapeutic communication techniques.

Apply the clinical judgment/cognitive skill, *generate solutions,* to this question. Remember to focus on the client's feelings, concerns, and fears and select the client-focused option. Review the following nursing responses:

1. "I know how you feel."—nontherapeutic and minimizes the client's feelings
2. "You will do just fine, just wait and see."—nontherapeutic and minimizes and avoids the client's feelings and provides false reassurance
3. "Don't worry about anything. You are in good hands!"—nontherapeutic; avoids the client's feelings and provides false reassurance
4. "Why do you still smoke when you know that you have cancer?"—nontherapeutic; demoralizes the client and also can make the client feel guilty, angry, anxious, or unsupported
5. "Let's talk more about why you are not following your diet."—therapeutic and uses the technique of focusing and exploring feelings
6. "You are feeling anxious because of the conversation that you had with your boss yesterday."—therapeutic and indicates the use of reflection; also encourages the client to verbalize feelings

▌▶ TIP FOR THE NURSING STUDENT

This question asks you to select the statements that reflect the use of therapeutic communication techniques. The use of therapeutic communication techniques promotes the communication process between the nurse and client. So think about these therapeutic techniques. You will learn about therapeutic and nontherapeutic techniques in your foundations of nursing course.

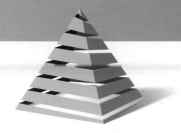

CHAPTER **11**

Pharmacology, Medication, and Intravenous Calculation Questions

Pharmacology is one of the most difficult nursing content areas to master. One reason it is so difficult is because of the enormous number of medications available. Another reason is the vast amount of information to know about each medication. The National Council Licensure Examination (NCLEX) Test Plan addresses pharmacological and parenteral therapies in the Physiological Integrity Client Needs category. The registered nurse (RN) Test Plan identifies 12% to 18% as the percentage of this type of test question that will possibly appear on the examination, and the licensed practical/vocational nurse (PN) Test Plan identifies pharmacological therapies as 10% to 16%. This means that if you took a 100-question examination, 12 to 18 of the questions (RN Test Plan) or 10 to 16 of the questions (PN Test Plan) would relate to pharmacology and parenteral therapies. Therefore, it is important to spend ample time reviewing pharmacology in preparation for the NCLEX exam, and it is best to do your review from a question-and-answer perspective. Thinking about the NGN, any of the six cognitive skills (recognize cues, analyze cues, prioritize hypotheses, generate solutions, take action, evaluate outcomes) could be tested with pharmacology questions.

This chapter provides the strategies for preparing to answer pharmacology questions and various general guidelines to use when attempting to answer the questions correctly. The pharmacology strategies are listed in the *Pharmacology Strategies* box. In addition, remember to read the question carefully, noting the strategic words, the data in the question, and the subject of the question, and always use the process of elimination to select the correct option. Think about the cognitive skill being tested. As with any type of question, it is best to use your nursing knowledge to answer the question. However, a question may appear on your examination that contains a medication name with which you are unfamiliar. When this occurs, the guidelines and the strategies to answer a pharmacology question correctly will be valuable. After you read this chapter, practice answering as many pharmacology questions as you can. Several resources are available that contain hundreds of pharmacology practice questions.

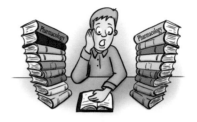

NCLEX® EXAM TIP

When a pharmacology question appears on the exam, note the name of the medication. The NCLEX exam will only identify the generic name of a medication. Focus on the medication name to determine the medication classification and its intended use. Also, use other pharmacology strategies and guidelines to answer the question.

Additional Pharmacology Practice Question Resources

For the RN student:
- *Saunders Comprehensive Review for the NCLEX-RN® Examination*
- *Saunders Q&A Review for the NCLEX-RN® Examination*
- *Saunders Q&A Review Cards for the NCLEX-RN® Examination*
- *HESI/Saunders Online Review Course for the NCLEX-RN® Examination*
- Skyscape Saunders Apps for the *Saunders Comprehensive Review for the NCLEX-RN® Examination and the Saunders Q&A Review for the NCLEX-RN® Examination*

For the PN student:
- *Saunders Comprehensive Review for the NCLEX-PN® Examination*
- *Saunders Q&A Review for the NCLEX-PN® Examination*
- *Saunders Review Cards for the NCLEX-PN® Examination*
- *HESI/Saunders Online Review Course for the NCLEX-PN® Examination*
- Skyscape Saunders Apps for the *Saunders Comprehensive Review for the NCLEX-PN® Examination and the Saunders Q&A Review for the NCLEX-PN® Examination*
  These products can be obtained at the Elsevier website (www.elsevierhealth.com).

SMART STUDY TIP

Student-to-Student

When answering questions about medications, look at the case event and the query very closely. If a disease process is mentioned, this information can help you answer the question correctly. Remember though, on the NCLEX a diagnosis may not be mentioned in a pharmacology question.

Pharmacology: General Guidelines to Follow

Some general guidelines to keep in mind as you are trying to select the correct option are given in the following list:

1. Medication absorption, distribution, metabolism, and excretion are affected by age and physiological processes; the older client and the neonate and infant are at greater risk for toxicity than an adult is.
2. Many medications are contraindicated in pregnancy and during breastfeeding.
3. Antacids are not usually administered with medication because the antacid will affect the absorption of the medication.
4. Grapefruit juice is not usually administered with medication because it contains a substance that will impede the absorption of the medication.
5. Enteric-coated and sustained-release tablets should not be crushed; also, capsules should not be opened.
6. Nursing interventions always include monitoring for intended effects, side effects, adverse effects, or toxic effects of the medication.
7. Nursing interventions sometimes include monitoring therapeutic serum medication levels and monitoring for signs and symptoms of toxicity.
8. Nursing interventions always include client education, and specifically the client should understand dosages, timing, diet modifications, safety considerations, and potential medication interactions.
9. The nurse or client should never adjust or change a medication dose, abruptly stop taking a medication, or discontinue a medication, unless prescribed parameters allow for these decisions to be made.
10. The nurse may withhold a medication if he or she suspects that the client is experiencing an adverse or toxic effect of a medication; the nurse must immediately contact the primary health care provider if either of these effects occurs. The nurse may also withhold the medication if specific parameters are prescribed and withholding the medication is indicated based on these parameters.
11. The client needs to avoid taking any over-the-counter medications or any other medications, such as herbal preparations, unless they are approved for use by the primary health care provider.
12. The client needs to know how to correctly administer the medication.
13. The client needs to be aware of the side effects and adverse effects of medications and how to check his or her own temperature, pulse, and blood pressure.
14. The client needs to take the prescribed dose for the prescribed length of therapy and understand the necessity of adherence.
15. The client needs to avoid consuming alcohol and avoid smoking.
16. The client should wear a Medic-Alert bracelet if he or she is taking medications such as, but not limited to, anticoagulants, oral hypoglycemics or insulin, certain cardiac medications, corticosteroids and glucocorticoids, antimyasthenic medications, anticonvulsants, and monoamine oxidase inhibitors.
17. The client needs to follow up with a primary health care provider as prescribed.
18. The nurse should be aware of multiple health care providers prescribing multiple medications and the potential for adverse and toxic effects due to polypharmacy. Medication reconciliation is an important step in ensuring medication safety.

The following sample pharmacology question illustrates how these general pharmacology guidelines may be helpful.

 ### SAMPLE QUESTION: General Pharmacology Guidelines

Case Event: A client taking amitriptyline calls the nurse at the primary health care provider's office and reports that he has an upset stomach whenever he takes the medication.
Question Query: What information would the nurse provide to the client?
1. Take the medication with food.
2. Take the medication with an antacid.
3. Take the medication on an empty stomach.
4. Stop the medication for 2 days and then resume the medication schedule.

ANSWER: 1

TEST-TAKING STRATEGY
Remember to read the question carefully, focusing on the data in the question, the client's complaint of an upset stomach. Apply the clinical judgment/cognitive skill, *generate solutions*. Recalling that antacids are not usually administered with medication and that the nurse would not tell a client to discontinue a medication will assist in eliminating options 2 and 4. From the remaining options, focusing on the data in the question will assist in eliminating option 3.

▮▶ TIP FOR THE NURSING STUDENT
Amitriptyline is a medication that is called a *tricyclic antidepressant*. It affects chemicals in the brain that may become unbalanced and is used to treat symptoms of depression. You will learn about this medication in your pharmacology nursing course and in your mental health nursing course.

Pharmacology: Assessment/Data Collection Guidelines

What Are the Pharmacology Assessment/Data Collection Guidelines, and How Will They Help in Answering a Pharmacology Question?

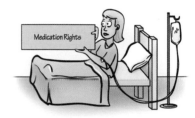

There are some specific assessment/data collection guidelines to follow when you administer medication to a client. In addition to using the medication rights when administering medications, these guidelines include client assessment and assessment of other factors related to the medication, such as checking certain laboratory values or vital signs; checking for potential interactions or contraindications related to the medication; client teaching; monitoring for intended effects, side effects, adverse effects, or toxic effects; and evaluating the client's response to the medication therapy. When you are presented with a pharmacology question and are trying to select the correct option, using the pharmacology assessment/data collection guidelines will assist you in eliminating incorrect options. Some of these guidelines are listed below.

Pharmacology: Assessment/Data Collection Guidelines to Follow

The following list gives pharmacology assessment/data collection guidelines to use when administering medication to a client:

1. Assess for client allergies or hypersensitivity to a medication.
2. Assess the client for existing health problems that are contraindicated with the administration of a prescribed medication.
3. Assess for potential interactions related to the medication.
4. Check pertinent laboratory results.
5. Check the client's vital signs, particularly if medications such as antihypertensive or cardiac medications are being administered.
6. Assess the client for intended effects, side effects, adverse effects, or toxic effects of the medication.
7. Assess the client's response to the medication.

These guidelines are particularly helpful if the question asks for the priority nursing action when administering a medication. The following is a sample pharmacology question illustrating how these assessment/data collection guidelines may be helpful.

Medication Rights

Right client
Right prescription and medication
Right reason and dose
Right time and frequency
Right route, approach, technique
Right assessment and indication
Right client education
Right to refuse
Right evaluation
Right documentation

SMART STUDY TIP

Scope of Practice

Remember that as a nurse, if you are questioning anything about a medication prescription, you can use the pharmacy as your resource to answer your questions. If you feel that the prescription requires further clarification, be sure to contact the primary health care provider before administering it.

SAMPLE QUESTION: Pharmacology

Case Event: The nurse notes that the primary health care provider has prescribed sulfa-methoxazole and trimethoprim for a client.
Question Query: Which **priority** action would the nurse take before administering this medication?
1. Ask the client about an allergy.
2. Call the pharmacy to obtain the medication.
3. Inform the client about the need to increase fluid intake.
4. Check the medication supply room to find out whether the medication needs to be obtained from the pharmacy.

ANSWER: 1

TEST-TAKING STRATEGY
Remember to read the question carefully, noting the subject and the strategic word. In this question the strategic word is *priority*, and the subject is the action that the nurse will take. Apply the clinical judgment/cognitive skill, *prioritize hypotheses*. Using the pharmacology assessment/data collection guidelines will direct you to option 1. In addition, use of the steps of the nursing process will direct you to the correct option because option 1 is the only one that addresses client assessment/data collection.

II▶ TIP FOR THE NURSING STUDENT
Sulfamethoxazole and trimethoprim is a combination antibiotic that treats different types of infection caused by bacteria. It is used to treat ear infections, urinary tract infections, bronchitis, *Pneumocystis jiroveci* pneumonia, and other types of infection. You will learn about this medication in your pharmacology nursing course and in your medical-surgical nursing course when you study the immune system.

 Medication Effects

What Are the Differences Between an Intended Effect, a Side Effect, an Adverse Effect, and a Toxic Effect of a Medication?

It is important to understand the differences between an intended effect, a side effect, an adverse effect, and a toxic effect; understanding them will assist in eliminating the incorrect options in a pharmacology question that asks about one of these effects. When you are presented with a question on the examination that asks about an effect of a medication, note the specific subject—is the subject of the question an intended effect, a side effect, an adverse effect, or a toxic effect? The differences are described in the following sections, and each section has a sample question related to the specific effect discussed in that section.

Intended Effect

An intended effect is the desired and expected effect of a medication. For example, the intended effect of morphine sulfate is pain relief. A sample question that asks about an intended effect is provided.

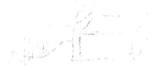 **SMART STUDY TIP**

Lifestyle Planning

Pharmacology is a difficult content area to study and retain information. When you know that you have an exam that includes pharmacology, or you are studying pharmacology for the NCLEX exam, it may be best to study this content area first when you begin your study session, when your mind is brightest.

INTENDED EFFECT: A desired effect

 SAMPLE QUESTION: Intended Effect

Case Event: Ibuprofen is prescribed for a client.
Question Query: On a follow-up visit to the primary health care provider's office, the nurse would ask the client whether the medication has provided relief from which symptom?

1. Diarrhea
2. Joint pain
3. Dyspepsia
4. Flatulence

ANSWER: 2

TEST-TAKING STRATEGY

Read the question carefully, noting the subject of the question. Apply the clinical judgment/cognitive skill, *evaluate outcomes*. In this question, the subject is an intended effect of ibuprofen and the noteworthy words are *provided relief from*. Also note that options 1, 3, and 4 are comparable or alike in that they all address gastrointestinal symptoms. When options are comparable or alike, it is best to eliminate those options because they are unlikely to be correct. In addition, options 1, 3, and 4 are side effects of ibuprofen, not intended effects.

▌▶ TIP FOR THE NURSING STUDENT

Ibuprofen is in a group of medications called *nonsteroidal anti-inflammatory drugs (NSAIDs)*. It works by reducing hormones that cause inflammation and pain in the body. It is used to reduce fever and treat pain or inflammation caused by many conditions, such as headache, toothache, back pain, arthritis, menstrual cramps, or minor injury. You will learn about this medication in your pharmacology course and in your medical-surgical nursing course.

Side Effect

A side effect is a physiological effect of a medication that is unrelated to the intended medication effects. For example, a side effect of an antihistamine medication is drowsiness. A side effect of a medication is not usually life threatening, and normally there are measures that will either eliminate the side effect or alleviate the discomfort associated with it. A sample question that asks about a side effect is provided.

> **SIDE EFFECT:** Not a desired effect, not usually life threatening, and can often be alleviated with specific measures

❓ SAMPLE QUESTION: Side Effect

Case Event: Azithromycin has been prescribed for a client.
Question Query: The nurse would tell the client that which frequent side effect can occur from this medication?
1. Severe diarrhea
2. Yellow-colored skin
3. Abdominal cramping
4. Yellow discoloration to the white part of the eye

ANSWER: 3

TEST-TAKING STRATEGY

Remember to read the question carefully, noting the subject of the question. In this question the subject is a side effect of the medication. Apply the clinical judgment/cognitive skill, *take action*. Eliminate options 2 and 4 first because they are comparable or alike and both indicate the presence of jaundice. From the remaining options, eliminate option 1 because of the word *severe*. Remember that the question asks about a side effect, not an adverse effect.

▌▶ TIP FOR THE NURSING STUDENT

Azithromycin is in a group of medications called *macrolide antibiotics*. Macrolide antibiotics slow the growth of, or sometimes kill, sensitive bacteria by reducing the production of important proteins needed by the bacteria to survive. Azithromycin is used to treat many different types of infections caused by bacteria. You will learn about this medication in your pharmacology course and in your medical-surgical nursing course when you study the immune system.

> **ADVERSE EFFECT:** More severe than a side effect, always an undesirable effect, and always reported to the primary health care provider

Adverse Effect

An adverse effect is more severe than a side effect and is always an undesirable effect. For example, an adverse effect of a sulfonamide is hypersensitivity that may be evidenced by a rash, fever, and shortness of breath. An adverse effect can range from a mild effect to a severe effect, such as anaphylaxis. Adverse effects are always reported to the primary health care provider. A sample question that asks about an adverse effect is provided.

SAMPLE QUESTION: Adverse Effect

Case Event: A client is receiving furosemide.
Question Query: The nurse would monitor the client for which manifestation indicating an adverse effect of the medication?
1. Nausea
2. Gastric upset
3. Muscle weakness
4. Increase in urinary output

ANSWER: 3

TEST-TAKING STRATEGY

Read the question carefully, noting the subject of the question. In this question the subject is an adverse effect of the medication. Apply the clinical judgment/cognitive skill, *recognize cues.* Eliminate options 1 and 2 first because they are comparable or alike and both relate to the gastrointestinal system. From the remaining options, eliminate option 4 because it is an intended effect of the medication. Also, recall that furosemide is a diuretic and can cause electrolyte imbalances and that muscle weakness is an indication of hypokalemia. Remember that the question asks about an adverse effect.

▶ TIP FOR THE NURSING STUDENT

Furosemide is a potent diuretic (water pill) that works by blocking the absorption of salt and fluid in the kidney tubules, causing a profound increase in urine output (diuresis). The diuretic effect of furosemide can cause body water and electrolyte depletion. It is used to treat excessive fluid accumulation and swelling (edema) of the body caused by heart failure, cirrhosis, chronic kidney disease, and nephrotic syndrome. It is sometimes used in conjunction with other blood pressure pills to treat high blood pressure. You will learn about this medication in your pharmacology course and in your medical-surgical nursing course when you study the cardiovascular system.

Toxic Effect

A toxic effect (toxicity) of a medication occurs when the medication level in the body exceeds the therapeutic level either from overdosing or medication accumulation. Always report toxic effects to the primary health care provider. Toxic effects are most often identified by monitoring the plasma (serum) therapeutic range of the medication. For example, some resources indicate the optimal therapeutic blood level range of digoxin is 0.5 to 2 ng/mL. Thus, if the blood level is greater than 2 ng/mL, the client experiences toxicity. The client will normally exhibit certain signs and symptoms (depending on the medication) that indicate toxicity, and the nurse needs to monitor for these. For example, in digoxin toxicity, the client may experience gastrointestinal disturbances, such as anorexia, nausea, and vomiting; or ocular disturbances, such as photophobia, light flashes, or halos around bright objects.

> **TOXIC EFFECT:** The medication level in the body exceeds the therapeutic level.

SAMPLE QUESTION: Toxic Effect

Case Event: The nurse reviews the results of a therapeutic blood level that was drawn from a client taking theophylline and notes that the level is 22 mcg/mL.

Question Query: The nurse would take which **most appropriate** action?

1. Report the result to the primary health care provider.
2. Administer the next scheduled dose of theophylline.
3. Ask the laboratory to draw another blood specimen to verify the result.
4. Place these normal results of the blood test in the client's medical record.

ANSWER: 1

TEST-TAKING STRATEGY

Remember to read the question carefully, noting the subject of the question and the strategic words. In this question, the strategic words are *most appropriate,* and the subject is a toxic effect of the medication. Apply the clinical judgment/cognitive skill, *take action.* Recalling that the therapeutic blood level range of theophylline is 10 to 20 mcg/mL will assist in determining that the client is experiencing toxicity. Remember that toxic effects are always reported to the primary health care provider.

▮▶ TIP FOR THE NURSING STUDENT

Theophylline is an oral bronchodilator medication used to treat symptoms of asthma, chronic bronchitis, and emphysema. It opens the airways by relaxing the smooth muscle of the airways and blood vessels in the lungs. It is indicated for the treatment of the symptoms of reversible airflow obstruction associated with chronic asthma and other chronic lung diseases, such as emphysema and chronic bronchitis. You will learn about this medication in your pharmacology course and in your medical-surgical nursing course when you study the respiratory system.

⛰ Medication Names

What Do You Need to Know About Medication Names?

During your nursing courses, you may learn both the generic name and the trade/brand name of a medication. There is only one generic name and this is the name that is the most reliable. However, there can be multiple trade/brand names for one medication. For example, a generic name is epoetin alfa, and two common trade/brand names used are Epogen and Procrit.

Nursing exams administered during nursing school may identify both names in a pharmacology question. The NCLEX examination will only identify the generic name in a pharmacology question. For example, a nursing school exam may present a question about furosemide (Lasix), a diuretic. The NCLEX examination testing the same medication will present the question using the generic name, furosemide, only. This is important information for you to know now as a nursing student. Focus on learning the generic names of medications when they are presented during your nursing program. Then you will be well prepared for the NCLEX examination!

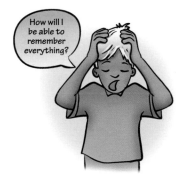

⛰ Medication Classifications

How Will It Help to Identify a Medication by Its Classification?

 Medications that belong to a particular classification have similar medication actions and usually have commonalities in their side effects and nursing interventions related to administration. It is nearly impossible to learn every feature about every individual medication. Learning medications by a "classification system method" groups several medications with similar properties together and makes the amount of information that needs to be learned condensed and manageable.

With regard to side, adverse, and toxic effects and nursing interventions, do not try to memorize every effect and every nursing intervention for every medication. It is best if you associate these effects with nursing interventions. Learn to recognize the common effects associated with each medication classification, and then relate the appropriate nursing interventions to each effect. For example, if a side effect is hypertension, then the associated nursing intervention would be to monitor blood pressure; if a side effect is hypokalemia, then the associated nursing interventions are to monitor the client for signs of hypokalemia and to monitor the client's potassium blood level. Again, this makes the vast amount of information that you need to remember manageable.

> **Relate nursing interventions to the side effects and potential adverse or toxic effects of a medication!**

 ## Commonalities in Medication Names

Learning commonalities in medication names that belong to a particular classification will also help in answering a question. If you note a medication name in a test question and are unfamiliar with the medication, if you can at least associate the medication with a classification, you will be able to determine the medication's action, side effects, and nursing interventions. Note the letters in the medication name, and look for those letters that identify a particular medication classification.

Sample questions follow.

1. Androgens: *Most* medication names end with the letters *-terone*, such as testosterone.
2. Angiotensin-converting enzyme (ACE) inhibitors: *Most* medication names end with the letters *-pril*, such as enalapril.
3. Antidiuretic hormones: *Most* medication names end with the letters *-pressin*, such as desmopressin.
4. Antilipemic medications: *Some* medication names end with the letters *-statin*, such as atorvastatin. Others have *-chole* or *-cole*, such as colestipol, and, *-fib*, such as gemfibrozil.
5. Antiviral medications: *Most* antiviral medications contain *vir* in their names, such as ritonavir.
6. Benzodiazepines: Benzodiazepines include alprazolam, chlordiazepoxide, clorazepate, and triazolam; *most* other benzodiazepine names end with the letters *-pam*, such as diazepam.
7. β-Adrenergic blockers: *Most* medication names end with the letters *-lol*, such as atenolol.
8. Calcium channel blockers: *Most* medication names end with the letters *-pine*, such as amlodipine; some exceptions include diltiazem and verapamil.
9. Carbonic anhydrase inhibitors: *Most* medication names end with the letters *-mide*, such as acetazolamide.
10. Estrogens: *Most* estrogen medications contain *est* in their names, such as conjugated estrogen.
11. Glucocorticoids and corticosteroids: *Most* medication names end with the letters *-sone*, such as prednisone.
12. Histamine H_2 receptor antagonists: *Most* medication names end with the letters *-dine*, such as cimetidine.
13. Nitrates: *Most* medications contain *nitr* in their names, such as nitroglycerin.
14. Pancreatic enzyme replacements: *Most* medications contain *pancre* in their names, such as pancrelipase.
15. Phenothiazines: *Most* medication names end with the letters *-zine*, such as chlorpromazine.
16. Proton pump inhibitors: *Most* medication names end with the letters *-zole*, such as lansoprazole.

17. Sulfonamides: *Most* medications include *sulf* in their names, such as sulfamethoxazole.

18. Sulfonylureas: *Most* medication names end with the letters *-mide,* such as chlorpropamide, or *-ide,* such as glimepiride.

19. Thiazide diuretics: *Most* medication names end with the letters *-zide,* such as hydrochlorothiazide.

20. Thrombolytic medications: *Most* medication names end with the letters *-ase,* such as alteplase.

21. Thyroid hormones: *Most* medications contain *thy* in their names, such as levothyroxine.

22. Xanthine bronchodilators: *Most* medication names end with the letters *-line,* such as theophylline. .

SAMPLE QUESTION: Commonalities in Medication Names

Case Event: A nurse is collecting data from a client who is taking pantoprazole.

Question Query: The nurse determines that the medication is **effective** if the client states relief of which symptom?

1. Heartburn
2. Constipation
3. A nighttime cough
4. Migraine headaches

ANSWER: 1

TEST-TAKING STRATEGY

Remember to read the question carefully, noting the subject of the question and the strategic word. Apply the clinical judgment/cognitive skill, *evaluate outcomes.* In this question the strategic word is *effective,* and the subject is an intended effect. Remembering that most proton pump inhibitor medication names end with the suffix *-zole* will direct you to option 1.

▐▶ TIP FOR THE NURSING STUDENT

Pantoprazole is in a group of medications called *proton pump inhibitors* that decrease the amount of acid produced in the stomach. It is used to treat erosive esophagitis (damage to the esophagus from stomach acid) and other conditions involving excess stomach acid, such as a condition known as *Zollinger-Ellison syndrome.* You will learn about this medication in your pharmacology course and in your medical-surgical nursing course when you study gastrointestinal disorders.

SAMPLE QUESTION: Commonalities in Medication Names

Case Event: The nurse is collecting a health history on a client seen at the primary health care clinic for the first time. When the nurse asks the client about current prescribed medications, the client tells the nurse that he takes indinavir twice daily.

Question Query: Based on this finding, the nurse would suspect the presence of which condition?

1. Diverticulitis
2. Peptic ulcer disease
3. Inflammatory bowel disease
4. Human immunodeficiency virus (HIV)

ANSWER: 4

TEST-TAKING STRATEGY

Remember to read the question carefully, focusing on the data in the question. Apply the clinical judgment/cognitive skill, *analyze cues*. Note the nurse's health history finding. Remembering that many antiviral medication names contain the letters *vir* will direct you to option 4. Also note that options 1, 2, and 3 are comparable or alike and relate to a gastrointestinal disorder.

 TIP FOR THE NURSING STUDENT

Indinavir is a protease inhibitor. Protease inhibitors block the part of HIV called *protease*. When protease is blocked or inhibited, HIV is unable to infect new cells. Protease inhibitors are almost always used in combination with at least two other anti-HIV medications. You will learn about this medication in your pharmacology course and in your medical-surgical nursing course when you study immune disorders.

? **SAMPLE QUESTION: Commonalities in Medication Names**

Case Event: The nurse is preparing to administer atenolol to a client.
Question Query: The nurse would check which item before administering the medication?
1. Temperature
2. Blood pressure
3. Potassium level
4. Blood glucose level

ANSWER: 2

TEST-TAKING STRATEGY

Remember to read the question carefully, noting the subject of the question. In this question the subject is an assessment before administration of the medication. Apply the clinical judgment/cognitive skill, *take action*. Note the name of the medication, *atenolol*. Recalling that most β-blocker medication names end with the letters *-lol* and that one intended effect of these medications is to control blood pressure will direct you to option 2.

 TIP FOR THE NURSING STUDENT

Atenolol is a β-adrenergic blocking agent that is used for treating high blood pressure, heart pain (angina pectoris), abnormal rhythms of the heart, and some neurological conditions, such as migraines. It blocks the action of the sympathetic nervous system by blocking beta receptors on sympathetic nerves. Because the sympathetic nervous system is responsible for increasing the heart rate, by blocking the action of these nerves, atenolol reduces the heart rate and is useful in treating abnormally rapid heart rhythms. Atenolol also reduces the force of contraction of heart muscle and thereby lowers blood pressure. You will learn about this medication in your pharmacology course and in your medical-surgical nursing course when you study the cardiovascular system.

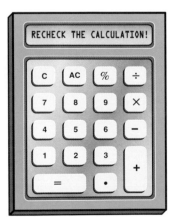

What Strategies Will Help When Answering Medication and Intravenous Calculation Questions?

When a medication or IV calculation question is presented, always use the appropriate formula to solve the problem. Shortcuts should not be used in making these calculations. The problem and the answer should be expressed in the correct units of measure. Always be careful with decimal points. It is important to place the decimal points in the correct places, or the answer will be incorrect and unsafe. When solving a medication calculation problem, always determine whether the answer is within reason and makes sense. Always use a calculator to confirm your answer. Following are two sample questions related to medication and IV calculations.

NCLEX® EXAM TIP

On the NCLEX exam, medication and IV calculation questions will most likely be in a fill-in-the-blank format. You are provided with an on-screen calculator for these medication and IV problems. Even if you use the calculator to calculate dosages and flow rates, it is important to recheck the calculation before typing the answer. Follow the formula, place the decimal points in the correct places, and check the accuracy of the calculation. Read the question carefully, because many of these questions will ask you to record your answer using one decimal place or to record your answer to the nearest whole number. Always follow the directions accompanying the question. In addition, if you are asked to round numbers, always round at the end of performing the calculation.

Medication and Intravenous Calculations

Follow the directions accompanying the question.
Use the on-screen calculator.
Apply the cognitive skill, *generate solutions*.
Convert the unit of measure if necessary.
Follow the formula.
Place the decimal point in the correct place.
Recheck the accuracy of the calculation.
If rounding is necessary, perform at the end of the calculation.

SAMPLE QUESTION: Medication Calculation

Case Event: A prescription reads phenytoin 0.2 g orally twice daily. The medication label states 100-mg capsules.
Question Query: The nurse prepares how many capsule(s) to administer one dose? **Fill in the blank.**

ANSWER: 2 capsules

TEST-TAKING STRATEGY

Focus on the data in the question. Apply the clinical judgment/cognitive skill, *generate solutions*. Use the medication calculation formula. In this medication calculation problem, it is necessary to first convert grams to milligrams. In the metric system, to convert a larger unit to a smaller unit multiply by 1000 or move the decimal 3 places to the right; therefore, 0.2 g = 200 mg.

FORMULA:

$$\frac{D\,(desired)}{A\,(available)} \times Q\,(quantity) = tablet\,(s)$$

$$\frac{200\ \text{mg}}{100\ \text{mg}} \times 1\ \text{tablet} = 2\ \text{tablets}$$

Use the on-screen calculator to perform the calculation, and then recheck your work, making sure that the answer makes sense and is a safe dose before typing it!

▐▶ TIP FOR THE NURSING STUDENT

You will learn about nursing math in your foundations of nursing course or in another course specifically designed to teach you about nursing math. You will be using nursing math to perform calculations when you prepare medications in the clinical setting. Be sure to learn the formulas including dimensional analysis and how to perform the calculations because the formulas are critical steps in the process of preparing a safe dose of a medication.

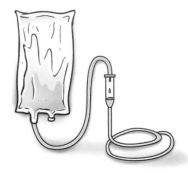

 SAMPLE QUESTION: Intravenous Calculation

Case Event: An intravenous solution of 1000 mL of 0.45% normal saline is prescribed to infuse over 8 hours. The drop factor is 15 gtt/mL.

Question Query:

The nurse would set the flow rate at how many drops per minute (gtt/min)? **Fill in the blank. Round answer to the nearest whole number.**

ANSWER: 31 gtt/min

TEST-TAKING STRATEGY

This question is in the fill-in-the-blank format. Apply the clinical judgment/cognitive skill, *generate solutions.* Use the formula for calculating IV flow rates when answering the question. Focus on the data in the question and note that the question asks you to round the answer to the nearest whole number. Also, be sure to change 8 hours to minutes.

FORMULA:

$$\frac{\text{Total volume to infuse} \times \text{Drop(gtt) factor}}{\text{Time in minutes}} = \text{Drops/minute}$$

$$\frac{1000 \times 15}{480 \left(8 \text{ hours} \times 60 \text{ minutes} \right)} = 31.25 \text{ or } 31 \text{ gtt/min}$$

Use the on-screen calculator. Remember to follow the formula, recheck your answer, and make sure that the answer makes sense and is safe before typing it. Also remember to round to the nearest whole number if asked to do so.

▐▶ TIP FOR THE NURSING STUDENT

You will learn about calculating IV flow rates in your foundations of nursing course or in another course specifically designed to teach you about IV therapy. You will be using this formula for calculating an IV flow rate in the clinical setting when you care for a client receiving IV therapy. Be sure to learn this formula and how to determine the accurate flow rate because it is critical for the safe administration of IV fluids to a client.

CHAPTER 12

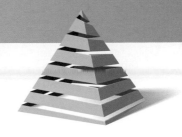

Additional Pyramid Strategies

In addition to all the test-taking strategies you have reviewed so far in this book, you can use other helpful strategies to assist in the process of elimination and answering questions correctly. This chapter reviews these helpful strategies and provides sample questions to illustrate how these strategies are used. Also included in this chapter are useful strategies for answering questions that relate to laboratory values, client positioning, and disaster planning. Some additional pyramid strategies include:

1. Eliminating options that contain closed-ended words
2. Eliminating options that contain medical rather than nursing interventions
3. Eliminating comparable or alike options
4. Ensuring that all components of an option are correct
5. Selecting the umbrella option
6. Visualizing the information in the case event, question query, and options
7. Looking for concepts in the question that are comparable or alike to a concept in one of the options

 ## Eliminating Options That Contain Closed-Ended Words: How Will This Help?

In most situations, if an option contains a closed-ended word, it is incorrect. As you read each option, if you note a word that is closed-ended, eliminate that option. Conversely, as you read an option and note an open-ended word, then that may be the correct option. A list of closed-ended and open-ended words follows.

Closed-Ended Words

All
Always
Cannot
Every
Must
Never
None
Not
Only
Will not

Open-Ended Words

Generally
May
Possibly
Usually

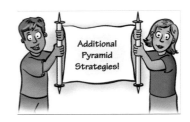

STUDY TIP

Lifestyle Planning

In addition to all of the strategies you have learned about so far in this text, remember that self-care is one of the most important factors that will lead to your success. Take the time to care for your own needs, and you will notice that you are able to focus much better on your schoolwork!

Closed-ended words may indicate an incorrect option!

Open-ended words may indicate a correct option!

Following are sample questions that illustrate the strategy of closed-ended versus open-ended words.

SAMPLE QUESTION: Eliminating Options That Contain Closed-Ended Words

Case Event: The nurse is providing dietary instructions to a client about a low-fat diet.
Question Query: The nurse would make which statement to the client?
1. "Never use butter for cooking."
2. "Drink fluids only if they are fat free."
3. "Eat foods that have less than 1% fat content only."
4. "Read the labels on food items to determine the fat content."

ANSWER: 4

TEST-TAKING STRATEGY

Read every word in each option carefully. Apply the clinical judgment/cognitive skill, *take action*. Note the closed-ended words *never* in option 1 and *only* in options 2 and 3. Remember that the use of a closed-ended word in an option will most likely make the option incorrect!

▐▌▶ TIP FOR THE NURSING STUDENT

For a regular healthy diet it is usually recommended that of the total calories eaten, no more than 30% should come from fat. A low-fat diet may require even greater restriction. Low-fat diets may be prescribed for a variety of conditions, including gastrointestinal disorders such as liver disease or gallbladder disease, cardiovascular disorders, or obesity. You will learn about the various types of diets in your foundations of nursing course or nutrition course and in your medical-surgical nursing course when you study nutrition for various health problems.

SAMPLE QUESTION: Selecting Options That Contain Open-Ended Words

Case Event: A client scheduled for a computerized tomography (CT) scan of the abdomen asks the nurse when the results of the test will be available.
Question Query: The nurse would make which **most appropriate** response to the client?
1. "Your doctor may have the results in about 3 days."
2. "The results will not be available for at least 1 week."
3. "You must ask the CT technician for that information."
4. "Every scan is read by a radiologist, and this process always takes 1 week."

ANSWER: 1

TEST-TAKING STRATEGY

Read every word in each option carefully, and note the strategic words, *most appropriate*. Apply the clinical judgment/cognitive skill, *take action*. If you were unable to answer this question using nursing knowledge, note the use of the open-ended word *may* in option 1. Also, note the closed-ended words *will not* in option 2, *must* in option 3, and *every* and *always* in option 4. Remember that the use of a closed-ended word in an option will most likely make the option incorrect, and the use of an open-ended word in an option tends to make the option correct.

▐▌▶ TIP FOR THE NURSING STUDENT

A CT scan is a procedure that combines x-ray images with the aid of a computer to generate cross-sectional views and, if needed, three-dimensional images of the internal organs and structures of the body. A CT scan is used to define normal and abnormal structures in the body and/or assist in procedures by helping accurately guide the placement of instruments or treatments. You will learn about this diagnostic procedure during your nursing education, most likely in your foundations and medical-surgical nursing course.

SMART STUDY TIP

Preparing for Clinical

When in clinical, you should be aware of any diagnostic procedures your assigned client(s) have recently undergone, what the results of these procedures are if they are available, and any related postprocedure care that needs to be followed. Additionally, you should be aware of any procedures your assigned client(s) are scheduled to undergo while you are caring for them, and ensure implementation of any specific preprocedure indications, such as diet prescriptions, withholding or administering certain medications, ensuring intravenous access, ensuring consent has been obtained, completing screening forms, reviewing laboratory results, or any other specific indications needed.

Eliminating Options That Contain Medical Rather Than Nursing Interventions: How Will This Help?

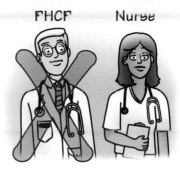

An important point to remember is that the NCLEX® exam is a nursing examination, not a medical one. Therefore, focus on nursing and select the option that relates to a nursing intervention rather than a medical one. The only situation in which you may need to select a medical intervention is if the question indicates to do so. For example, if the question query states, "Which intervention does the nurse anticipate to be prescribed?" then you may need to select the option that contains a medical action or prescription. Following is a review of sample questions that illustrate this strategy.

> Focus on nursing rather than medical interventions!

 ### SAMPLE QUESTION: Eliminating Options That Contain Medical Rather Than Nursing Interventions

Case Event: The nurse is caring for a client with a diagnosis of heart failure who suddenly experiences severe dyspnea and suspects that pulmonary edema has developed.

Question Query: What is the **immediate** nursing action?

1. Insert a Foley catheter.
2. Place the client in high Fowler's position.
3. Obtain a vial of furosemide and a syringe.
4. Obtain a dose of morphine sulfate from the opioid medication drawer.

ANSWER: 2

TEST-TAKING STRATEGY

Note the strategic word, *immediate*, and note the subject of the question, a nursing action, and apply the clinical judgment/cognitive skill, *take action*. Although options 1, 3, and 4 are interventions that may be done in this situation, they all relate to a medical intervention rather than a nursing one. Option 2 is a nursing action that will assist to alleviate dyspnea. Remember, your exams are nursing examinations, not medical examinations!

▌▶ TIP FOR THE NURSING STUDENT

Heart failure is an inability of the heart to maintain adequate circulation to meet the metabolic needs of the body because of an impaired pumping ability. Heart failure can progress to pulmonary edema, a condition in which fluid accumulates in lung tissue and the lung tissue becomes swollen. This is detectable on radiology of the chest. This is a medical emergency. If this occurs, the immediate action of the nurse is to place the client in an upright (high Fowler's) position. Other actions, such as administration of oxygen, administration of diuretics, and insertion of a Foley catheter, are important, and frequent monitoring of vital signs and urine output is important. You will learn about heart failure and pulmonary edema when you learn about cardiac disorders in your medical-surgical nursing course. One important thing to remember is that with all clients, airway is the priority.

SMART STUDY TIP

Scope of Practice

Be sure to be familiar with the scope of nursing practice with regard to various aspects of client care. Knowing this information will help you with questions that relate to scope of practice and require you to differentiate between medical actions and nursing actions.

 ### SAMPLE QUESTION: Selecting an Option That Indicates a Medical Intervention

Case Event: The nurse is admitting an infant to the pediatric unit with a diagnosis of respiratory syncytial virus (RSV).

Question Query: The nurse anticipates that the primary health care provider will prescribe which measure?

1. Ribavirin
2. A private room
3. Contact precautions
4. Strict handwashing procedures

ANSWER: 1

TEST-TAKING STRATEGY

Note the subject of the question, the intervention that the primary health care provider will prescribe. Apply the clinical judgment/cognitive skill, *analyze cues*. Although the primary health care provider may document options 2, 3, and 4 on the medical prescription sheet, these are interventions that the nurse can implement for an infant with RSV. That is, these are nursing interventions and a prescription is not required. Remember that your exam is a nursing examination, not a medical examination, and the only situation in which you may need to select a medical intervention is if the question indicates to do so!

TIP FOR THE NURSING STUDENT

RSV is a viral infection that is a common cause of acute bronchiolitis, bronchopneumonia, and the common cold in infants and young children. Symptoms include fever, cough, and severe malaise. Treatment includes rest, humidity, adequate fluid intake, oxygen, and the administration of ribavirin. You will learn about this virus when you study respiratory infections in your pediatrics course.

Eliminating Comparable or Alike Options: How Will This Help?

Eliminate comparable or alike options!

An important point for you to remember is that multiple-choice and some multiple response questions have only one correct option. As you read the options, if you note ones that are comparable or alike with regard to their context, eliminate these options. The correct answer to the question will be the option that is different. Following is a sample question that illustrates this strategy of eliminating comparable or alike options.

SAMPLE QUESTION: Eliminating Comparable or Alike Options

Case Event: The nurse is creating a plan of care for a client who will be receiving a blood transfusion.

Question Query: The nurse would write which intervention in the plan that relates to monitoring for a transfusion reaction?

1. Weigh the client before and after the transfusion.
2. Check the client's lung sounds hourly for crackles.
3. Monitor the client's temperature during the transfusion.
4. Monitor the client's intake and output during the transfusion.

ANSWER: 3

TEST-TAKING STRATEGY

Note the subject of the question, a transfusion reaction. Apply the clinical judgment/cognitive skill, *generate solutions*. If you know the signs of a transfusion reaction, you can answer this question easily. If you do not know these signs, read the options carefully. Note that options 1, 2, and 4 are comparable or alike in that they relate to the complication of fluid overload. Because they are all comparable or alike, they are incorrect and need to be eliminated. Remember that the correct answer to the question will be the option that is different!

TIP FOR THE NURSING STUDENT

A blood transfusion involves the IV administration of a component of blood, such as packed red blood cells, to replace blood or one of its components lost as a result of trauma, surgery, or a disease. One complication that can occur when administering blood is a blood transfusion reaction. Some signs and symptoms of this complication include fever; facial flushing; rapid, thready pulse; cold, clammy skin; itching; dizziness; difficulty breathing; or low back or chest pain. You will learn about blood transfusions, the complications, and the nursing care involved with the administration of blood during your medical-surgical nursing course when you study hematological disorders.

Ensuring That All Parts of an Option Are Correct: How Will This Help?

Some questions on exams or on the NCLEX exam may contain options that include two parts, and each part of the option is separated by the word *and*. Read the question carefully, note the strategic words, and focus on the subject. As you read the options, read both parts of the option. If you note that one part of the option is incorrect, then the entire option is incorrect; therefore, eliminate that option. In these types of questions, it is important to ensure that both parts of the option are correct. Following is a sample question that illustrates this strategy of ensuring that all parts of an option are correct.

? SAMPLE QUESTION: Ensuring That All Parts of an Option Are Correct

Case Event: The nurse is collecting data from a client diagnosed with a cataract of the right eye.

Question Query: The nurse would expect to obtain which finding on data collection?
1. Reports of eye pain and a cloudy white pupil
2. Reports of a frontal headache and photophobia
3. Reports of a gradual loss of vision and photophobia
4. Reports of blurred vision and excessive tearing of the eye

ANSWER: 3

TEST-TAKING STRATEGY

The options in this question contain two parts, and each part of the option is separated by the word *and*. Noteworthy words are *expect to obtain*, and the subject of the question is data noted in a client with a cataract. Apply the clinical judgment/cognitive skill, *recognize cues*. In this question, knowledge regarding the differences between the signs and symptoms of a cataract versus glaucoma will assist in answering the question correctly. Although a cloudy white pupil and photophobia occur in a client with a cataract, eye pain and frontal headaches do not. Therefore, options 1 and 2 are not entirely correct and need to be eliminated. Eye pain and frontal headaches occur in the client with glaucoma. From the remaining two options, recalling that excessive tearing occurs in the client with glaucoma, not the client with a cataract, will assist in eliminating option 4. Remember that all parts of the option need to be correct for the option to be correct!

⏩ TIP FOR THE NURSING STUDENT

Cataract is a condition that affects the lens of the eye. On data collection the nurse would note a cloudy white pupil. Symptoms include a gradual loss of vision, photophobia, painless blurring and distortion of objects, and glare from bright lights. You will learn about cataracts, their treatment, and the nursing care involved during your medical-surgical nursing course when you study eye disorders.

Selecting the Umbrella Option: How Will This Help?

The umbrella option is a general statement that may incorporate the content of the other options within it. When you are answering a question and note that more than one option appears to be correct, look for the umbrella option.

SMART STUDY TIP

Student-to-Student

Watch for comparable or alike options when answering exam questions, and if you encounter them, eliminate them because it is not possible for both of them to be correct. Additionally, look for options that are opposite. It is likely that one of the opposite options is the correct one!

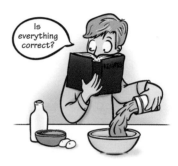

Ensure that all parts of an option are correct!

SMART STUDY TIP

Student-to-Student

When preparing for nursing exams, remember that many questions will be related to nursing assessment/data collection. When studying certain health problems, it may be helpful for you to look at images or animations of expected findings associated with these conditions, especially if you are a visual learner!

Look for the umbrella option!

The umbrella option will be the correct answer. Following is a sample question that illustrates this strategy.

❓ SAMPLE QUESTION: Selecting the Umbrella Option

Case Event: In a telephone call from emergency medical services, the nurse in the emergency department is told that several victims who survived a plane crash and are suffering from cold exposure will be transported to the hospital.

Question Query: What is the **initial** nursing action by the emergency department nurse?

1. Call the nursing supervisor to activate the agency disaster plan.
2. Supply the trauma rooms with bottles of sterile water and normal saline.
3. Call the intensive care unit to request that nurses be sent to the emergency department.
4. Call the laundry department to request as many warm blankets as possible for the emergency department.

ANSWER: 1

TEST-TAKING STRATEGY

Note the strategic word, *initial,* and focus on the subject, the nursing action in the event of a disaster. Apply the clinical judgment/cognitive skill, *take action.* As you read each option, you will note that all options are correct. In this type of question, look for the umbrella option. Option 1 is the umbrella option. Activating the agency disaster plan will ensure that the interventions in options 2, 3, and 4 will occur. Remember that the umbrella option incorporates the ideas of the other options within it.

▐▶ TIP FOR THE NURSING STUDENT

A disaster preparedness plan is a structured and formal plan of action that is implemented when a disaster occurs in the health care agency or external to the agency, such as in the community. The plan provides a coordinated plan of action for all members of the health care team. You will learn about disasters and disaster preparedness plans during your community nursing course.

LEARN NORMAL LABORATORY VALUES!

▲ What Strategies Will Help When Answering Questions Related to Laboratory Values?

The questions on a nursing exam or the NCLEX exam related to laboratory values require you to identify whether the laboratory value is normal or abnormal and then to think critically about the effects of the laboratory value in terms of the client. If you know the normal values, you will be able to determine if an abnormality exists when a laboratory value is presented in a question.

Refer to the detailed NCLEX Test Plan for the laboratory tests most likely to appear on the NCLEX exam. Create your own flash cards for learning about these laboratory tests. Points to note are the normal values for the most common laboratory tests, what it means if the value is higher than normal or lower than normal, and determination of the need to implement specific actions based on the findings. Remember that most blood specimens should not be drawn during hemodialysis or from an extremity that has an IV solution running. Another point to note is that on the NCLEX examination, some laboratory test questions will provide you with the normal ranges of the laboratory values. If so, this will be helpful to you.

When a question is presented on your exams regarding a specific laboratory value, note the health problem presented in the question and the associated body organ that is affected. This will help you determine the correct option. For example, if the question asks you about the immune status of a client receiving chemotherapy, assessment of laboratory values will focus on the white blood cell count. You will need to analyze the results as possibly being low and determine the specific client need, which in this case would be the risk for infection. In the client receiving chemotherapy who has a low white blood cell count, your plan should center on the immune system, specifically protecting that client from infection. Interventions focus on preventive actions related to infection, perhaps even protective isolation measures, such as neutropenic precautions. Evaluation may focus on maintaining a normal temperature in the client. Following is a sample question that relates to a laboratory test.

> **Laboratory Values**
>
> Note the health problem presented in the question.
> Identify the associated body organ that is affected as a result of the health problem.
> Identify whether the laboratory value is normal or abnormal.

SAMPLE QUESTION: Laboratory Values

Case Event: A client with a diagnosis of sepsis is receiving antibiotics by the intravenous (IV) route.
Question Query: The nurse checks for nephrotoxicity by monitoring which laboratory value **most** closely?
1. Lipase level
2. Platelet count
3. Creatinine level
4. White blood cell count

ANSWER: 3

TEST-TAKING STRATEGY

Note the strategic word, *most*. Focus on the data in the question, and note that the subject is nephrotoxicity. Apply the clinical judgment/cognitive skill, *analyze cues*. Read each option carefully, and note that option 3 is the only option that relates to kidney function. Option 1 relates to pancreatic function. Option 2 relates to the hematological system. Option 4 relates to the immune system. Remember to note the disorder presented in the question and the associated body organ that is affected as a result!

▐▶ TIP FOR THE NURSING STUDENT

Sepsis refers to a systemic infection that can occur as a result of a localized or other type of infection in the body. This serious infection needs to be treated aggressively with antibiotics, and usually blood cultures are done to determine the antibiotic of choice. Nephrotoxicity, which refers to the destruction of kidney cells, is a complication that can occur with the use of antibiotics. To monitor for nephrotoxicity, the nurse would check the results of the blood urea nitrogen and creatinine levels, which are kidney function tests. You will learn about antibiotics in a pharmacology course or in your medical-surgical nursing course when you study infections and immune disorders.

▲ Visualizing the Information in the Case Event, Question Query, and Options: How Will This Help?

As you read the question, it is helpful to visualize the case event. Forming a mental image of the situation places you as the nurse into the scenario. This may be useful because as you create the mental image, you may recall a similar situation that you experienced in the actual clinical area and recall what you or another nurse did in the situation. In addition, visualize each option as you read it. Visualizing and relating the case event to a similar clinical experience can be a valuable strategy as you attempt to eliminate incorrect options. Following is a sample question that illustrates this strategy of visualizing the information.

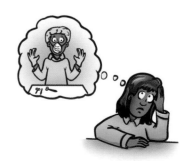

Visualize the information!

SAMPLE QUESTION: Visualizing the Information in the Case Event, Question Query, and Options

Case Event: The nurse prepares to perform a sterile dressing change on an abdominal incision.

Question Query: The nurse explains the procedure to the client, washes her hands, and sets up the sterile field. The nurse would take which action **next?**

1. Don sterile gloves.
2. Assess the integrity of the abdominal incision.
3. Don clean gloves and remove the old dressing.
4. Clean the wound with povidone–iodine solution as prescribed.

ANSWER: 3

TEST-TAKING STRATEGY

Note the strategic word, *next*. Apply the clinical judgment/cognitive skill, *take action*. Form a mental image of this procedure and visualize the steps that you would take. You cannot clean the wound or assess the wound unless you remove the old dressing; therefore, eliminate options 2 and 4. From the remaining options, recall that sterile gloves are necessary for cleaning and dressing the incision once the old dressing is removed. This will direct you to option 3. Remember that visualizing and relating the case event to a similar clinical experience can be a valuable strategy as you attempt to eliminate incorrect options!

Ⅲ▶ TIP FOR THE NURSING STUDENT

A sterile procedure, such as a sterile dressing change, is one that involves taking measures so that no microorganisms come in contact with the wound or anything that is used to perform the procedure. A special technique is used to maintain sterility when performing this procedure; you will learn this technique and how to perform sterile dressing changes during your foundations of nursing course.

Looking for Concepts in the Question That Are Comparable or Alike to a Concept in One of the Options: How Will This Help?

> Look for a concept in the question that is comparable or alike to a concept in one of the options!

Read the question carefully, noting the strategic words and the subject of the question. As you read each option, look for the one that contains comparable or alike concepts or has a relationship to those identified in the question. This strategy may help as you are eliminating the incorrect options. Following is a sample question that illustrates this strategy of looking for comparable or alike concepts.

SAMPLE QUESTION: Looking for Comparable or Alike Concepts in the Question and in One of the Options

Case Event: A client is admitted to the hospital with a diagnosis of pericarditis.

Question Query: The nurse assesses the client for which manifestation that differentiates pericarditis from other cardiopulmonary problems?

1. Anterior chest pain
2. Pericardial friction rub
3. Weakness and irritability
4. Chest pain that worsens on inspiration

ANSWER: 2

TEST-TAKING STRATEGY

Note the word *differentiates*, and focus on the subject, a manifestation that differentiates pericarditis from other cardiopulmonary problems. Apply the clinical judgment/cognitive skill, *recognize cues*. This tells you that the correct option will be one that is unique to this health problem. Note the relationship between the word *pericarditis* in the question and the word *pericardial* in the correct option. Also recall that a pericardial friction rub is heard when there is inflammation of the pericardial sac during the inflammatory phase of pericarditis. Remember to look for the option that contains a comparable or alike concept or has a relationship to the information in the question!

▮▶ TIP FOR THE NURSING STUDENT

Pericarditis is an inflammation of the pericardium (the sac that surrounds the heart) and can be associated with trauma, infection, myocardial infarction, malignant disease, or other disorders. The client exhibits fever, substernal chest pain, difficulty breathing, a dry nonproductive cough, and a rapid pulse rate. On auscultation of the lungs and chest, a pericardial friction rub and a muffled heartbeat over the apex of the heart would be heard. You will learn about auscultation of the lungs and chest during your health and physical assessment course and about pericarditis during your medical-surgical nursing course when you study cardiac disorders.

 ## What Strategies Will Help When Answering Questions Related to Client Positioning?

Nursing responsibility includes positioning clients in a safe and appropriate manner to provide safety and comfort. Knowledge regarding the client position required for a certain procedure or condition is expected. It is the nurse's responsibility to reduce the likelihood and prevent the development of complications related to an existing condition, prescribed treatment, or medical or surgical procedure. It is imperative that the nurse review the health care provider's prescriptions after treatments or procedures and take note of instructions regarding positioning and mobility.

When you are presented with a question that relates to positioning a client, focus on the data in the question, the client's diagnosis, and the anatomical location of the client's diagnosis, and consider the pathophysiology of the disorder and the goals of care. That is, think about what complications you want to prevent. Some guidelines to remember when answering questions related to positioning are listed next.

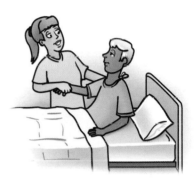

Client Positioning
Always review the primary health care provider's or surgeon's prescriptions.
Focus on the client's diagnosis.
Identify the anatomical location of the client's disorder.
Consider the pathophysiology of the disorder and the goals of care.
Think about what complications you want to prevent.

Guidelines Related to Positioning

- Always review the primary health care provider's or surgeon's prescriptions regarding positioning.
- Elevation of an affected body part reduces edema.
- Clients who have had neck or head surgery are placed in semi-Fowler's or Fowler's position.
- After a liver biopsy, the client is placed in a right lateral (side-lying) position to provide pressure to the site and prevent bleeding.
- Clients receiving irrigations or feedings through a nasogastric, gastrostomy, or jejunostomy tube are placed in semi-Fowler's or Fowler's position to prevent aspiration.
- The left Sims' position is used to administer a rectal enema or irrigation to allow the solution to flow by gravity in the natural direction of the colon.
- Clients with a respiratory disorder or cardiovascular disorder are usually placed in semi-Fowler's or Fowler's position.
- Clients with peripheral arterial disease may be advised to elevate their feet and legs at rest, because swelling can prevent arterial blood flow, but they should not raise their legs above the level of the heart because extreme elevation slows arterial blood flow; some clients may be advised to maintain a slightly dependent position to promote perfusion.

- Clients with peripheral venous disease are usually advised to elevate their feet and legs above heart level.
- Clients with a head injury are placed in semi-Fowler's or Fowler's position.
- If a client develops autonomic dysreflexia, the head of the bed is elevated.
- In clients with hemorrhagic strokes, the head of the bed is usually elevated to 30 degrees to reduce intracranial pressure and to facilitate venous drainage.
- For clients with ischemic strokes, the head of the bed is usually kept flat.
- After craniotomy the client should NOT be positioned on the operated site, especially if the bone flap has been removed, because the brain has no bony covering on the affected site; semi-Fowler's to Fowler's position is maintained with the head in a midline, neutral position to facilitate venous drainage from the head, and extreme hip and neck flexion is avoided.
- With increased intracranial pressure, the client is placed in semi-Fowler's to Fowler's position; the head is maintained in a midline, neutral position to facilitate venous drainage from the head, and extreme hip and neck flexion is avoided.
- In a spinal cord injury the client is immobilized on a spinal backboard, with the head in a neutral position, to prevent incomplete injury from becoming complete; a neck collar is applied and head flexion, rotation, or extension is avoided; and the client is logrolled.
- In the client who underwent a total hip arthroplasty, positioning will depend on the surgical techniques used, the method of implantation, the prosthesis, and the surgeon's preference; extreme internal and external rotation and adduction are avoided; and side-lying on the operative side is usually not allowed (unless specifically prescribed by the surgeon).

The following question relates to positioning a client.

? SAMPLE QUESTION: Client Positioning

Case Event: The nurse assists in performing a liver biopsy.
Question Query: After the biopsy, the nurse plans to place the client in which position?
1. Prone
2. Supine
3. A left side-lying position with a small pillow or folded towel under the puncture site
4. A right side-lying position with a small pillow or folded towel under the puncture site

ANSWER: 4

TEST-TAKING STRATEGY

Focus on the subject, positioning after liver biopsy, and think about the anatomical location of the procedure and what complication you want to prevent. Apply the clinical judgment/cognitive skill, *generate solutions*. In this situation you want to prevent bleeding. Remember that the liver is on the right side of the body and that the application of pressure on the right side will minimize the escape of blood or bile through the puncture site, because this position compresses the liver against the chest wall at the biopsy site. Also, note that options 3 and 4 are opposite positions (left or right side), indicating that one of these options may be the correct one. Remember to focus on the subject of the question, the client's diagnosis, and the anatomical location of the client's diagnosis, and consider the pathophysiology of the disorder and the goals of care!

▌▶ TIP FOR THE NURSING STUDENT

A liver biopsy is a diagnostic procedure in which local anesthesia is administered followed by the introduction of a special needle into the liver to obtain a specimen for pathological examination. Bleeding is a concern after the procedure, and this is the reason why the client will be placed on the right side. This position provides pressure at the biopsy site by compressing the liver against the chest wall. You will learn about a liver biopsy in your medical-surgical nursing course when you study gastrointestinal disorders.

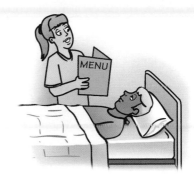

What Strategies Will Help When Answering Questions Related to Therapeutic Diets?

On nursing examinations, you may be asked questions about diet therapy and certain food items that are allowed with certain diets. You may also be asked about a particular diet that may be prescribed for a client with a certain health problem. Therefore, nutritional therapy and knowing the nutritional components of various food items are essential. Some strategies that you can use to help you answer these questions are noted next.

Strategies for Answering Questions Related to Therapeutic Diets

1. Focus on the data in the question.
2. Note the subject of the question: Is the question asking about a specific diet or a specific food item?
3. Note the diagnosis of the client, and think about the organ system that is affected.
4. Think about the pathophysiology associated with the client's health problem.
5. Look at the options that are provided, and try to relate the client's health problem to the correct option.

 SAMPLE QUESTION: Therapeutic Diet

Case Event: The nurse is providing dietary instructions to a client who is immobile and experiencing frequent episodes of constipation. The client complains that the constipation is uncomfortable.

Question Query: The nurse would tell the client that which food item would be **most** helpful to include in the diet?

1. Pasta
2. Cabbage
3. White bread
4. Whole-grain bread

ANSWER: 4

TEST-TAKING STRATEGY

Note the strategic word, *most.* Focus on the data in the question, and note the client complains of constipation. Apply the clinical judgment/cognitive skill, *generate solutions.* Think about the body organ affected in this condition and the associated pathophysiology. A client with constipation needs to include high-fiber foods in the diet. The only food item that is high in fiber is whole grains. Also note that options 1 and 3 are comparable or alike in that they are low-fiber foods. Option 2 is a gas-forming food and needs to be avoided because it will increase any discomfort that the client may be experiencing. Remember to focus on the data in the question, note the client's health problem or complaint, and think about the body organ affected and the associated pathophysiology.

▐▶ TIP FOR THE BEGINNING NURSING STUDENT

Constipation is a condition in which the client is having difficulty passing stool or is experiencing the incomplete or infrequent passage of hard stool. One intervention is to include adequate amounts of fiber and fluids in the diet. You will learn about constipation in your foundations of nursing course when you study elimination patterns and in your medical-surgical nursing course when you study gastrointestinal health problems.

What Strategies Will Help When Answering Questions Related to Disasters?

A disaster is any human-made or natural event that causes destruction and devastation and requires assistance from others. For a health care agency, a disaster can be external or internal. External disasters include those that occur outside the health care agency, and internal disasters include those that occur inside the health care agency. If a disaster or mass casualty event occurs, the agency disaster preparedness plan (emergency response plan) is immediately activated by the health care agency, and the nurse responds by following the directions identified in the plan. In the community setting, if the nurse is the first responder to a disaster, the nurse cares for the victims by attending to those with life-threatening problems first; once rescue workers arrive at the scene, immediate plans for triage should begin.

Natural Disasters

Blizzards
Communicable disease
  epidemics and pandemics
Cyclones
Droughts
Earthquakes
Floods
Forest fires
Hailstorms
Hurricanes
Landslides
Mudslides
Tornadoes
Tsunamis (tidal waves)
Volcanic eruptions

Human-Made Disasters

Dam failures resulting in flooding
Hazardous substance accidents, such as pollution, chemical spills, or toxic gas leaks
Accidents that result in the release of radiological materials
Resource shortages, such as food, water, and electricity
Structural collapse, fire, or explosions
Terrorist attacks, such as bombings, riots, and bioterrorism
Transportation accidents

The NCLEX exam may contain questions about disasters and mass casualty events that focus on nursing interventions. Questions about communicable diseases and epidemics and pandemics and safely managing these crisis situations and caring for many ill clients will also be a part of the NCLEX. A disaster question may identify the nurse as the first responder to a disaster site and ask you to identify the victim that the nurse should attend to first. If the question identifies a site outside the hospital environment, select the option that identifies a victim that the nurse could realistically save. Think about survivability and ask yourself, "Who can I save?" Also use prioritizing skills. Ask yourself, "Which victims sustained injuries that are not critical or life threatening and could wait to be cared for?"

An NCLEX question may also identify the nurse as the leader of a nursing unit and ask which clients in the unit could be discharged to free up beds for victims of a mass casualty event or epidemic or pandemic brought to the emergency department who need to be admitted to the hospital. In this situation, read each client's description carefully and determine if the client can safely return home and if there are home care and community resources that could care for the client and meet the client's needs. These types of questions require the use of prioritizing skills.

When triaging victims of a disaster at a disaster site, think survivability. Determine which victims sustained life-threatening injuries and need immediate treatment to sustain life.

SAMPLE QUESTION: Human-Made Disaster

Case Event: The nurse is the first responder to the site of a disaster in which several people were injured in a train crash.
Question Query: Which victim of the crash would the nurse attend to **first?**
1. A victim with a fractured arm
2. A victim with multiple bruises on the legs
3. A victim with a severe head injury who is not breathing
4. A victim with an upper leg injury who is bleeding profusely

ANSWER: 4

TEST-TAKING STRATEGY

Note the strategic word, *first*. Focus on the data in the question, and note that the disaster site is outside the hospital environment. Apply the clinical judgment/cognitive skill, *prioritize hypotheses*. Therefore, determine which victim has a life-threatening injury and requires immediate treatment to sustain life. Think survivability. The victims described in options 1 and 2 sustained injuries that are not critical or life threatening and could wait for care. Outside the hospital environment, resources are limited. Therefore, it is unlikely that the nurse could help the victim with a severe head injury who is not breathing. The nurse could apply pressure to the leg of the victim who is bleeding profusely and could save this victim's life.

▋▶ TIP FOR THE NURSING STUDENT

Disaster management is an important role of the nurse. An important point to remember is that the nurse needs to use prioritizing skills to determine how best to proceed in a disaster situation. Many types of disasters can occur, but the principles of care remain the same. The immediate priority of the nurse is to attend to the victim who has immediate and life-threatening needs and who could be saved. You will learn about mass casualty events and disaster management and the nurse's roles and responsibilities in your community nursing course.

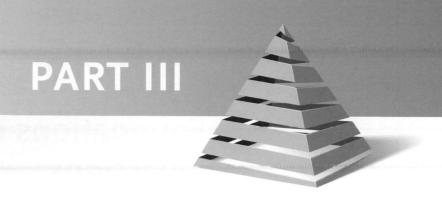

PART III

Practice Tests

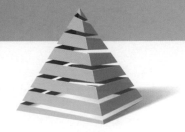

CHAPTER 13

Foundations of Care Questions

1. The nurse creates a plan of care for a newly hospitalized client who reports difficulty sleeping. The nurse plans to implement which **best initial** intervention?
   1 Offer the client a sleeping pill at night.
   2 Provide the client with a snack at bedtime.
   3 Ask the client what she or he does to prepare for sleep.
   4 Leave the television on in the client's room at a very low volume.

Level of Cognitive Ability: Creating
Client Needs: Physiological Integrity
Clinical Judgment/Cognitive Skills: Generate Solutions
Integrated Process: Nursing Process/ Planning
Content Area: Foundations of Care
Priority Concepts: Caregiving; Health Promotion
Level of Nursing Student: Beginning

ANSWER: 3
Rationale: The best initial intervention is to ask what the client does to prepare for sleep. The nurse needs to assess habits that are beneficial to the client compared with those that disturb sleep. Options 1, 2, and 4 provide interventions without initially assessing what measures would be helpful to the client.

Test-Taking Strategy: Apply the clinical judgment/cognitive skill, *generate solutions.* Note the strategic words, *best* and *initial.* Use the steps of the nursing process when determining the best answer, remembering that assessment/data collection would be done initially. This will direct you to the correct option. **Review:** Care of the client experiencing difficulty **sleeping.**

Tip for the Nursing Student: Determine what measures the client takes at home to sleep; then incorporate these measures into the plan of care during hospitalization.

---

2. The nurse notes documentation in a client's medical record that the client is experiencing anuria. The nurse plans care based on which interpretation?
   1 The client is unable to produce urine.
   2 The client has a diminished capacity to form urine.
   3 The client has difficulty having a bowel movement.
   4 The client has episodes of alternating constipation and diarrhea.

Level of Cognitive Ability: Applying
Client Needs: Physiological Integrity
Clinical Judgment/Cognitive Skills: Generate Solutions
Integrated Process: Nursing Process/Planning
Content Area: Foundations of Care
Priority Concepts: Elimination; Fluids and Electrolytes
Level of Nursing Student: Beginning

ANSWER: 1
Rationale: Anuria is the term used to describe an inability to produce urine. Oliguria is a diminished capacity to produce urine and is most likely the result of decrease in renal perfusion. Options 3 and 4 do not relate to urinary tract dysfunction.

Test-Taking Strategy: Apply the clinical judgment/cognitive skill, *generate solutions.* Focus on the subject, the definition of anuria. Use medical terminology skills to answer the question. Recalling that the prefix *an-* refers to *absence* and that the suffix *-uria* refers to *urine* will direct you to the correct option. **Review:** The definition of **anuria.**

Tip for the Nursing Student: Remember that the client should maintain a urinary output of at least 30 mL/hour and that the nurse would monitor for this occurrence. A decline in urinary output could indicate kidney dysfunction or failure, hypovolemia, or an obstruction in the renal system. This occurrence needs to be reported.

3. The nurse is caring for a client who has a fever and is diaphoretic. The nurse monitors the client's intake and output and expects to note which finding?
   1 The client's urine is diluted.
   2 The client's output is decreased.
   3 The client's urine production is increased.
   4 The majority of the client's fluid loss is through the skin.

Level of Cognitive Ability: Applying
Client Needs: Physiological Integrity
Clinical Judgment/Cognitive Skills: Recognize Cues
Integrated Process: Nursing Process/ Assessment/Data Collection
Content Area: Foundations of Care
Priority Concepts: Fluids and Electrolytes; Thermoregulation
Level of Nursing Student: Beginning

ANSWER: **2**
Rationale: Febrile conditions affect urine production. The client who is diaphoretic loses fluids through insensible water loss, which decreases urine production. However, the increased body temperature associated with fever increases the accumulation of body wastes. Although the volume of urine may be reduced, it is highly concentrated. Some fluid (not the majority) will be lost through the skin.

Test-Taking Strategy: Apply the clinical judgment/cognitive skill, *recognize cues.* Focus on the subject, care of the client experiencing a fever and diaphoresis. Think about the physiological response of the body to fever and diaphoresis. This will direct you to the correct option. Also remember that although some fluid is lost through the skin, the majority of fluid loss is not lost through this system. **Review:** Conditions that affect **fluid imbalance.**

Tip for the Nursing Student: Fluid can be lost through the skin, the lungs during breathing, the kidneys, and the gastrointestinal tract. Most fluid is lost through the kidneys. If the client has a fever and is diaphoretic (sweating), the normal daily amount of fluid loss through the skin will be increased.

---

4. The nurse provides instructions to a female client regarding the procedure for collecting a midstream urine sample. The nurse would tell the client to perform which action?
   1 Douche before collecting the specimen.
   2 Cleanse the perineum from front to back.
   3 Collect the urine in the cup as soon as the urine flow begins.
   4 Collect the specimen before bedtime, and bring it to the laboratory the next morning.

Level of Cognitive Ability: Applying
Client Needs: Safe and Effective Care Environment
Clinical Judgment/Cognitive Skills: Take Action
Integrated Process: Teaching and Learning
Content Area: Foundations of Care
Priority Concepts: Client Education; Elimination
Level of Nursing Student: Beginning

ANSWER: **2**
Rationale: As part of correct procedure, the client should cleanse the perineum from front to back with the antiseptic wipes that are packaged with the specimen kit. The client would begin the flow of urine then stop the flow and then begin to urinate again to collect the midstream sample. The specimen would be sent to the laboratory as soon as possible and not allowed to stand. Improper specimen collection can yield inaccurate test results. It is not normal procedure to douche before collecting the specimen.

Test-Taking Strategy: Apply the clinical judgment/cognitive skill, *take action.* Focus on the subject, urine collection for laboratory analysis. Noting the name of the type of sample—*midstream*—will assist in eliminating option 3. Recalling that the specimen should be sent or brought to the laboratory immediately after collection will assist in eliminating option 4. From the remaining options, use basic principles related to hygiene and infection control to assist in directing you to the correct option. **Review:** The procedure for **midstream urine collection.**

Tip for the Nursing Student: The female client is taught to always wipe or cleanse the perineum from front to back to prevent the spread of microorganisms from the rectal area to the labial area, which could result in a urinary tract infection. Additionally, the male client is instructed to cleanse the penis with the towelettes from the meatus outward and to gently retract the foreskin, if present, for cleansing.

5. The nurse provides dietary instructions to a client diagnosed with iron-deficiency anemia. The nurse would tell the client to increase the intake of which food item?
   1 Plums
   2 Red apples
   3 Egg whites
   4 Kidney beans

Level of Cognitive Ability: Applying
Client Needs: Physiological Integrity
Clinical Judgment/Cognitive Skills: Take Action
Integrated Process: Teaching and Learning
Content Area: Foundations of Care
Priority Concepts: Client Education; Nutrition
Level of Nursing Student: Beginning

ANSWER: 4
Rationale: The client with iron-deficiency anemia would increase intake of foods that are naturally high in iron, including kidney beans, soybeans, chickpeas, lima beans, cooked Swiss chard, red meat, liver and other organ meats, blackstrap molasses, lentils, egg yolk, spinach, kale, turnip tops, beet greens, carrots, raisins, and apricots. The food items in options 1, 2, and 3 are not high in iron.

Test-Taking Strategy: Apply the clinical judgment/cognitive skill, *take action*. Focus on the subject, a food high in iron. Eliminate options 1 and 2 first because they are comparable or alike options and are fruit items. From the remaining options, recall either that beans are high in iron or that egg yolk (not egg white) is high in iron. This will direct you to the correct option. **Review: Iron-rich foods.**

Tip for the Nursing Student: Iron-deficiency anemia is a condition in which the client lacks sufficient red blood cells. One cause is an insufficient intake of dietary iron. These food items are important to know because you will be teaching your client about a high-iron diet.

6. A client asks the nurse about the use of a complementary or alternative measure that will assist in promoting sleep. The nurse would make which suggestion?
   1 Herbal therapy
   2 Acupuncture sessions
   3 Muscle relaxation techniques
   4 Traditional Chinese medicine sessions

Level of Cognitive Ability: Applying
Client Needs: Physiological Integrity
Clinical Judgment/Cognitive Skills: Take Action
Integrated Process: Nursing Process/ Implementation
Content Area: Foundations of Care
Priority Concepts: Health Promotion; Stress and Coping
Level of Nursing Student: Beginning

ANSWER: 3
Rationale: A simple relaxation technique, such as muscle relaxation, can help reduce anxiety and promote sleep. Herbal therapy involves the use of herbs (plant or a plant part). Some herbs have been determined to be safe, but other herbs, even in small amounts, can be toxic, and the nurse would not recommend their use to a client. The client who is taking prescription medications would consult the primary health care provider regarding the use of herbs because serious interactions between herbs and medications can occur. Acupuncture is an invasive procedure that stimulates certain points on the body by the insertion of special needles to modify the perception of pain, normalize physiological functions, or treat or prevent disease. Traditional Chinese medicine focuses on restoring and maintaining a balanced flow of vital energy; interventions include acupressure, acupuncture, herbal therapies, diet, meditation, and tai chi and qi gong (exercise that focuses on breathing, visualization, and movement). Any invasive therapy requires a prescription from the primary health care provider.

Test-Taking Strategy: Apply the clinical judgment/cognitive skill, *take action*. The subject of the question is a method to promote relaxation and sleep. Note that options 1, 2, and 4 are comparable or alike options in that they involve invasive measures. **Review: Complementary and alternative therapies.**

Tip for the Nursing Student: Complementary and alternative therapies must be prescribed by the primary health care provider. An important point to remember is that the nurse would not recommend the use of these treatments, especially invasive ones, without first consulting the primary health care provider. Some of these therapies can harm the client.

7. The nurse instructs a client taking a potassium-sparing diuretic about foods high in potassium that need to be avoided. The nurse determines that the client **needs further instruction** if the client states that which food is high in potassium?
   1 Kiwi
   2 Celery
   3 Oranges
   4 Dried fruit

Level of Cognitive Ability: Evaluating
Client Needs: Physiological Integrity
Clinical Judgment/Cognitive Skills: Evaluate Outcomes
Integrated Process: Teaching and Learning
Content Area: Foundations of Care
Priority Concepts: Fluids and Electrolytes; Nutrition
Level of Nursing Student: Beginning

ANSWER: 2
Rationale: Meats, some dairy products, dried fruits, bananas, cantaloupe, kiwi, and oranges are high in potassium. Vegetables that are high in potassium include avocados, broccoli, dried beans or peas, lima beans, mushrooms, potatoes, seaweed, soybeans, and spinach. Celery is a vegetable that is low in potassium.

Test-Taking Strategy: Apply the clinical judgment/cognitive skill, *evaluate outcomes*. Note the strategic words, *needs further instruction*. These words indicate a negative event query and indicate that an incorrect response needs to be selected. Eliminate options 1, 3, and 4 because they are comparable or alike options and are fruit items. **Review:** High- and low-**potassium foods.**

Tip for the Nursing Student: A diuretic is a medication that promotes the formation and excretion of urine and leads to an increase in urine output. These medications are used for clients with excess body fluid, such as those with hypertension or heart failure. Many diuretics cause the loss of potassium in the urine. A potassium-sparing diuretic does not, and the client tends to retain potassium rather than lose it. The client is taught about diet and the foods that are high and low in potassium. Both a low potassium level and a high potassium level can cause serious problems for the client; therefore, potassium imbalances are important to learn.

---

8. A clear liquid diet has been prescribed for a client. The nurse would offer which item to the client?
   1 Apple juice
   2 Orange juice
   3 Tomato juice
   4 Ice cream without nuts

Level of Cognitive Ability: Applying
Client Needs: Physiological Integrity
Clinical Judgment/Cognitive Skills: Take Action
Integrated Process: Nursing Process/ Implementation
Content Area: Foundations of Care
Priority Concepts: Fluids and Electrolytes; Nutrition
Level of Nursing Student: Beginning

ANSWER: 1
Rationale: A clear liquid diet consists of foods that are relatively transparent. The food items in options 2, 3, and 4 would be included in a full liquid diet.

Test-Taking Strategy: Apply the clinical judgment/cognitive skill, *take action*. Eliminate options 2, 3, and 4 because they are comparable or alike options and are items allowed on a full liquid diet. Remember that a clear liquid diet consists of foods that are relatively transparent. Option 1 is the only food item that is transparent. **Review:** Food items allowed on a **clear liquid diet.**

Tip for the Nursing Student: A clear liquid diet may be prescribed to provide fluids to treat or prevent dehydration, to provide complete bowel rest, to feed a malnourished person or a person who has not had any oral intake for some time, in preparation for surgery or tests, or as a postsurgical diet. A clear liquid diet consists of foods that are relatively transparent.

9. Oxygen by nasal cannula at 4 L/minute is prescribed for a hospitalized client. The nurse would perform which actions in the care of the client? **Select all that apply.**

   ☐ **1** Humidify the oxygen.

   ☐ **2** Apply water-soluble lubricant to the nares.

   ☐ **3** Instruct the client to breathe only through the nose.

   ☐ **4** Instruct the client and family about the purpose of the oxygen.

   ☐ **5** Increase the oxygen flow if the client complains of dryness in the nares.

Level of Cognitive Ability: Applying
Client Needs: Physiological Integrity
Clinical Judgment/Cognitive Skills: Take
   Action
Integrated Process: Nursing Process/
   Implementation
Content Area: Foundations of Care
Priority Concepts: Caregiving; Gas Exchange
Level of Nursing Student: Beginning

ANSWER: 1, 2, 4
Rationale: The nasal cannula provides for lower concentrations of oxygen and can even be used with mouth breathers because movement of air through the oropharynx pulls oxygen from the nasopharynx. The nurse would humidify the oxygen and apply water-soluble lubricant to the nares to prevent and treat dryness. The nurse would also instruct the client and family regarding the purpose of the oxygen. It is unnecessary to instruct a client to breathe only through the nose. It is unnecessary and potentially harmful to increase the oxygen flow. Additionally, increasing the flow of oxygen will contribute further to dryness of the nares.

Test-Taking Strategy: Apply the clinical judgment/cognitive skill, *take action*. Focus on the subject, care of the client receiving oxygen via nasal cannula. Noting that option 3 contains the closed-ended word "only" will assist in eliminating this option. Additionally, recalling the scope of nursing practice will assist in eliminating option 5. **Review:** Care of the client receiving **oxygen.**

Tip for the Nursing Student: Oxygen therapy is a treatment measure that needs to be prescribed by the primary health care provider. It is used when a client is unable to take in sufficient oxygen on her or his own to adequately provide nutrients to the cells of the body.

10. The nurse is preparing to care for a client who is diagnosed with a terminal disease. The nurse would plan which appropriate interventions in the care of the client? **Select all that apply.**

   ☐ **1** Offer to contact the clergy to support the client's spiritual needs.

   ☐ **2** Make referrals to other disciplines based on the client's stated needs.

   ☐ **3** Balance the client's need for assistance with that for independence.

   ☐ **4** Provide extremely thorough answers to each question asked by the client or family.

   ☐ **5** Ask the client about goals for the treatment plan and how she or he can best be assisted in achieving these goals.

Level of Cognitive Ability: Applying
Client Needs: Psychosocial Integrity
Clinical Judgment/Cognitive Skills: Generate
   Solutions
Integrated Process: Caring
Content Area: Foundations of Care
Priority Concepts: Care Coordination;
   Palliative Care
Level of Nursing Student: Intermediate

ANSWER: 1, 2, 3, 5
Rationale: In planning care for the client diagnosed with a terminal disease, the nurse provides information and answers questions to the extent most helpful to the client and family; extremely thorough answers may be overwhelming at this time. The nurse makes referrals to other disciplines and clergy based on an identified need and tries to balance the client's need for assistance with the need to maintain some measure of independence. It is also very helpful to spend time with the client and to ask the client about treatment goals and the best way these goals can be achieved; this involves the client in planning her or his own care and allows the client to maintain a sense of control at this vulnerable time.

Test-Taking Strategy: Apply the clinical judgment/cognitive skill, *generate solutions*. Focus on the subject, care of the client with a terminal disease. Note the closed-ended word "extremely" in option 4 to assist in eliminating this option. **Review:** The psychosocial needs of the **dying client.**

Tip for the Nursing Student: The client who is diagnosed with a terminal disease may have many physical and psychosocial needs. Remember that the client's family may also need some supportive care. Simply letting the family know that you are there to assist them if they should need anything can be quite supportive. Use therapeutic communication techniques to focus on the client's and family's feelings.

11. The nurse is calculating the client's fluid intake during a 12-hour period. The client consumed 4 oz of juice, 8 oz of coffee, and 6 oz of milk at breakfast. At lunchtime the client consumed 8 oz of iced tea and 6 oz of water. At dinnertime the client consumed 8 oz of coffee and 6 oz of lemonade. The client also consumed 4 oz of water at 10:00 AM, at 2:00 PM, and again at 6:00 PM when receiving oral medications. At 8:00 AM and 2:00 PM the client received an intravenous antibiotic diluted in 50 mL of normal saline. What would the nurse document as the client's total intake in milliliters? **Fill in the blank.**

Answer: _____ mL

Level of Cognitive Ability: Applying
Client Needs: Physiological Integrity
Clinical Judgment/Cognitive Skills: Take Action
Integrated Process: Nursing Process/ Implementation
Content Area: Foundations of Care
Priority Concepts: Clinical Judgment; Fluids and Electrolytes
Level of Nursing Student: Beginning

ANSWER: 1840 ML

Rationale: There are 30 mL in 1 oz. The client consumed 4 oz of juice, 8 oz of coffee, and 6 oz of milk at breakfast. This totals 18 oz and equals 540 mL. At lunchtime the client consumed 8 oz of iced tea and 6 oz of water. This totals 14 oz and equals 420 mL. At dinnertime the client consumed 8 oz of coffee and 6 oz of lemonade. This totals 14 oz and equals 420 mL. The client also consumed 4 oz of water at 10:00 AM, at 2:00 PM, and again at 6:00 PM when receiving oral medications. This totals 12 oz and equals 360 mL. At 8:00 AM and 2:00 PM, the client received an intravenous antibiotic diluted in 50 mL of normal saline. This totals 100 mL. Therefore, adding 540 mL, 420 mL, 420 mL, 360 mL, and 100 mL equals 1840 mL.

Test-Taking Strategy: Apply the clinical judgment/cognitive skill, *take action.* Focus on the subject, calculation of client intake. Note that the question requires you to convert ounces to milliliters. Remember that there are 30 mL in 1 oz. Read the question carefully, note the amount of oral intake in ounces, and then convert the total to milliliters. Use a calculator to assist in answering the question. Also remember to add the amount of intravenous intake. **Review:** The procedure for **calculating fluid intake.**

Tip for the Nursing Student: Calculating intake and output will be a nursing measure that you will be implementing for many of your clients. It involves knowing how many milliliters are contained in various eating and drinking utensils and knowing that there are 30 mL in 1 oz. If you can remember this conversion and learn about the amount of milliliters in various eating and drinking utensils, then simple addition will be all that is necessary to determine intake and output.

---

12. The nurse is teaching a client about a low-fat diet. The nurse would tell the client that it is acceptable to consume which food items? **Select all that apply.**
☐ 1 Lentil soup
☐ 2 Watermelon
☐ 3 Tomato soup
☐ 4 Low-fat yogurt
☐ 5 Cream of mushroom soup

Level of Cognitive Ability: Applying
Client Needs: Physiological Integrity
Clinical Judgment/Cognitive Skills: Take Action
Integrated Process: Teaching and Learning
Content Area: Foundations of Care
Priority Concepts: Health Promotion; Nutrition
Level of Nursing Student: Beginning

ANSWER: 1, 2, 3, 4

Rationale: One cup of cream of mushroom soup contains 14 g of fat, whereas lentil soup contains 4 g and tomato soup contains 2 g. Low-fat yogurt contains 2 g of fat. Fresh fruits and vegetables are low in fat.

Test-Taking Strategy: Apply the clinical judgment/cognitive skill, *take action.* Focus on the subject, food items low in fat. The word *cream* in option 5 indicates a high-fat food group. **Review: High-fat food** groups.

Tip for the Nursing Student: Remember that most fruits and vegetables are low in fat. Also, some protein foods such as chicken and turkey are low in fat, whereas red meats tend to contain a higher fat content.

13. An antibiotic is diluted in 100 mL normal saline (NS) and is to be administered piggyback over 30 minutes. The drop factor is 10 drops (gtt)/mL. The nurse would plan to set the flow rate at how many drops per minute? **Fill in the blank. Round to the nearest whole number.**

Level of Cognitive Ability: Applying
Client Needs: Physiological Integrity
Clinical Judgment/Cognitive Skills: Generate Solutions
Integrated Process: Nursing Process/ Planning
Content Area: Foundations of Care
Priority Concepts: Clinical Judgment; Safety
Level of Nursing Student: Beginning

ANSWER: 33 gtt/minute
Rationale: Use the intravenous (IV) flow rate formula:

$$\frac{\text{Total volume} \times \text{drop factor}}{\text{Time in minutes}} = \text{Drops / minute}$$

$$\frac{100\,\text{mL} \times 10\,\text{gtt}}{30\,\text{minutes}} = \frac{1000}{30} = 33.3, \text{or } 33\,\text{gtt / minute}$$

Test-Taking Strategy: Apply the clinical judgment/cognitive skill, *generate solutions*. Focus on the subject, a medication calculation. Use the formula for calculating IV flow rates. Use a calculator, follow the formula, recheck your answer, and make sure that it makes sense before documenting the answer. Remember to round the answer to the nearest whole number. **Review: Medication calculations.**

Tip for the Nursing Student: You will be using this formula for calculating an IV flow rate in the clinical setting when you care for a client receiving IV therapy. Be sure to learn this formula and how to determine the accurate flow rate because it is critical for the safe administration of IV fluids to a client.

---

14. The nurse is preparing to assist in performing a venipuncture to initiate continuous intravenous (IV) therapy with 0.9% normal saline solution. The nurse gathers the needed supplies and plans to perform which action before beginning the venipuncture?
   1 Applying a tourniquet below the chosen venipuncture site
   2 Placing an armboard at the joint located above the venipuncture site
   3 Placing cool compresses over the vein to be used for the venipuncture
   4 Inspecting the 0.9% normal saline solution for particles or contamination

Level of Cognitive Ability: Applying
Client Needs: Physiological Integrity
Clinical Judgment/Cognitive Skills: Generate Solutions
Integrated Process: Nursing Process/ Planning
Content Area: Foundations of Care
Priority Concepts: Clinical Judgment; Safety
Level of Nursing Student: Intermediate

ANSWER: 4
Rationale: All IV solutions must be free of particles or precipitates. A tourniquet is applied above the chosen venipuncture site, not below. Cool compresses cause vasoconstriction, making the vein less visible. Warm compresses will help to vasodilate. Armboards are applied only if necessary and after the IV line is started.

Test-Taking Strategy: Apply the clinical judgment/cognitive skill, *generate solutions*. Note the subject, the procedure for performing a venipuncture. Visualizing the procedure for preparing to initiate an IV infusion will help eliminate options 1 and 2. From the remaining options, use principles related to heat and cold to eliminate option 3. **Review:** The procedure for **IV insertion.**

Tip for the Nursing Student: A venipuncture is the insertion of a special needle or cannula into a client's vein to provide access for administering fluids and medications. One extremely important point to remember when you are preparing to infuse or administer any solution by the IV route is that you need to inspect the solution for particles or precipitates. If these are noted, then you would not use the solution for administration and would contact the pharmacy and return the solution to the department.

---

15. The physician prescribes 25 mg of hydroxyzine hydrochloride intramuscularly. The nurse reads the label on the medication vial and administers how many milliliters to the client? **Refer to figure. Fill in the blank.**

ANSWER: 0.5 mL
Rationale: Use the following formula for calculating medication doses.

(Adapted from Ogden S, Fluharty L: *Calculation of drug dosages*, ed 9, St Louis, 2012, Mosby.)

Answer: _____ mL

Level of Cognitive Ability: Applying
Client Needs: Physiological Integrity
Clinical Judgment/Cognitive Skills: Take Action
Integrated Process: Nursing Process/ Implementation
Content Area: Foundations of Care
Priority Concepts: Clinical Judgment; Safety
Level of Nursing Student: Beginning

$$\frac{\text{Desired}}{\text{Available}} \times mL = mL \text{ per dose}$$

$$\frac{25\,mg}{50\,mg} \times 1\,mL = 0.5\,mL$$

Test-Taking Strategy: Apply the clinical judgment/cognitive skill, *take action*. Note the subject, a medication calculation question. Follow the formula for the calculation of the correct dose. It is not necessary to perform a conversion with this problem. Label the formula, including the answer. Remember to use a calculator, follow the formula, recheck your answer, and make sure that it makes sense before documenting the answer. **Review: Medication calculations.**

Tip for the Nursing Student: You will use nursing math to perform calculations when you prepare medications in the clinical setting. Be sure to learn the formulas and how to perform the calculations because the formulas are critical steps in preparing a safe dose of a medication.

---

16. The nurse receives a telephone call from the hospital admission office and is told that a client with human immunodeficiency virus (HIV) will be admitted to the nursing unit. In planning infection control measures for the client, which is the **best** type of isolation precaution that the nurse would prepare?
    1 Droplet precautions
    2 Contact precautions
    3 Standard precautions
    4 Airborne precautions

Level of Cognitive Ability: Applying
Client Needs: Safe and Effective Care Environment
Clinical Judgment/Cognitive Skills: Generate Solutions
Integrated Process: Nursing Process/ Planning
Content Area: Foundations of Care
Priority Concepts: Infection; Safety
Level of Nursing Student: Beginning

ANSWER: 3
Rationale: HIV is a retrovirus that can cause acquired immunodeficiency syndrome (AIDS). HIV is transmitted through anal or oral sexual contact with infected semen or vaginal secretions, through contact with infected blood or blood products, by transmission of the virus from mother to fetus during childbirth, through breastfeeding, or from any other infected body fluids. Standard precautions, which include blood and body fluid precautions, will prevent contact with infectious matter and protect a health care provider from contracting the virus when providing care. Droplet, contact, and airborne precautions are more specific types of precautions and are known as *transmission-based precautions*. Droplet precautions require the use of a mask and are used when organisms can be spread by respiratory droplets but are unable to remain in the air farther than 3 feet (1 meter) (e.g., influenza). Contact precautions are used when caring for clients who have an infection that can be spread by direct or indirect contact (e.g., draining wounds, splashes). Airborne precautions require the use of a special particulate filter mask. These precautions are used to prevent infection when infectious organisms remain in the air for prolonged periods and can be transported in the air for distances greater than 3 feet (1 meter) (e.g., tuberculosis). No data in the question indicate that these types of precautions alone are necessary.

Test-Taking Strategy: Apply the clinical judgment/cognitive skill, *generate solutions*. Note the strategic word, *best*. Read each option carefully. Think about the pathophysiology of HIV and its transmission. Also, note that option 3 is the umbrella option. **Review: The methods of transmission of human immunodeficiency virus (HIV).**

Tip for the Nursing Student: Standard precautions are actions developed by the Centers for Disease Control and Prevention (CDC) that include hand hygiene and the use of other barrier precautions designed to reduce the transmission of infectious organisms. These actions are used for the care of every client, regardless of whether an infection is present. Standard precautions are specific to the task and include the use of gloves, water-impermeable gowns, masks, and eye protection.

---

17. A client with heart disease says to the nurse, "I guess I'll never be able to eat ice cream again." Which response would the nurse make to the client?
    1 "Why do you say that?"
    2 "There are lots of other foods you can eat."
    3 "You do not think you will be able to eat ice cream at all?"
    4 "Ice cream has too much fat content, so why would you even want to eat it?"

Level of Cognitive Ability: Applying
Client Needs: Psychosocial Integrity
Clinical Judgment/Cognitive Skills: Take Action
Integrated Process: Communication and Documentation
Content Area: Foundations of Care
Priority Concepts: Communication; Nutrition
Level of Nursing Student: Beginning

ANSWER: 3
Rationale: The nurse most appropriately responds by rephrasing the client's statement. Option 3 is a therapeutic response and rephrases the client's statement. Options 1, 2, and 4 are examples of nontherapeutic communication techniques. Option 1 requests an explanation from the client. Options 2 and 4 give advice. In addition, option 4 lectures the client.

Test-Taking Strategy: Apply the clinical judgment/cognitive skill, *take action*. Use therapeutic communication techniques. Option 3 is the only therapeutic response and rephrases the client's statement. **Review: Therapeutic communication techniques**

Tip for the Nursing Student: Therapeutic communication techniques promote and encourage the client to communicate and share feelings with the nurse. Nontherapeutic communication techniques block the communication process and are not methods that the nurse would use when caring for a client.

---

18. A client scheduled for an operative procedure states to the nurse, "I am not sure if I should have this surgery." Which response would the nurse make to the client?
    1 "It is your decision."
    2 "Do not worry. Everything will be fine."
    3 "Why do you not want to have this surgery?"
    4 "Tell me what concerns you have about the surgery."

Level of Cognitive Ability: Applying
Client Needs: Psychosocial Integrity
Clinical Judgment/Cognitive Skills: Take Action
Integrated Process: Communication and Documentation
Content Area: Foundations of Care
Priority Concepts: Anxiety; Communication
Level of Nursing Student: Beginning

ANSWER: 4
Rationale: The nurse needs to gather more data and assist the client in exploring feelings about the surgery. Options 1, 2, and 3 are nontherapeutic. Option 1 is a blunt response and does not address the client's concern. Option 2 provides false reassurance. Option 3 can make the client feel defensive.

Test-Taking Strategy: Apply the clinical judgment/cognitive skill, *take action*. Use therapeutic communication techniques. Option 4 is the only option that addresses the client's concern. **Review: Therapeutic communication techniques.**

Tip for the Nursing Student: Regardless of the type of surgery the client is having, the nurse needs to address any concerns that the client may have. Always focus on the client's feelings and concerns. The nurse would use therapeutic communication techniques to promote and encourage the client to communicate and share her or his feelings with the nurse. Nontherapeutic communication techniques block the communication process and are not methods that the nurse would use when caring for a client.

19. A 15-year-old seeks treatment for a sexually transmitted infection at a local clinic. With regard to informed consent, the nurse would perform which action?

1 Ask the client to sign the informed consent form.

2 Tell the client that a court order for treatment is needed.

3 Tell the client that parental consent for treatment is needed.

4 Call the client's mother to obtain telephone consent for treatment.

Level of Cognitive Ability: Applying
Client Needs: Safe and Effective Care Environment
Clinical Judgment/Cognitive Skills: Take Action
Integrated Process: Nursing Process/ Implementation
Content Area: Foundations of Care
Priority Concepts: Health Care Law; Infection
Level of Nursing Student: Beginning

ANSWER: 1

Rationale: Parents normally must give informed consent for treatment of a minor. Some exceptions to this include the need for emergency treatment; when the consent of the minor is sufficient, such as for treatment of a sexually transmitted infection; or when a court order or other legal authorization has been made. Therefore, options 2, 3, and 4 are incorrect.

Test-Taking Strategy: Apply the clinical judgment/cognitive skill, *take action*. Note the words *15-year-old* and *sexually transmitted infection*. Eliminate options 2, 3, and 4 because they are comparable or alike options and indicate the need for informed consent from someone other than the client. **Review: Informed consent** for the treatment of **minors.**

Tip for the Nursing Student: Informed consent involves obtaining permission from the client to perform a treatment or procedure. Some types of informed consent include those needed to administer anesthesia, perform surgery, or administer blood; it is the primary health care provider's responsibility to explain the treatment or procedure to the client. The legal issues surrounding informed consent in the health care environment are extremely important ones, and knowledge of when a minor can provide informed consent is one of these areas.

---

20. A client will be receiving long-term, continuous total parenteral nutrition (TPN) at home. The nurse would incorporate which **priority** client problem in the plan of care?

1 Lack of hope

2 Social isolation

3 Inability to cope effectively

4 Low self-esteem related to current situation

Level of Cognitive Ability: Analyzing
Client Needs: Psychosocial Integrity
Clinical Judgment/Cognitive Skills: Prioritize Hypotheses
Integrated Process: Nursing Process/Analysis
Content Area: Foundations of Care
Priority Concepts: Adherence; Stress and Coping
Level of Nursing Student: Beginning

ANSWER: 2

Rationale: The client will be receiving long-term, continuous TPN at home. Therefore, the client will be socially isolated from stimuli outside the home. Social isolation indicates that the client's ability to socialize with others will be limited as a result of the client's condition. No data in the question support options 1, 3, or 4.

Test-Taking Strategy: Apply the clinical judgment/cognitive skill, *prioritize hypotheses*. Focus on the strategic word, *priority*, and note the subject, care of the client receiving TPN. Focus on the data in the question, and note the words *long-term*, *continuous*, and *at home*. Eliminate options 1, 3, and 4 because no data in the question support these options. **Review:** Care of the client receiving **TPN.**

Tip for the Nursing Student: TPN is a solution containing a high concentration of nutrients and glucose. It is administered intravenously (usually through the subclavian vein) to a client who has a disorder in which she or he is unable to obtain adequate nutrition orally.

21. The nurse is having a conversation with a client and responds to the client's statement by saying, "You say that your mother left you when you were 6 years old." The nurse is using which therapeutic communication technique?

1 Focusing
2 Restating
3 Summarizing
4 Sharing observations

Level of Cognitive Ability: Applying
Client Needs: Psychosocial Integrity
Clinical Judgment/Cognitive Skills: Take Action
Integrated Process: Communication and Documentation
Content Area: Foundations of Care
Priority Concepts: Communication; Family Dynamics
Level of Nursing Student: Beginning

ANSWER: 2
Rationale: In restating, the nurse repeats the main thought that the client expressed. This therapeutic communication technique indicates that the nurse is listening to the client. In this technique, the nurse validates, reinforces, or calls attention to something important that the client said. Therefore, options 1, 3, and 4 are incorrect.

Test-Taking Strategy: Apply the clinical judgment/cognitive skill, *take action.* Use your knowledge regarding therapeutic communication techniques. Focus on the nursing statement. Noting the words *"You say that..."* in the nursing statement will assist in identifying the technique that the nurse is using as restating. **Review: Therapeutic communication techniques.**

Tip for the Nursing Student: Therapeutic communication techniques promote and encourage the client to communicate and share feelings with the nurse. Nontherapeutic communication techniques block the communication process and are not methods that the nurse would use when caring for a client.

---

22. A physician's prescription reads morphine sulfate 7.5 mg intramuscularly stat. The medication ampule reads "morphine sulfate 10 mg per mL." The nurse would prepare how many milliliters to administer the correct dose? **Fill in the blank.**
Answer: _____ mL

Level of Cognitive Ability: Applying
Client Needs: Physiological Integrity
Clinical Judgment/Cognitive Skills: Generate Solutions
Integrated Process: Nursing Process/ Planning
Content Area: Foundations of Care
Priority Concepts: Clinical Judgment; Safety
Level of Nursing Student: Beginning

ANSWER: 0.75 mL
Rationale: Use the formula to calculate the correct dose.

Formula:

$$\frac{\text{Desired}}{\text{Available}} \times mL = mL \, per \, dose$$

$$\frac{7.5\,mg}{10\,mg} \times 1\,mL = 0.75\,mL$$

Test-Taking Strategy: Apply the clinical judgment/cognitive skill, *generate solutions.* Focus on the subject, a medication calculation. Next, use a calculator and follow the formula for the calculation of the correct dose. Recheck your work, making sure that the answer makes sense. **Review: Medication calculations.**

Tip for the Nursing Student: You will be using nursing math to perform calculations when you prepare medications in the clinical setting. Be sure to learn the formulas and how to perform the calculations because the formulas are critical steps in the process of preparing a safe dose of a medication.

---

23. The nurse instructs a client on a tyramine-restricted diet about foods that are acceptable to consume. The nurse tells the client to consume which items in the diet? **Select all that apply.**
☐ 1 Pizza
☐ 2 Apples
☐ 3 Chicken
☐ 4 Tomatoes
☐ 5 Homemade bread

ANSWER: 2, 3, 4
Rationale: Some foods that are naturally high in tyramine include aged cheeses, yogurt, canned meats, beef or chicken liver, sausage, dried fish, beer and some wines, sherry, and chocolate. The client should also avoid yeast and any products made with yeast, such as pizza and homemade bread. Most fruits and vegetables are acceptable. The fruits and vegetables that should be avoided are bananas, figs, broadleaf beans and pea pods, eggplant, and mixed Chinese vegetables.

Level of Cognitive Ability: Applying
Client Needs: Physiological Integrity
Clinical Judgment/Cognitive Skills: Take
Action
Integrated Process: Teaching and Learning
Content Area: Foundations of Care
Priority Concepts: Nutrition; Client
Education
Level of Nursing Student: Beginning

Test-Taking Strategy: Apply the clinical judgment/cognitive skill, *take action*. Note the subject, foods acceptable to consume in a tyramine-restricted diet. Eliminate options 1 and 5 because they are foods that contain yeast. **Review:** Food items that contain **tyramine.**

Tip for the Nursing Student: A healthy and balanced diet is important for all individuals. In the clinical setting, a major responsibility will be to ensure that your clients are receiving adequate nutrition to heal and to maintain health. Many times, specific diets are prescribed for clients, and you will be responsible for teaching the client about the diet, what can be eaten, and what food items should be restricted. Tyramine is an amino acid that stimulates the release of the catecholamines epinephrine and norepinephrine. Tyramine may be restricted in certain disorders, and it is very important that individuals taking monoamine oxidase inhibitors avoid the ingestion of foods and beverages containing tyramine.

---

24. A client's medication is available for injection in an ampule. Which action would the nurse take when drawing up this medication?
    1 Shake the ampule gently to mix the contents.
    2 Snap the top of the ampule so that it opens toward the nurse.
    3 Wipe the neck of the ampule with gauze after snapping it open.
    4 Place an alcohol wipe around the neck of the ampule before snapping it open.

Level of Cognitive Ability: Applying
Client Needs: Safe and Effective Care
Environment
Clinical Judgment/Cognitive Skills: Take
Action
Integrated Process: Nursing Process/
Implementation
Content Area: Foundations of Care
Priority Concepts: Clinical Judgment; Safety
Level of Nursing Student: Beginning

ANSWER: 4
Rationale: Basic procedure for drawing up medication from an ampule involves tapping the top chamber until the medication lies in the lower area, placing an alcohol wipe around the neck of the ampule, snapping the top so that it opens away from the nurse, and withdrawing the medication without injecting air into the ampule. Snapping the ampule so that it opens away from the nurse prevents injury from possible shattered glass fragments. The neck is not wiped with the gauze after it is opened because, first, it is unnecessary and could contaminate the contents of the ampule, and second, it could injure the nurse's fingers from sharp glass edges.

Test-Taking Strategy: Apply the clinical judgment/cognitive skill, *take action*. Focus on the subject, medication preparation from an ampule. Visualize this procedure and each of the options. Eliminate option 1 because of the word *shake*. Next, eliminate option 2 because it is unsafe and could harm the nurse. From the remaining options, use principles of both asepsis and safety to direct you to the correct option. **Review:** Preparing medication from an **ampule.**

Tip for the Nursing Student: An ampule is a small container usually made of glass that contains a single dose of a medication. You will be administering injections and drawing medication from ampules and other types of containers to prepare injections in the clinical setting.

---

25. The client has a platelet count of 60,000 mm³ (60×10^9/L). The nurse implements which measure in the care of this client?
    1 Using a razor for shaving the client
    2 Providing vigorous skin care and avoiding the use of lotions
    3 Measuring the temperature using a temporal thermometer
    4 Encouraging the client to use a firm-bristle toothbrush for mouth care

ANSWER: 3
Rationale: The client with a low platelet count is at risk for bleeding. Therefore, the nurse institutes measures that will minimize the risk of injury or bleeding. The nurse must avoid vigorous washing or rubbing of the skin to avoid causing ecchymosis and would use lotions to prevent dryness and cracking of the skin. The nurse would avoid the use of razors or firm-bristle toothbrushes, which could also cause bleeding. In addition, the nurse would measure the temperature using a temporal thermometer. Rectal thermometers are avoided because of the risk of bleeding, and oral thermometers are avoided if there is oral soreness or bleeding.

Level of Cognitive Ability: Applying
Client Needs: Safe and Effective Care
  Environment
Clinical Judgment/Cognitive Skills: Take
  Action
Integrated Process: Nursing Process/
  Implementation
Content Area: Foundations of Care
Priority Concepts: Perfusion; Safety
Level of Nursing Student: Beginning

Test-Taking Strategy: Apply the clinical judgment/cognitive skill, *take action*. Focus on the subject, a platelet count of 60,000 mm^3 (60×10^9/L). Recalling the normal platelet count and determining that a platelet count of 60,000 mm^3 (60×10^9/L) is low, placing the client at risk for bleeding, will assist in eliminating options 1, 2, and 4. Also, noting the words *razor, vigorous,* and *firm* in these options, respectively, will assist in eliminating them. **Review: Bleeding precautions.**

Tip for the Nursing Student: Platelets are a component of the blood and are formed in the bone marrow. They are essential for the coagulation of blood and in the maintenance of hemostasis. Therefore, if the platelet count is low, the coagulation of blood will not occur as it should, and the client is at risk for bleeding. The normal platelet count is 150,000 to 400,000 mm^3 (150 to 400 $\times 10^9$/L). If the count is low, then the nurse institutes measures to protect the client from injury and resultant bleeding.

CHAPTER 14

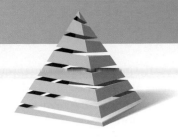

Adult Health Questions

1. The nurse is monitoring a client who underwent a pleural biopsy. The nurse determines that the client is experiencing a complication if the client exhibits which manifestation?
   1 Diaphoresis
   2 Warm, dry skin
   3 Mild pain at the biopsy site
   4 Capillary refill of 2 seconds

   Level of Cognitive Ability: Analyzing
   Client Needs: Physiological Integrity
   Clinical Judgment/Cognitive Skills: Recognize Cues
   Integrated Process: Nursing Process/ Assessment/Data Collection
   Content Area: Adult Health
   Priority Concepts: Clinical Judgment; Safety
   Level of Nursing Student: Intermediate

   ANSWER: 1
   Rationale: The nurse observes the client for dyspnea (difficulty breathing), excessive pain, pallor, or diaphoresis (profuse sweating) after pleural biopsy. These signs could indicate the presence of complications, such as pneumothorax, hemothorax, or intercostal nerve injury. Options 2 and 4 are normal findings. Mild pain is expected, because the procedure itself is painful. Abnormal signs and symptoms should be reported to the primary health care provider.

   Test-Taking Strategy: Apply the clinical judgment/cognitive skill, *recognize cues.* Focus on the subject, a complication associated with pleural biopsy. Eliminate options 2 and 4 because they are comparable or alike options and are normal findings. From the remaining options, noting the word *mild* in option 3 will assist in eliminating this option. **Review:** The complications associated with a **pleural biopsy**.

   Tip for the Nursing Student: A pleural biopsy is an invasive procedure that involves the insertion of a needle into the pleural cavity or pleural space to obtain tissue or fluid for pathological examination. This procedure is diagnostic and may be done if suspicious lesions are present. The nurse monitors for signs of respiratory distress or bleeding after a biopsy, which would indicate a complication.

2. The nurse caring for a client after a bowel resection notes that the client is restless. The nurse takes the client's vital signs and notes that the pulse rate has increased and that the blood pressure has dropped significantly since the previous readings. The nurse suspects that the client is going into shock and would take which **immediate** action?
   1 Check the client's oxygen saturation level.
   2 Recheck the vital signs to verify the findings.
   3 Raise the client's legs above the level of the heart.
   4 Slow the rate of the intravenous (IV) fluid infusing.

   ANSWER: 1
   Rationale: In addition to hypotension, manifestations of shock include tachycardia; restlessness and apprehension; and cold, moist, pale, or cyanotic skin. If a client develops signs of shock, the nurse would check the oxygen saturation, because as a result of decreased circulating volume, oxygenation may be inadequate and supplemental oxygenation may be required. The nurse would also increase the rate of IV fluids (unless contraindicated), administer medications as prescribed, and continue to monitor the client and the client's response to interventions. It is not recommended to place the client in Trendelenburg's position (legs above the level of the heart), because there is no definitive research to support that placing the client in this position assists in perfusion. Additionally, the client may have conditions such as compromised pulmonary function and increased intracranial pressure, so this position would be potentially detrimental.

Level of Cognitive Ability: Applying
Client Needs: Physiological Integrity
Clinical Judgment/Cognitive Skills: Take
   Action
Integrated Process: Nursing Process/
   Implementation
Content Area: Adult Health
Priority Concepts: Clinical Judgment; Perfusion
Level of Nursing Student: Intermediate

Test-Taking Strategy: Apply the clinical judgment/cognitive skill, *take action*. Note the strategic word, *immediate*. Use the ABCs—airway, breathing, and circulation—to answer the question. This will direct you to the correct option. **Review:** Interventions for **shock**.

Tip for the Nursing Student: Shock is an abnormal condition of inadequate blood flow to the body's tissues, resulting in an inadequate delivery of oxygen and nutrients to the tissues. There are different types of shock, but the most common is hypovolemic shock. It is caused by any condition that results in hypovolemia, such as with hemorrhage. Oxygenation is necessary, and fluid volume must be restored immediately to oxygenate perfusion-deprived tissues. This condition can be life threatening if not immediately treated.

---

3. The nurse is performing an assessment on a client with a diagnosis of a brain tumor that is located in the brainstem and notes that the client is assuming the posture in the figure. The nurse contacts the primary health care provider and reports that the client is exhibiting which assessment finding? **Refer to figure.**

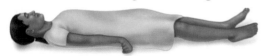

   1 Opisthotonos
   2 Flaccid quadriplegia
   3 Decorticate posturing
   4 Decerebrate posturing

Level of Cognitive Ability: Analyzing
Client Needs: Physiological Integrity
Clinical Judgment/Cognitive Skills: Recognize
   Cues
Integrated Process: Nursing Process/
   Assessment/Data Collection
Content Area: Adult Health
Priority Concepts: Clinical Judgment;
   Intracranial Regulation
Level of Nursing Student: Advanced

ANSWER: 4
Rationale: In decerebrate posturing the upper extremities are stiffly extended and adducted with internal rotation and pronation of the palms. The lower extremities are stiffly extended with plantar flexion. The teeth are clenched, and the back is hyperextended. Decerebrate posturing indicates a lesion in the brainstem at the midbrain or upper pons. Opisthotonos is a prolonged arching of the back with the head and heels bent backward. It indicates meningeal irritation. Flaccid quadriplegia is complete loss of muscle tone and paralysis of all 4 extremities, indicating a completely nonfunctional brainstem. In decorticate posturing the upper extremities (arms, wrists, and fingers) are flexed with adduction of the arms. The lower extremities are extended with internal rotation and plantar flexion. Decorticate posturing indicates a hemispheric lesion of the cerebral cortex.

Test-Taking Strategy: Apply the clinical judgment/cognitive skill, *recognize cues*. Focus on the subject, assessment findings in the client with a brain tumor. Note the position of the client and that the extremities are stiffly extended. Also, noting the client's diagnosis and recalling that this posture indicates a lesion in the brainstem at the midbrain or upper pons will assist in answering the question. **Review: Decerebrate posturing.**

Tip for the Nursing Student: A brain tumor refers to a lesion in the brain. The clinical manifestations that the client exhibits depend on the location of the tumor. If a client has a tumor in the brain, 1 concern is increased intracranial pressure occurring because of the tumor. Another concern is deterioration in the client's condition as a result of the tumor pressing on structures in the brain. The nurse needs to monitor the neurological status of the client closely. If the nurse notes posturing, this indicates deterioration in the client's condition and needs to be reported immediately.

4. A client newly diagnosed with type 1 diabetes mellitus is taking an intermediate-acting insulin at 0700 daily. The nurse would monitor the client closely for which signs and symptoms in the late afternoon?
1 Increased appetite and abdominal pain
2 Hunger; shakiness; and cool, clammy skin
3 Thirst; red, dry skin; and fruity breath odor
4 Increased urination and rapid deep breathing

Level of Cognitive Ability: Analyzing
Client Needs: Physiological Integrity
Clinical Judgment/Cognitive Skills: Recognize Cues
Integrated Process: Nursing Process/Assessment/Data Collection
Content Area: Adult Health
Priority Concepts: Clinical Judgment; Glucose Regulation
Level of Nursing Student: Intermediate

ANSWER. 2

Rationale: The client taking an intermediate-acting insulin would experience peak effects of the medication from approximately 4 to 12 hours after administration. At this time, the client is at risk for hypoglycemia if food intake is insufficient. The nurse would teach the client to watch for signs and symptoms of hypoglycemia during this time frame, which include hunger, shakiness, cold sweating, headache, anxiety, increased pulse, blurred vision, confusion, and difficulty in concentrating. The other options list various manifestations of hyperglycemia.

Test-Taking Strategy: Apply the clinical judgment/cognitive skill, *recognize cues.* Focus on the subject, that the client is taking an intermediate-acting insulin at 0700. Also note the words *signs and symptoms in the late afternoon.* Recall that hypoglycemic reactions can occur at peak insulin times. Recall that an intermediate-acting insulin peaks during the afternoon. Therefore, you are looking for the option that identifies signs and symptoms of a hypoglycemic reaction. Also, eliminate options 1, 3, and 4 because they are comparable or alike options and identify signs and symptoms of hyperglycemia. Remember the *3 Ps* of hyperglycemia: polyuria, polydipsia, and polyphagia. **Review:** The signs and symptoms of **hypoglycemia**.

Tip for the Nursing Student: Both injectable insulin and oral hypoglycemic medications are used to treat the client with diabetes mellitus, and these medications can cause hypoglycemia. Two important complications of diabetes mellitus are hypoglycemia and hyperglycemia. It is important to know the signs and symptoms of each and the interventions needed if either occurs and to teach this information to the client.

---

5. The nurse is creating a teaching plan for a client with viral hepatitis. The nurse would list which item in the plan?
1 Consume 3 large meals daily.
2 The diet should be low in calories.
3 Activity should be limited to prevent fatigue.
4 Alcohol intake should be limited to 2 oz (60 mL) per day.

Level of Cognitive Ability: Creating
Client Needs: Physiological Integrity
Clinical Judgment/Cognitive Skills: Generate Solutions
Integrated Process: Teaching and Learning
Content Area: Adult Health
Priority Concepts: Infection; Inflammation
Level of Nursing Student: Intermediate

ANSWER: 3

Rationale: The client with viral hepatitis should limit activity to avoid fatigue during the recuperation period. The client should take in several small meals per day rather than 3 large meals. The diet should be optimal in calories, protein, and carbohydrates. Alcohol is restricted, not limited.

Test-Taking Strategy: Apply the clinical judgment/cognitive skill, *generate solutions.* Note the subject, care of the client with viral hepatitis. Eliminate option 4 first, using general principles related to client teaching. Next, focus on the client's diagnosis, and recall that the liver needs rest during the healing process. This will direct you to the correct option. **Review:** Care of the client with **hepatitis**.

Tip for the Nursing Student: Viral hepatitis is a viral inflammatory disease of the liver caused by 1 of the hepatitis viruses. It can be transmitted orally, sexually, through contaminated water or food, or through exposure to infected blood; the mode of transmission varies, depending on the type of hepatitis virus.

6. The nurse is reading the results of the client's tuberculin skin test and palpates a 4-mm area of induration at the test site. The nurse would document which result?
 1 Confirms tuberculosis
 2 Is positive for tuberculosis
 3 Is negative for tuberculosis
 4 Provides a conclusive determination of tuberculosis

Level of Cognitive Ability: Analyzing
Client Needs: Physiological Integrity
Clinical Judgment/Cognitive Skills: Analyze Cues
Integrated Process: Communication and Documentation
Content Area: Adult Health
Priority Concepts: Clinical Judgment; Immunity
Level of Nursing Student: Intermediate

ANSWER: 3
Rationale: More than 10 mm of induration indicates exposure to and infection with tuberculosis. However, the infection may not be an active one, and the result could indicate the presence of inactive (dormant) disease. More than 5 mm of induration is considered a positive result for clients with known or suspected human immunodeficiency virus infection, intravenous drug users, people in close contact with a known case of tuberculosis, or clients with a chest radiograph suggestive of previous tuberculosis.

Test-Taking Strategy: Apply the clinical judgment/cognitive skill, *analyze cues.* Eliminate options 1, 2, and 4 because they are comparable or alike options and indicate that tuberculosis is present. **Review:** The **tuberculin skin test**.

Tip for the Nursing Student: Tuberculosis is an infection caused by an acid-fast bacillus known as *Mycobacterium tuberculosis*. It is usually transmitted by the inhalation or ingestion of infected droplets and usually affects the lungs. The tuberculin skin test is a test that consists of an intradermal injection of a purified protein derivative of the tubercle bacillus. This test is used to assist in establishing a diagnosis of tuberculosis.

---

7. The nurse is preparing to conduct a training session on cardiopulmonary resuscitation (CPR). The nurse would incorporate which guideline in the session?
 1 Stop CPR once fatigue is felt.
 2 Look, listen, and feel for breathing.
 3 Give compressions first, then address airway and breathing.
 4 Determine cardiac arrest based on unresponsiveness only.

Level of Cognitive Ability: Applying
Client Needs: Physiological Integrity
Clinical Judgment/Cognitive Skills: Generate Solutions
Integrated Process: Teaching and Learning
Content Area: Adult Health
Priority Concepts: Gas Exchange; Perfusion
Level of Nursing Student: Beginning

ANSWER: 3
Rationale: The American Heart Association sets forth guidelines for effective CPR. The current sequence for CPR is compressions, then airway, and then breathing (CAB). The health care provider would continue CPR until the return of spontaneous circulation or resuscitative efforts are terminated, not once fatigue is felt. Ideally, additional personnel would be available to assist in resuscitative efforts. "Look, listen, and feel" is not currently a part of CPR procedures. Cardiac arrest is determined based on unresponsiveness and absence of a heartbeat and breathing.

Test-Taking Strategy: Apply the clinical judgment/cognitive skill, *generate solutions.* Note the subject, guidelines of CPR. Begin by eliminating option 4, noting the closed-ended word "only." From the remaining options, recall that the current guidelines implement CAB. **Review: CPR** guidelines.

Tip for the Nursing Student: Review the guidelines for performing CPR to ensure that you are ready to perform the procedure if an emergency situation arises. Remember that CAB is the sequence to follow and that if the client is a victim of injury, such as from a motor vehicle crash or a fall from a ladder, and you suspect a neck injury, the jaw thrust maneuver is used to open the airway. As a nurse, you will be required to remain current with your CPR certification.

8. The client has been diagnosed with poly-cystic kidney disease. The nurse would assess the client for which manifestation that is **most** common for this disorder?
   1 Headache
   2 Hypotension
   3 Flank pain and hematuria
   4 Complaints of low pelvic pain

Level of Cognitive Ability: Analyzing
Client Needs: Physiological Integrity
Clinical Judgment/Cognitive Skills: Recognize Cues
Integrated Process: Nursing Process/ Assessment/Data Collection
Content Area: Adult Health
Priority Concepts: Elimination; Tissue Integrity
Level of Nursing Student: Intermediate

ANSWER: 3
Rationale: The most common findings with polycystic kidney disease are hematuria and flank or lumbar pain that is either colicky in nature or dull and aching. Other common findings include protein-uria, calculi, uremia, and palpable kidney masses. Hypertension is another common finding and may be associated with cardiomegaly and heart failure. The client may complain of a headache, but this is not a specific assessment finding in polycystic kidney disease.

Test-Taking Strategy: Apply the clinical judgment/cognitive skill, *recognize cues*. Note the strategic word, *most*. Note the relationship between the word *kidney* in the name of the disorder and the word *flank* in the correct option. **Review:** The manifestations of **polycys-tic kidney disease**.

Tip for the Nursing Student: Polycystic kidney disease is an abnor-mal condition in which the kidneys are enlarged and contain many cysts. The 3 forms of the disease are childhood polycystic disease, congenital polycystic disease, and adult polycystic disease. Kidney failure can result, which can progress to uremia and death. Treat-ment is symptomatic or may include dialysis or renal transplant.

---

9. A client is tested for human immuno-deficiency virus (HIV) with an enzyme-linked immunosorbent assay (ELISA) test, and the test result is positive. The client is very upset and asks the nurse if this means that she or he definitely has HIV. How would the nurse respond to the client?
   1 "Yes, you definitely have HIV."
   2 "Another test will be done to deter-mine whether you have HIV."
   3 "False-positive results are reported all of the time, and you should not be worried."
   4 "A positive test means that the infec-tion was diagnosed early in the initial infection period."

Level of Cognitive Ability: Applying
Client Needs: Physiological Integrity
Clinical Judgment/Cognitive Skills: Take Action
Integrated Process: Communication and Documentation
Content Area: Adult Health
Priority Concepts: Client Education; Infection
Level of Nursing Student: Beginning

ANSWER: 2
Rationale: The normal value for an ELISA test is negative. If the ELISA is positive, a second test, the Western blot, is performed to confirm a positive HIV status. The other options are incorrect. In addition, the nurse would not tell a client that she or he "should not be worried." If testing is performed too early in the initial infec-tion period, a false negative result may occur.

Test-Taking Strategy: Apply the clinical judgment/cognitive skill, *take action*. Use therapeutic communication techniques to elimi-nate options 1 and 3. Next, careful reading of option 4 will assist in eliminating this option. Remember that if testing is performed too early in the initial infection period, a false-negative result may occur. **Review:** Interpretations of results of an **ELISA** test.

Tip for the Nursing Student: HIV is a retrovirus that causes acquired immunodeficiency syndrome (AIDS). The HIV virus is transmitted through anal or oral sexual contact with infected semen or vaginal secretions, through contact with infected blood or blood products, by transmission of the virus from mother to fetus during childbirth, through breast-feeding, or through other infected body fluids. Vari-ous blood tests done to confirm the diagnosis include the ELISA and the Western blot.

10. The nurse monitors for which acid–base disorder that can likely occur in a client with an ileostomy?

   1 Metabolic acidosis
   2 Metabolic alkalosis
   3 Respiratory acidosis
   4 Respiratory alkalosis

Level of Cognitive Ability: Applying
Client Needs: Physiological Integrity
Clinical Judgment/Cognitive Skills: Recognize Cues
Integrated Process: Nursing Process/ Assessment/Data Collection
Content Area: Adult Health
Priority Concepts: Acid-Base Balance; Clinical Judgment
Level of Nursing Student: Intermediate

ANSWER: 1

Rationale: Intestinal secretions are high in bicarbonate because of the effects of pancreatic secretions. These fluids may be lost from the body before they can be reabsorbed with conditions such as diarrhea or creation of an ileostomy. The decreased bicarbonate level creates the actual base deficit of metabolic acidosis. The client with an ileostomy is not at risk for developing the acid–base disorders identified in the other options.

Test-Taking Strategy: Apply the clinical judgment/cognitive skill, *recognize cues.* Focus on the subject, acid–base disorders. Note that the client has an ileostomy. Because the client does not have a respiratory condition, eliminate options 3 and 4. Next, recall that intestinal fluids are alkaline; therefore, alkaline secretions are lost in a client with an ileostomy, resulting in an acidotic condition. **Review:** Causes of **metabolic acidosis**.

Tip for the Nursing Student: An ileostomy is a surgical formation of an opening of the ileum onto the surface of the abdomen, through which fecal matter is emptied. This surgical procedure is performed for conditions such as advanced or recurrent ulcerative colitis, Crohn's disease, or cancer of the large bowel.

---

11. The nurse provides instructions to a client who is being discharged after undergoing a percutaneous renal biopsy. Which statement by the client indicates a **need to reinforce the instructions?**

   1 "A fever is normal after this procedure."
   2 "I should not work out at the gym for about 2 weeks."
   3 "I need to avoid any strenuous lifting for about 2 weeks."
   4 "I will call my health care provider if my urine becomes bloody."

Level of Cognitive Ability: Evaluating
Client Needs: Physiological Integrity
Clinical Judgment/Cognitive Skills: Evaluate Outcomes
Integrated Process: Teaching and Learning
Content Area: Adult Health
Priority Concepts: Client Education; Infection
Level of Nursing Student: Intermediate

ANSWER: 1

Rationale: After percutaneous renal biopsy, the client is instructed to immediately report fever, increasing pain levels (back, flank, or shoulder), bleeding from the puncture site, weakness, dizziness, grossly bloody urine, or dysuria. Activity needs to be restricted if blood is seen in the urine. The client is also instructed to avoid strenuous lifting, physical exertion, or trauma to the biopsy site for up to 2 weeks after discharge.

Test-Taking Strategy: Apply the clinical judgment/cognitive skill, *evaluate outcomes.* Note the strategic words, *need to reinforce the instructions.* These words indicate a negative event query and the need to select the option that identifies an incorrect client statement. Eliminate options 2 and 3 first because they are comparable or alike options. From the remaining options, recall the complications of this procedure. This will direct you to the correct option. **Review:** Client instructions after a percutaneous **renal biopsy**.

Tip for the Nursing Student: A percutaneous renal biopsy is performed by inserting a needle through the skin into the kidney to obtain a piece of tissue for pathological analysis. Infection and bleeding are concerns after this procedure, and the nurse monitors the client closely for these complications.

12. A client being treated for respiratory failure has the following arterial blood gas (ABG) results: pH 7.30, $Paco_2$ 58 mm Hg, Pao_2 75 mm Hg, HCO_3- 27 mEq/L. The nurse interprets that the client has which acid–base disturbance?
1 Metabolic acidosis
2 Metabolic alkalosis
3 Respiratory acidosis
4 Respiratory alkalosis

Level of Cognitive Ability: Analyzing
Client Needs: Physiological Integrity
Clinical Judgment/Cognitive Skills: Analyze Cues
Integrated Process: Nursing Process/Analyze Cues
Content Area: Adult Health
Priority Concepts: Acid-Base Balance; Gas Exchange
Level of Nursing Student: Advanced

ANSWER: 3
Rationale: Acidosis is defined as a pH of less than 7.35, whereas alkalosis is defined as a pH of greater than 7.45. In a respiratory condition, an opposite effect will be seen between the pH and the $Paco_2$. In respiratory acidosis, the pH is decreased and the $Paco_2$ is elevated. The normal HCO_3- is 22 to 27 mm Hg. Metabolic acidosis is present when the HCO_3- is less than 22 mEq/L and the pH is less than 7.35, whereas metabolic alkalosis is present when the HCO_3- is greater than 27 mEq/L and the pH is greater than 7.45. This client's ABG results are consistent with respiratory acidosis.

Test-Taking Strategy: Apply the clinical judgment/cognitive skill, *analyze cues.* Note the subject, interpretation of ABG values. Focus on the client's diagnosis, and recall that this client will have difficulty exchanging oxygen and carbon dioxide. This will assist in eliminating options 1 and 2. From the remaining options, remember that the pH is decreased with acidosis. This will direct you to the correct option. **Review:** The steps related to reading **ABG values**.

Tip for the Nursing Student: Respiratory failure is the inability of the cardiovascular and pulmonary system to maintain an adequate exchange of oxygen and carbon dioxide in the lungs. Respiratory failure can be caused by various conditions that affect oxygenation or ventilation, such as emphysema, infection, pneumonia, or lung cancer.

---

13. A client with a family history of cervical cancer has made an appointment to have a Papanicolaou test done. The nurse who schedules the appointment would make which statement to the client?
1 "Sexual intercourse needs to be avoided for 24 hours before the test."
2 "If you are menstruating, douching will be required right before the test."
3 "A vaginal hygiene spray should be used for 2 consecutive days before the scheduled test."
4 "The test is very uncomfortable, but a local anesthetic will be injected into the vaginal area."

Level of Cognitive Ability: Applying
Client Needs: Health Promotion and Maintenance
Clinical Judgment/Cognitive Skills: Take Action
Integrated Process: Teaching and Learning
Content Area: Adult Health
Priority Concepts: Client Education; Health Promotion
Level of Nursing Student: Intermediate

ANSWER: 1
Rationale: A Papanicolaou test cannot be performed during menstruation. The test is usually painless but may be slightly uncomfortable with placement of the speculum or while a cervical scraping is obtained. A local anesthetic is not injected into the vaginal area. The client is instructed to avoid sexual intercourse, douching, or using vaginal hygiene sprays or deodorants for 24 hours before the test.

Test-Taking Strategy: Apply the clinical judgment/cognitive skill, *take action.* Focus on the subject, client instructions for a Papanicolaou test. Eliminate option 4 first because of the words *very uncomfortable.* From the remaining options, think about the test and its purpose to direct you to the correct option. **Review:** Client preparation for a **Papanicolaou test**.

Tip for the Nursing Student: A Papanicolaou test is a simple procedure in which cells are scraped from the cervix to obtain a specimen for examination for early diagnosis of cervical cancer.

14. A client with a diagnosis of multiple myeloma is admitted to the hospital. When collecting data from the client, the nurse would ask which question that specifically relates to a clinical manifestation of this disorder?
    1 "Do you have diarrhea?"
    2 "Are you having any bone pain?"
    3 "Have you noticed an increase in appetite?"
    4 "Do you have feelings of anxiety and nervousness, along with difficulty sleeping?"

Level of Cognitive Ability: Applying
Client Needs: Physiological Integrity
Clinical Judgment/Cognitive Skills: Recognize Cues
Integrated Process: Nursing Process/Assessment/Data Collection
Content Area: Adult Health
Priority Concepts: Cellular Regulation; Pain
Level of Nursing Student: Intermediate

ANSWER: 2

Rationale: Multiple myeloma is characterized by an abnormal proliferation of plasma B cells. These cells infiltrate the bone marrow and produce abnormal and excessive amounts of immunoglobulin. The most common presenting complaint is bone pain. Hypercalcemia occurs as a result of release of calcium from the deteriorating bone tissue, and subsequently the client presents with confusion, somnolence, constipation, nausea, and thirst.

Test-Taking Strategy: Apply the clinical judgment/cognitive skill, *recognize cues.* Note the subject, clinical manifestations associated with multiple myeloma. Focus on the client's diagnosis, and use medical terminology to answer the question. Also, recalling the pathophysiology of multiple myeloma and the effects it produces on the body will direct you to the correct option. **Review:** The manifestations associated with **multiple myeloma**.

Tip for the Nursing Student: Multiple myeloma is a malignant tumor of the bone marrow. The tumor disrupts normal bone marrow function; destroys osseous tissue; and causes pain, fractures, hypercalcemia, and skeletal deformities.

15. The nurse has provided instructions to a client scheduled for an exercise electrocardiogram (ECG) (stress test) at 0900 on the following day. The nurse determines that the client **needs additional instructions** if the client makes which statement?
    1 "I should not go to the gym to work out today."
    2 "I should wear sneakers when I come for the test."
    3 "I will wear light, loose, comfortable clothing for the procedure."
    4 "I cannot eat for 24 hours before the procedure; I should only drink water."

Level of Cognitive Ability: Evaluating
Client Needs: Physiological Integrity
Clinical Judgment/Cognitive Skills: Evaluate Outcomes
Integrated Process: Teaching and Learning
Content Area: Adult Health
Priority Concepts: Client Education; Safety
Level of Nursing Student: Intermediate

ANSWER: 4

Rationale: The client needs to eat a light meal 1 to 2 hours before this procedure, but caffeine should be avoided. In addition, the client would wear rubber-soled, supportive shoes, such as sneakers, and light, loose, comfortable clothing. A shirt that buttons in front is helpful for ECG lead placement. A workout at the gym the day before the procedure is acceptable as long as the workout is at least 12 hours before testing and there are no existing cardiac disorders contraindicating this type of activity.

Test-Taking Strategy: Apply the clinical judgment/cognitive skill, *evaluate outcomes.* Note the strategic words, *needs additional instructions.* These words indicate a negative event query and the need to select the option that is an incorrect client statement. Recall what this test entails. Because the test requires physical activity, not eating for 24 hours before the procedure could be harmful to the client. **Review:** Client teaching related to a **stress test**.

Tip for the Nursing Student: An exercise ECG (stress test) measures the function of the cardiopulmonary system as the body is subjected to carefully controlled amounts of physiological stress. In this test, a cardiac monitoring device is attached to the client and the cardiopulmonary system is monitored while the client performs some type of exercise, such as walking on a treadmill. The results of this test provide valuable information for the primary health care provider to determine cardiopulmonary problems or the effectiveness of medications or other treatments.

16. A client has undergone pericardiocentesis to treat cardiac tamponade. The nurse would monitor the client for which sign to determine whether the tamponade is recurring?
1 Facial flushing
2 Decreasing pulse
3 Paradoxical pulse
4 Rising blood pressure

Level of Cognitive Ability: Applying
Client Needs: Physiological Integrity
Clinical Judgment/Cognitive Skills: Recognize Cues
Integrated Process: Nursing Process/ Assessment/Data Collection
Content Area: Adult Health
Priority Concepts: Clinical Judgment; Perfusion
Level of Nursing Student: Advanced

ANSWER: 3

Rationale: Cardiac tamponade is a life-threatening situation caused by the accumulation of fluid in the pericardium. The fluid accumulates rapidly and in sufficient quantity to compress the heart and restrict blood flow in and out of the ventricles. Hypotension, tachycardia, jugular vein distention, cyanosis of the lips and nails, dyspnea, muffled heart sounds, diaphoresis, and paradoxical pulse (a decrease in systolic arterial pressure greater than 10 mm Hg during inspiration) are indications of this emergency situation. The emergency intervention of choice is pericardiocentesis, a procedure in which fluid is aspirated from the pericardial sac. Options 1, 2, and 4 are not indications of cardiac tamponade.

Test-Taking Strategy: Apply the clinical judgment/cognitive skill, *recognize cues.* Focus on the subject, signs of cardiac tamponade. Note the word *recurring.* This tells you that the correct option is a symptom of the original problem, which is cardiac tamponade. Recalling the pathophysiology associated with cardiac tamponade will direct you to option 3. **Review:** Signs of **cardiac tamponade**.

Tip for the Nursing Student: When cardiac tamponade occurs, the heart becomes compressed by the accumulation of fluid in the pericardium. To sustain life, this fluid needs to be removed. Pericardiocentesis involves a surgical puncture into the pericardial space between the serous membranes for aspiration of the fluid from the pericardial sac.

17 A client has undergone cardiac catheterization using the right femoral artery for access. The nurse determines that the client is experiencing a complication of the procedure if which finding is noted?
1 Urine output 40 mL/hour
2 Blood pressure 118/76 mm Hg
3 Pallor and coolness of the right leg
4 Respirations 18 breaths per minute

Level of Cognitive Ability: Analyzing
Client Needs: Physiological Integrity
Clinical Judgment/Cognitive Skills: Recognize Cues
Integrated Process: Nursing Process/ Assessment/Data Collection
Content Area: Adult Health
Priority Concepts: Clinical Judgment; Perfusion
Level of Nursing Student: Intermediate

ANSWER: 3

Rationale: Potential complications after cardiac catheterization include allergic reaction to the dye; cardiac dysrhythmias; and a number of vascular complications such as hemorrhage, thrombosis, or embolism. The nurse detects these complications by monitoring for signs and symptoms of allergic reaction, decreased urine output, hematoma or hemorrhage at the insertion site, or signs of decreased circulation to the affected leg. Options 1, 2, and 4 are normal findings.

Test-Taking Strategy: Apply the clinical judgment/cognitive skill, *recognize cues.* Note the words *experiencing a complication.* This tells you that the correct option is an abnormal piece of assessment data. Eliminate options 1, 2, and 4 because they are comparable or alike options and are normal findings. Pallor and coolness indicate thrombosis or hematoma and need to be further assessed and reported. **Review:** The signs of complications after a **cardiac catheterization**.

Tip for the Nursing Student: A cardiac catheterization is a diagnostic procedure in which a catheter is introduced through an incision into a large blood vessel and threaded through the circulatory system of the heart. This procedure is primarily done to assess the status of the coronary arteries in the heart and to determine whether any blockage is present and, if so, the extent of the blockage. Postprocedure monitoring for complications is a primary nursing responsibility.

18. The nurse in the emergency department is performing an assessment on a client who sustained a right finger laceration from a fish hook while fishing. The nurse would ask the client which **priority** question?

1 "When was your last physical examination?"

2 "Have you had a chest x-ray in the last year?"

3 "When did you receive your last tetanus immunization?"

4 "Have you ever sustained this type of injury in the past?"

Level of Cognitive Ability: Applying
Client Needs: Physiological Integrity
Clinical Judgment/Cognitive Skills: Take Action
Integrated Process: Nursing Process/ Assessment/Data Collection
Content Area: Adult Health
Priority Concepts: Immunity; Tissue Integrity
Level of Nursing Student: Intermediate

ANSWER: 3

Rationale: A client who sustains a laceration is at risk for developing complications such as osteomyelitis, gas gangrene, and tetanus. During the assessment, the nurse would ask the client about the date of the last tetanus immunization to ensure that the client has tetanus prophylaxis. Although options 1 and 4 may be components of the assessment, these questions are not the priority. Option 2 is unrelated to the data in the question.

Test-Taking Strategy: Apply the clinical judgment/cognitive skill, *take action.* Note the strategic word, *priority.* Focusing on the data in the question will assist in eliminating option 2. From the remaining options, noting the word *laceration* will direct you to option 3. **Review:** Emergency care for the client who sustains a **laceration**.

Tip for the Nursing Student: Tetanus toxoid is an active immunizing agent prepared from detoxified tetanus toxin that produces an antigenic response in the body. It provides immunity to tetanus, an acute, potentially fatal infection of the central nervous system caused by an anaerobic bacillus, *Clostridium tetani.* The bacillus may enter the body through a wound, such as a laceration. If a client sustains an injury that involves a laceration or other type of wound, a booster shot of tetanus toxoid is given if the client was previously immunized. People known to have been adequately immunized within 5 years of the injury (or a period determined by the primary health care provider) do not usually require immunization.

---

19. A client has been admitted to the hospital with a fractured pelvis sustained in a motor vehicle crash. The nurse monitors for complications and would assess the client closely for which finding in the **early** posttrauma period?

1 Pain

2 Fever

3 Hematuria

4 Bradycardia

Level of Cognitive Ability: Analyzing
Client Needs: Physiological Integrity
Clinical Judgment/Cognitive Skills: Prioritize Hypotheses
Integrated Process: Nursing Process/Analysis
Content Area: Adult Health
Priority Concepts: Inflammation; Perfusion
Level of Nursing Student: Intermediate

ANSWER: 3

Rationale: One complication of a pelvic fracture is damage to the kidneys and lower urinary tract. Therefore, the nurse would monitor for signs of this complication, which includes bloody urine. This client is also at risk for hypovolemic shock. Bone fragments can damage blood vessels, leading to hemorrhage into the abdominal cavity and the thigh area. Signs of hypovolemic shock include tachycardia and hypotension. Pain is an expected finding. Although infection is also a complication (indicated by a fever), it is not generally noted in the early posttrauma period.

Test-Taking Strategy: Apply the clinical judgment/cognitive skill, *prioritize hypotheses.* Note the strategic word, *early.* Focus on the subject, complications after this type of injury. Noting the strategic word will assist in eliminating option 2. Next, focus on the anatomical location of the injury to direct you to the correct option from the remaining options. **Review:** The complications after **pelvic fracture**.

Tip for the Nursing Student: Pelvic fractures usually occur as a result of motor vehicle crashes, falls, and crush injuries. Hemorrhage is a primary concern, because the force from the impact can rupture blood vessels surrounding the pelvic ring.

20. A client has just had a plaster cast removed from the right arm. The nurse assesses the skin to ensure intactness and then would perform which action?
1 Soak the arm in warm water for 1 hour.
2 Wash the skin gently and apply skin lotion.
3 Scrub the skin vigorously with soap and water.
4 Instruct the client that continuous skin soaking will be necessary for the next 24 hours.

Level of Cognitive Ability: Applying
Client Needs: Physiological Integrity
Clinical Judgment/Cognitive Skills: Take Action
Integrated Process: Nursing Process/ Implementation
Content Area: Adult Health
Priority Concepts: Caregiving; Tissue Integrity
Level of Nursing Student: Beginning

ANSWER: 2
Rationale: The skin under a casted area may be discolored and crusted with dead skin layers. Once the skin is inspected for intactness, the nurse should gently wash the skin and apply a generous coating of lotion, gently massaging it into the skin. The client is instructed that it may take several days for the entire residue and debris to be removed from the skin. Lengthy or continuous soaks may cause excessive skin softening that could result in skin breakdown.

Test-Taking Strategy: Apply the clinical judgment/cognitive skill, *take action.* Eliminate option 3 first because of the word *vigorously.* Next eliminate options 1 and 4 because they are comparable or alike options and would lead to excessive skin softening that could result in skin breakdown. Also, noting the word *gently* will direct you to the correct option. **Review:** Client instructions regarding skin care after removal of a **cast**.

Tip for the Nursing Student: A plaster cast is a solid and stiff dressing formed with plaster of Paris around a limb or other body part to immobilize it.

---

21. The home care nurse is assessing a client who began using peritoneal dialysis 1 week ago. The nurse would suspect the onset of peritonitis if which finding is noted on assessment?
1 Anorexia
2 Cloudy dialysate output
3 Mild abdominal discomfort
4 Oral temperature of 99.0°F (37°C)

Level of Cognitive Ability: Analyzing
Client Needs: Physiological Integrity
Clinical Judgment/Cognitive Skills: Recognize Cues
Integrated Process: Nursing Process/ Assessment/Data Collection
Content Area: Adult Health
Priority Concepts: Infection; Inflammation
Level of Nursing Student: Advanced

ANSWER: 2
Rationale: Typical symptoms of peritonitis include fever, nausea, malaise, rebound abdominal tenderness, and cloudy dialysate output. The complaint of anorexia is too vague to indicate peritonitis. Some mild abdominal discomfort may occur initially with peritoneal dialysis. The very slight temperature elevation in option 4 is not the clearest indicator of infection. Peritonitis would cause cloudy dialysate output.

Test-Taking Strategy: Apply the clinical judgment/cognitive skill, *recognize cues.* Focus on the subject, peritonitis. Use medical terminology to recall that the suffix *-itis* indicates inflammation or infection. Eliminate option 1 first because it is a vague symptom. Next eliminate option 3 because of the word *mild.* From the remaining options, note that the temperature is only slightly elevated, and recall that infection would cause white blood cells to be present in the dialysate output, which would yield cloudiness. **Review:** The signs of **peritonitis** in the client receiving **peritoneal dialysis**.

Tip for the Nursing Student: Peritoneal dialysis is a procedure used for clients with acute kidney injury or chronic kidney disease to remove toxins and other wastes that are normally removed by the kidneys from the body. It is a procedure that uses the peritoneum (membrane that lines the abdominal cavity) as the membrane to filter out these toxins and wastes. Fluid (dialysate) flows into the abdominal cavity, filters out these toxins and wastes, and flows out. One complication of peritoneal dialysis is peritonitis, an inflammation and infection of the peritoneum. One indication of peritonitis is cloudy output because output should be clear.

22. After cataract surgery on the right eye, a client is taught to avoid strain on the operative eye. Which statement by the client indicates a **need for further teaching**?

1 "I should not rub my eye."
2 "I can lie on my right side to sleep at night."
3 "I need to take stool softeners to prevent straining."
4 "I should avoid bending over lower than my waist level."

Level of Cognitive Ability: Evaluating
Client Needs: Physiological Integrity
Clinical Judgment/Cognitive Skills: Evaluate Outcomes
Integrated Process: Teaching and Learning
Content Area: Adult Health
Priority Concepts: Client Education; Sensory Perception
Level of Nursing Student: Intermediate

ANSWER: 2

Rationale: After cataract surgery, the client needs to be instructed to lie on the nonoperative side to prevent swelling and pressure in the operated area. Options 1, 3, and 4 are correct measures to take after cataract surgery to reduce strain on the operated eye.

Test-Taking Strategy: Apply the clinical judgment/cognitive skill, *evaluate outcomes*. Note the strategic words, *need for further teaching*. These words indicate a negative event query and the need to select the option that is an incorrect client statement. Recalling that it is necessary to prevent pressure and strain on the operated site will assist in directing you to the correct option. **Review:** Postoperative care to the client after **cataract surgery**.

Tip for the Nursing Student: A cataract is an abnormal progressive clouding of the lens of the eye that leads to visual loss if untreated. Surgical removal of the lens is done only after vision is compromised. Lens implants may be inserted to restore vision. After surgery, teaching focuses on proper use and administration of eye medications, protecting the eye, activity restrictions, and preventing infection.

---

23. The wife of a man who sustained an eye injury calls the emergency department and speaks to the nurse. The wife reports that her husband was hit in the eye area by a piece of board while building a shed in the backyard. The nurse would advise the wife to take which **immediate** action?

1 Call an ambulance.
2 Apply ice to the affected eye.
3 Irrigate the eye with cool water.
4 Bring the husband to the emergency department.

Level of Cognitive Ability: Applying
Client Needs: Physiological Integrity
Clinical Judgment/Cognitive Skills: Take Action
Integrated Process: Nursing Process/ Implementation
Content Area: Adult Health
Priority Concepts: Inflammation; Sensory Perception
Level of Nursing Student: Intermediate

ANSWER: 2

Rationale: Treatment for a contusion ideally begins at the time of injury and includes applying ice to the site. The husband would also receive a thorough eye examination to rule out the presence of other injuries, but this is not the immediate action. Irrigating the eye with cool water may be implemented for injuries that involve a splash of an irritant into the eye. It is not necessary to call an ambulance.

Test-Taking Strategy: Apply the clinical judgment/cognitive skill, *take action*. Note the strategic word, *immediate*. Eliminate options 1 and 4 first because they are comparable or alike options. From the remaining options, focusing on the type of injury sustained will direct you to the correct option. Exposure to an irritant would require an eye irrigation. **Review:** Initial treatment after an **eye contusion**.

Tip for the Nursing Student: An eye contusion is an injury caused by a blow to the eye area. A contusion does not disrupt the integrity of the skin but causes swelling, pain, and bruising. Ice is immediately applied to limit swelling, pain, and bruising.

24. The nurse employed in an eye clinic checks a client's intraocular pressure and notes that the pressure is 16 mm Hg in the right eye and 18 mm Hg in the left eye. The nurse would tell the client that the pressure is indicative of which result?

1 Normal in both eyes
2 Elevated in the left eye
3 Elevated in the right eye
4 Low in both eyes, requiring treatment to increase it

Level of Cognitive Ability: Applying
Client Needs: Health Promotion and Maintenance
Clinical Judgment/Cognitive Skills: Take Action
Integrated Process: Nursing Process/ Implementation
Content Area: Adult Health
Priority Concepts: Clinical Judgment; Sensory Perception
Level of Nursing Student: Intermediate

ANSWER: 1
Rationale: Normal intraocular pressure ranges from 10 to 21 mm Hg. Therefore, the client's intraocular pressure is normal, and options 2, 3, and 4 are incorrect.

Test-Taking Strategy: Apply the clinical judgment/cognitive skill, *take action*. Note the subject, normal intraocular pressure. Focus on the data in the question. Recalling that normal intraocular pressure ranges from 10 to 21 mm Hg will direct you to the correct option. **Review: Intraocular pressure.**

Tip for the Nursing Student: Intraocular pressure is the pressure within the eye and is regulated by the flow of aqueous humor through the trabecular meshwork. An increase in intraocular pressure is associated with a condition known as glaucoma. If glaucoma is untreated, complete and permanent blindness can result.

---

25. A stapedectomy is performed on a client with otosclerosis. The nurse prepares the client for discharge and would provide the client with which home care instruction?

1 Expect acute vertigo to occur.
2 Delay plans for air travel for at least 1 month.
3 Lie on the operative ear with the head of the bed flat.
4 You can sneeze or blow your nose as you usually do.

Level of Cognitive Ability: Applying
Client Needs: Physiological Integrity
Clinical Judgment/Cognitive Skills: Take Action
Integrated Process: Teaching and Learning
Content Area: Adult Health
Priority Concepts: Client Education; Sensory Perception
Level of Nursing Student: Intermediate

ANSWER: 2
Rationale: After stapedectomy, no air travel is allowed for 1 month. The acute onset of vertigo needs to be reported to the surgeon because this could be indicative of a complication. The client is instructed to lie on the nonoperative ear with the head of the bed elevated. The client would also avoid excessive exercise, straining, and activities that might lead to head trauma. If the client needs to blow the nose, it needs to be done gently, one nostril at a time, and the client should sneeze with the mouth open.

Test-Taking Strategy: Apply the clinical judgment/cognitive skill, *take action*. Note the subject, client instructions after stapedectomy. Focus on the surgical procedure and its location to direct you to the correct option. Also, eliminate option 1 because of the words *acute vertigo*, option 3 because of the words *lie on the operative ear with the head of the bed flat*, and option 4 because of the words *as you usually do*. **Review: Postoperative care after stapedectomy.**

Tip for the Nursing Student: Apply the clinical judgment/cognitive skill, *take action*. Otosclerosis is a condition in which ossification occurs in the ossicles of the middle ear (especially the stapes), leading to hearing loss. Stapedectomy is the removal of the fixed stapes. Insertion of a graft and prosthesis is done to restore hearing.

26. The nurse is teaching the client taking medications by inhalation about the advantages of a spacer device. The nurse would tell the client that the spacer serves which purpose?
    1 Disperses medication more deeply and uniformly
    2 Reduces the frequency of medication use to only once per day
    3 Requires coordinating timing between pressing the inhaler and inhaling
    4 Totally eliminates the chance of developing a yeast infection in the mouth

Level of Cognitive Ability: Applying
Client Needs: Physiological Integrity
Clinical Judgment/Cognitive Skills: Take Action
Integrated Process: Teaching and Learning
Content Area: Adult Health
Priority Concepts: Client Education; Gas Exchange
Level of Nursing Student: Beginning

ANSWER: 1
Rationale: There are key advantages to the use of a spacer device for medications administered by inhalation. One is that the medication is dispersed more deeply and uniformly than without a spacer. Another advantage is that it reduces (but does not totally eliminate) the incidence of yeast infections because large medication droplets are not deposited on oral tissues. The use of a spacer may decrease either the number or the volume of the puffs taken but does not reduce the daily frequency for use. Finally, there is less need to coordinate the effort of inhalation with pressing on the canister of the inhaler.

Test-Taking Strategy: Apply the clinical judgment/cognitive skill, *take action*. Eliminate option 2 because of the closed-ended word "only." Next eliminate option 4 because of the closed-ended words "totally eliminates." From the remaining options visualize this device to assist in eliminating option 3. **Review:** The advantages of the use of the **spacer** with inhaled medications.

Tip for the Nursing Student: Some medications, particularly respiratory medications, are administered by the inhalation route. To accomplish administration by this route, special inhalation devices may be used. A spacer device is a small piece of equipment that can be attached to the inhalation device to make the administration of the medication more effective and easier for the client. Teaching the client how to use these devices is an important nursing intervention.

---

27. A client diagnosed with acquired immunodeficiency syndrome (AIDS) is hospitalized. The nurse develops a plan of care and determines that which intervention is the **priority**?
    1 Providing emotional support to the client
    2 Instituting measures to prevent infection in the client
    3 Identifying the ways that AIDS can be contracted by others
    4 Discussing the ways that the client contracted the AIDS virus

Level of Cognitive Ability: Analyzing
Client Needs: Physiological Integrity
Clinical Judgment/Cognitive Skills: Generate Solutions
Integrated Process: Nursing Process/Planning
Content Area: Adult Health
Priority Concepts: Infection; Safety
Level of Nursing Student: Intermediate

ANSWER: 2
Rationale: The client with AIDS has inadequate immune bodies and is at risk for infection. The priority nursing intervention would be to protect the client from infection. The nurse would also provide emotional support to the client, but this is not the priority from the options provided. Discussing the ways that the client contracted the AIDS virus and the ways others can contract AIDS are inappropriate priority interventions.

Test-Taking Strategy: Apply the clinical judgment/cognitive skill, *generate solutions*. Note the strategic word, *priority*. Eliminate options 3 and 4 first because they are comparable or alike options. Also use Maslow's Hierarchy of Needs theory to remember that physiological needs are the priority. This will direct you to the correct option. **Review:** The priority needs of a client with **AIDS**.

Tip for the Nursing Student: AIDS is a syndrome that is caused by the human immunodeficiency virus (HIV), a retrovirus that attacks and kills CD4+ lymphocytes (T helper cells). This results in a weakening of the immune system's ability to prevent infection.

28. A client who is recovering from a stroke has residual dysphagia. To assist in assessing the client's swallowing ability, the nurse would ask the client to perform which action?
1 Swallow some water.
2 Produce an audible cough.
3 Suck on a piece of hard candy.
4 Swallow a teaspoon of applesauce.

Level of Cognitive Ability: Applying
Client Needs: Safe and Effective Care Environment
Clinical Judgment/Cognitive Skills: Take Action
Integrated Process: Nursing Process/ Implementation
Content Area: Adult Health
Priority Concepts: Intracranial Regulation; Safety
Level of Nursing Student: Intermediate

ANSWER: 2
Rationale: To assess the client's readiness and ability to swallow, the nurse would assess the client's level of consciousness (client needs to be alert), check for a gag reflex (gag reflex must be present), have the client produce an audible cough (client must be able to produce an audible cough), and ask the client to produce a voluntary swallow (client must be able to do this). The nurse would not give the client a liquid or food item and would not ask the client to suck on a piece of hard candy or any other item because of the risk of aspiration.

Test-Taking Strategy: Apply the clinical judgment/cognitive skill, *take action.* Eliminate options 1, 3, and 4 first because they are comparable or alike options and would place the client at risk for aspiration. Also, use the ABCs—airway, breathing, and circulation—to direct you to the correct option. **Review:** Care of the client with residual **dysphagia**.

Tip for the Nursing Student: A stroke is an abnormal condition of the brain that is caused by an occlusion from a thrombus, embolus, vasospasm, or hemorrhage. Dysphagia refers to difficulty with swallowing and can occur as a result of the stroke. It places the client at risk for aspiration.

---

29. A client with chronic kidney disease returns to the nursing unit after receiving a second hemodialysis treatment. The nurse monitors the client closely for which sign of disequilibrium syndrome?
1 Irritability
2 Tachycardia
3 Hypothermia
4 Mental confusion

Level of Cognitive Ability: Applying
Client Needs: Physiological Integrity
Clinical Judgment/Cognitive Skills: Recognize Cues
Integrated Process: Nursing Process/ Assessment/Data Collection
Content Area: Adult Health
Priority Concepts: Clinical Judgment; Fluids and Electrolytes
Level of Nursing Student: Advanced

ANSWER: 4
Rationale: Disequilibrium syndrome most often occurs in clients who are new to hemodialysis. It is characterized by headache, mental confusion, decreasing level of consciousness, nausea, vomiting, twitching, and possible seizure activity. It results from rapid removal of solutes from the body during hemodialysis and a higher residual concentration gradient in the brain because of the blood–brain barrier. Water goes into cerebral cells because of the osmotic gradient, causing brain swelling and onset of symptoms. It is prevented by dialyzing for shorter times or at reduced blood flow rates. The signs in options 1, 2, and 3 are not associated with disequilibrium syndrome.

Test-Taking Strategy: Apply the clinical judgment/cognitive skill, *recognize cues.* Note the subject, signs of disequilibrium syndrome. Focusing on the name of the syndrome will direct you to the correct option. This is the only option that addresses a neurological sign. **Review:** The signs of **disequilibrium syndrome**.

Tip for the Nursing Student: Chronic kidney disease is a condition in which the kidneys are unable to excrete wastes, concentrate urine, and conserve electrolytes. A component of treatment is hemodialysis. Hemodialysis requires the use of a dialyzer that is connected to a shunt, fistula, or other device that allows access to the client's bloodstream. The client's blood is transported from the body through the dialyzer, which removes wastes and excess fluids from the blood. The cleaned blood is then returned to the client's body. Disequilibrium syndrome is one complication that can occur as a result of hemodialysis.

30. The nurse is planning home care instructions to a client with Parkinson's disease about measures to control a right-sided hand tremor. What instruction would the nurse give to the client?

1 Sleep on the unaffected side.
2 Use the left hand only to perform tasks.
3 Use the right hand only to perform tasks.
4 Squeeze a rubber ball with the right hand.

Level of Cognitive Ability: Applying
Client Needs: Physiological Integrity
Clinical Judgment/Cognitive Skills: Generate Solutions
Integrated Process: Teaching and Learning
Content Area: Adult Health
Priority Concepts: Client Education; Mobility
Level of Nursing Student: Intermediate

ANSWER: 4

Rationale: The client with a tremor is instructed to use both hands to accomplish a task. The client is also instructed to hold change in a pocket or to squeeze a rubber ball with the affected hand. The client should sleep on the side that has the tremor to control it.

Test-Taking Strategy: Apply the clinical judgment/cognitive skill, *generate solutions.* Eliminate options 2 and 3 first because of the closed-ended word "only." From the remaining options visualize each and think about each effect in terms of controlling the tremor. This will direct you to the correct option. **Review:** Client teaching points for **Parkinson's disease**.

Tip for the Nursing Student: Parkinson's disease is a progressive neurological disorder that is caused by a depletion of the neurotransmitter dopamine in the brain tissue. It is characterized by resting tremor, pill rolling of the fingers, shuffling gait, masklike facies, forward flexion of the trunk, muscle rigidity and weakness, and loss of postural reflexes.

---

31. The nurse answers the call bell of a client who has an internal cervical radiation implant. The client states that she or he thinks that the implant fell out. The nurse checks the client and sees the implant lying in the bed. The nurse immediately uses long-handled forceps to pick up the implant and places the implant into the lead container in the client's room. Which action would the nurse take **next?**

1 Ask another nurse to assist in reinserting the implant.
2 Contact the radiation therapist and radiation safety officer.
3 Call for a transport personnel to deliver the lead container to the radiation department.
4 Call a security officer, and ask the officer to send someone to guard the client's room until the situation is resolved.

Level of Cognitive Ability: Applying
Client Needs: Safe and Effective Care Environment
Clinical Judgment/Cognitive Skills: Take Action
Integrated Process: Nursing Process/ Implementation
Content Area: Adult Health
Priority Concepts: Clinical Judgment; Safety
Level of Nursing Student: Intermediate

ANSWER: 2

Rationale: A lead container and long-handled forceps would be kept in the client's room at all times during internal radiation therapy. If the implant becomes dislodged, the nurse would pick up the implant with long-handled forceps and place it in the lead container. The radiation therapist and radiation safety officer are notified immediately of the situation so that they can retrieve and secure the radiation source. The primary health care provider is also called after taking action to maintain the safety of the client and others. The nurse does not reinsert a radiation implant device. Options 3 and 4 are incorrect and can expose individuals to the radiation.

Test-Taking Strategy: Apply the clinical judgment/cognitive skill, *take action.* Note the strategic word, *next.* Option 1 can be eliminated first because inserting a radiation device is not a nursing activity. Recalling that the nurse needs to protect herself or himself and others from exposure to the radiation will help eliminate options 3 and 4. Also, these options are comparable or alike options. **Review:** The measures related to a dislodged **radiation implant**.

Tip for the Nursing Student: A cervical radiation implant is a device that is placed in the area of the cervix and emits radiation to the body area. It is a treatment measure for cervical cancer. Because exposure to radiation can be harmful, special precautions are taken to prevent exposure to other individuals.

32. The nurse is caring for a hospitalized client with a diagnosis of acute pancreatitis. The nurse would assist the client to which position that will decrease the abdominal pain?

1 Prone
2 Supine with the legs straight
3 Side lying with the head of the bed flat
4 Upright in a sitting position with the trunk flexed

Level of Cognitive Ability: Applying
Client Needs: Physiological Integrity
Clinical Judgment/Cognitive Skills: Take Action
Integrated Process: Nursing Process/ Implementation
Content Area: Adult Health
Priority Concepts: Caregiving; Pain
Level of Nursing Student: Intermediate

ANSWER: 4

Rationale: Correct positioning will assist in providing comfort to the client with acute pancreatitis. These positions include a side-lying position with the knees curled up to the chest and a pillow pressed against the abdomen or upright in a sitting position with the trunk flexed. Options 1, 2, and 3 are incorrect positions and will not alleviate discomfort.

Test-Taking Strategy: Apply the clinical judgment/cognitive skill, *take action*. Focus on the client's diagnosis, and evaluate each option in terms of the amount of stretching or flexing of the abdominal wall that the action will cause. Also note that options 1, 2, and 3 are comparable or alike options in that they are flat positions. **Review:** The positions that will reduce pain in the client with **acute pancreatitis**.

Tip for the Nursing Student: Pancreatitis is an inflammatory condition of the pancreas and can be acute or chronic. It is characterized by severe epigastric or upper-left-quadrant abdominal pain radiating to the back, fever, anorexia, nausea, and vomiting.

33. The nurse provides home care instructions to a client diagnosed with viral hepatitis. The nurse determines that the client understands the instructions if the client makes which statement?

1 "I need to limit my intake of alcohol."
2 "I need to remain in bed for the next 6 weeks."
3 "I can take acetaminophen for any discomfort."
4 "I need to eat small frequent meals that are low in fat and protein."

Level of Cognitive Ability: Evaluating
Client Needs: Physiological Integrity
Clinical Judgment/Cognitive Skills: Evaluate Outcomes
Integrated Process: Nursing Process/ Evaluation
Content Area: Adult Health
Priority Concepts: Client Education; Inflammation
Level of Nursing Student: Intermediate

ANSWER: 4

Rationale: Fatigue is a normal response to hepatic cellular damage. During the acute stage, rest is an essential intervention to reduce the liver's metabolic demands and increase its blood supply, but bed rest for 6 weeks is unnecessary. The client needs to avoid all alcohol consumption because of hepatotoxicity. The client should avoid taking all medications, including acetaminophen (which is hepatotoxic), unless prescribed by the primary health care provider. The client should consume small frequent meals that are low in fat and protein to reduce the workload of the liver.

Test-Taking Strategy: Apply the clinical judgment/cognitive skill, *evaluate outcomes*. Note the subject, client understanding of home care for viral hepatitis. Eliminate option 1 first, recalling that the client needs to avoid (not limit) alcohol intake. Next eliminate option 2 because of the words *next 6 weeks*. From the remaining options, recalling that acetaminophen is hepatotoxic will assist in eliminating option 3. **Review:** Instructions for the client with **viral hepatitis**.

Tip for the Nursing Student: Viral hepatitis is an inflammatory disease of the liver caused by one of the hepatitis viruses. It is characterized by jaundice, anorexia, abdominal and gastric discomfort, hepatomegaly, clay-colored stools, and tea-colored urine. The liver is usually able to regenerate its tissue, and rest is an essential component of therapy.

34. A hospitalized client with chronic kidney disease has returned to the nursing unit after a hemodialysis treatment. The nurse would check predialysis and postdialysis documentation of which parameters to determine the **effectiveness** of the procedure?
1 Blood pressure and weight
2 Weight and blood urea nitrogen
3 Potassium level and creatinine levels
4 Blood urea nitrogen and creatinine levels

Level of Cognitive Ability: Evaluating
Client Needs: Physiological Integrity
Clinical Judgment/Cognitive Skills: Evaluate Outcomes
Integrated Process: Nursing Process/ Evaluation
Content Area: Adult Health
Priority Concepts: Clinical Judgment; Fluids and Electrolytes
Level of Nursing Student: Intermediate

ANSWER: 1

Rationale: After hemodialysis the client's vital signs are monitored to determine whether the client is remaining hemodynamically stable and for comparison to predialysis measurements. The client's blood pressure and weight are expected to be reduced as a result of fluid removal. Laboratory studies are done as per protocol, but are not necessarily done after the hemodialysis treatment has ended.

Test-Taking Strategy: Apply the clinical judgment/cognitive skill, *evaluate outcomes*. Note the strategic word, *effectiveness*, and focus on the subject, determining the effectiveness of hemodialysis. Note that this is an evaluation-type question. Also remember that when options contain two parts, both parts need to be correct for the option to be the correct one. Knowing that weight is an important variable allows you to eliminate options 3 and 4. From the remaining options, recalling that vital signs reflect hemodynamic stability will direct you to the correct option. **Review:** The parameters that will determine the effectiveness of **hemodialysis**.

Tip for the Nursing Student: Chronic kidney disease is a condition in which the kidneys are unable to excrete wastes, concentrate urine, and conserve electrolytes. A component of treatment is hemodialysis. Hemodialysis requires the use of a dialyzer that is connected to a shunt, fistula, or other device that allows access to the client's bloodstream. The client's blood is transported from the body through the dialyzer, which removes wastes and excess fluids from the blood. The cleaned blood is then returned to the client's body.

---

35. The nurse is creating a plan of care for a client who is experiencing homonymous hemianopsia after a stroke. The nurse documents interventions that will promote a safe environment, knowing that in this disorder the client experiences which symptom?
1 Has a visual loss in the same half of the visual field of each eye
2 Has lost the ability to recognize familiar objects through the senses
3 Is unable to carry out a skilled act, such as dressing, in the absence of paralysis
4 Has paralysis of the sympathetic nerves of the eye, causing ocular manifestations

Level of Cognitive Ability: Creating
Client Needs: Safe and Effective Care Environment
Clinical Judgment/Cognitive Skills: Generate Solutions
Integrated Process: Nursing Process/Planning
Content Area: Adult Health
Priority Concepts: Intracranial Regulation; Safety
Level of Nursing Student: Intermediate

ANSWER: 1

Rationale: Homonymous hemianopsia is a visual loss in the same half of the visual field of each eye, so the client has only half of normal vision. Option 2 describes agnosia. Option 3 describes apraxia. Option 4 describes Horner's syndrome.

Test-Taking Strategy: Apply the clinical judgment/cognitive skill, *generate solutions*. Focus on the subject, homonymous hemianopsia. Use medical terminology, noting that *hemi-* means *half* and *-op-* refers to the eye. This will direct you to the correct option. **Review:** Care for the client with **homonymous hemianopsia**.

Tip for the Nursing Student: A stroke is an abnormal condition of the brain that is caused by an occlusion from a thrombus, embolus, vasospasm, or hemorrhage. Homonymous hemianopsia is a visual loss in the same half of the visual field of each eye, so the client has only half of normal vision. This disorder can occur as a result of the stroke and places the client at risk for injury.

CHAPTER 15

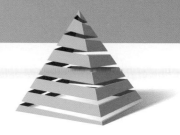

Mental Health Questions

1. The nurse helps a client with a diagnosis of obsessive-compulsive disorder prepare for bed. One hour later, the client calls the nurse and says he is feeling anxious and asks the nurse to sit and talk for a while. The nurse would take which **most appropriate** action?
   1 Sit and talk with the client.
   2 Have assistive personnel (AP) sit with the client.
   3 Ask the client if he would like an anti-anxiety medication.
   4 Tell the client that it is time for sleep and that they will talk tomorrow.

Level of Cognitive Ability: Applying
Client Needs: Psychosocial Integrity
Clinical Judgment/Cognitive Skills: Take Action
Integrated Process: Caring
Content Area: Mental Health
Priority Concepts: Anxiety; Caregiving
Level of Nursing Student: Intermediate

ANSWER: 1
Rationale: The most appropriate nursing action is to sit and talk if the client is expressing anxiety. Antianxiety medication may be necessary, but this is not the most appropriate nursing action. An AP may not be able to alleviate the client's anxiety. Option 4 is an inappropriate action and places the client's feelings on hold.

Test-Taking Strategy: Apply the clinical judgment skill/cognitive skill, *take action*. Note the strategic words, *most appropriate,* and use therapeutic communication techniques. Recalling that it is best to address the client's feelings assists in directing you to the correct option. **Review:** Care of the client with **obsessive-compulsive disorder**.

Tip for the Nursing Student: Obsessive-compulsive disorder is an anxiety disorder that is characterized by obsessions (ideas, emotions, or impulses that repetitively and insistently force themselves into consciousness) or compulsions (recurrent irresistible impulses to perform some act) that interfere with the individual's normal routine.

2. The nurse is performing an admission interview on a client being admitted to the mental health unit and discovers that the client experienced a severe emotional trauma 1 month ago and is now experiencing paralysis of the right arm. The nurse would plan for which **priority** intervention?
   1 Referring the client to group therapy
   2 Encouraging the client to move and use the arm
   3 Encouraging the client to talk about her or his feelings
   4 Checking the client for physiological causes of the paralysis

Level of Cognitive Ability: Analyzing
Client Needs: Physiological Integrity

ANSWER: 4
Rationale: The priority intervention is to check the client for any physiological cause of the paralysis. Although the client may be referred to group therapy, this is not the priority. Although a component of the plan of care is to encourage the client to discuss feelings, this also is not the priority. It is inappropriate to encourage the client to use the arm without ruling out a physiological cause of the paralysis.

Test-Taking Strategy: Apply the clinical judgment/cognitive skill, *generate solutions.* Note the strategic word, *priority.* Use Maslow's Hierarchy of Needs theory to remember that physiological needs are the first priority. Also use the steps of the nursing process. The correct option is the only one that addresses a physiological need and assessment/data collection, the first step in the nursing process. **Review: Conversion disorder**.

Clinical Judgment/Cognitive Skills: Generate
 Solutions
Integrated Process: Nursing Process/
 Planning
Content Area: Mental Health
Priority Concepts: Anxiety; Stress and
 Coping
Level of Nursing Student: Intermediate

Tip for the Nursing Student: A conversion disorder is a somatoform disorder characterized by a loss or alteration of physical functioning without evidence of physiological impairment. A conversion disorder can result after a traumatic experience.

---

3. The nurse is developing a plan of care for a client admitted to the mental health unit. The client has a diagnosis of obsessive-compulsive disorder and is experiencing severe anxiety. What would the nurse identify as the **priority** intervention in the plan of care?
 1 Monitor for repetitive behavior.
 2 Encourage active participation in care.
 3 Educate the client about self-care demands.
 4 Establish a trusting and therapeutic nurse–client relationship.

Level of Cognitive Ability: Applying
Client Needs: Psychosocial Integrity
Clinical Judgment/Cognitive Skills: Generate
 Solutions
Integrated Process: Caring
Content Area: Mental Health
Priority Concepts: Anxiety; Caregiving
Level of Nursing Student: Intermediate

ANSWER: 4
Rationale: The priority nursing intervention is to establish a trusting and therapeutic relationship with the client. The remaining options are appropriate components of the plan of care but are not the priority. A trusting nurse–client relationship needs to be established first.

Test-Taking Strategy: Apply the clinical judgment/cognitive skill, *generate solutions.* Focus on the strategic word, *priority,* and note that the client is being admitted to the mental health unit. Recalling that a nurse–client relationship needs to be developed first assists in directing you to the correct option. **Review:** Care to the client with **obsessive-compulsive disorder**.

Tip for the Nursing Student: Obsessive-compulsive disorder is an anxiety disorder that is characterized by obsessions (ideas, emotions, or impulses that repetitively and insistently force themselves into consciousness) or compulsions (recurrent irresistible impulses to perform some act) that interfere with the individual's normal routine. The first step in providing therapeutic care for the client is to establish a trusting and therapeutic relationship. If trust is established, the client is more likely to communicate with the nurse.

---

4. The nurse is preparing to care for a client admitted to the mental health unit with a diagnosis of dementia and notes that the client has difficulty carrying out activities of daily living effectively. The nurse would plan for which outcome in caring for the client?
 1 The client will feed self with cueing within 24 hours.
 2 The client will be oriented to place by the time of discharge.
 3 The client will be free of hallucinations by the time of discharge.
 4 The client will correctly identify objects in the room by the time of discharge.

Level of Cognitive Ability: Analyzing
Client Needs: Physiological Integrity
Clinical Judgment/Cognitive Skills: Generate
 Solutions
Integrated Process: Nursing Process/Planning
Content Area: Mental Health
Priority Concepts: Caregiving; Cognition
Level of Nursing Student: Intermediate

ANSWER: 1
Rationale: Option 1 identifies an outcome directly related to the client's ability to care for self. Options 2, 3, and 4 are not related to carrying out activities of daily living.

Test-Taking Strategy: Apply the clinical judgment/cognitive skill, *generate solutions.* Note the relationship between the subject, the client experiencing difficulty carrying out activities of daily living, and the correct option. Noting that options 2, 3, and 4 are comparable or alike options, addressing the time of discharge, will assist in eliminating these options. Also, use Maslow's Hierarchy of Needs theory. The correct option addresses a physiological need. **Review:** Care of the client with **dementia**.

Tip for the Nursing Student: Dementia is a term that describes an organic mental disorder characterized by cognitive impairments that are generally of gradual onset and are irreversible. Activities of daily living are activities performed during the course of a normal day, such as bathing, dressing, and eating.

5. A client experiencing delusions of being poisoned is admitted to the hospital. The client shows no evidence of dehydration and malnutrition at this time. The nurse creates a plan of care for the client and would include which client need as the **priority?**
1 Self-esteem
2 Physiological needs
3 Safety and security
4 Love and belonging

Level of Cognitive Ability: Analyzing
Client Needs: Safe and Effective Care Environment
Clinical Judgment/Cognitive Skills: Prioritize Hypotheses
Integrated Process: Nursing Process/ Analysis
Content Area: Mental Health
Priority Concepts: Cognition; Psychosis
Level of Nursing Student: Intermediate

ANSWER: 3
Rationale: The maintenance of safety is an important consideration when working with clients who have delusions. No data in the question indicate that options 1, 2, and 4 require immediate attention.

Test-Taking Strategy: Apply the clinical judgment/cognitive skill, *prioritize hypotheses.* Note the strategic word, *priority,* and note the words *shows no evidence of dehydration and malnutrition.* Use Maslow's Hierarchy of Needs theory. Safety takes precedence if a physiological need does not exist. This will direct you to the correct option. **Review:** Care of the client experiencing **delusions.**

Tip for the Nursing Student: A delusion is a false belief that is firmly maintained by a client even though the belief is not shared by others. The nurse would not attempt to obtain a logical explanation about the delusion from the client. Only the client understands the logic behind the delusion, yet she or he is not able to express it until the delusion has reached conscious awareness.

6. An older woman is admitted to the acute psychiatric unit with a diagnosis of moderate depression. The client is unclean, her hair is uncombed, and she is inappropriately dressed. She is accompanied by her adult daughter, who is very upset about her mother's lack of interest in her appearance. The nurse appropriately alleviates the daughter's concern by making which statement?
1 "Hygiene is not important to those who are depressed."
2 "Client self-esteem needs take priority over appearances."
3 "Group peer pressure on the unit will soon have your mother attending to her hygiene needs."
4 "The nurses will assist your mother in meeting hygiene needs until she is able to resume self-care."

Level of Cognitive Ability: Applying
Client Needs: Psychosocial Integrity
Clinical Judgment/Cognitive Skills: Take Action
Integrated Process: Caring
Content Area: Mental Health
Priority Concepts: Functional Ability; Mood and Affect
Level of Nursing Student: Intermediate

ANSWER: 4
Rationale: The client is experiencing psychomotor retardation and decreased energy at this time and requires assistance. Both the client and her family need to know that the nurse will assist the client until the client can resume self-care activities. Options 1, 2, and 3 will not alleviate the daughter's concern.

Test-Taking Strategy: Apply the clinical judgment/cognitive skill, *take action.* Note the data in the question, and focus on the subject, alleviating the concern of the client's daughter. Also, use Maslow's Hierarchy of Needs theory. Only the correct option addresses the client's physiological needs. **Review:** Care of the client with **depression.**

Tip for the Nursing Student: Depression is a state of sadness or grief and can range from mild and moderate states to severe states. The potential for suicidal behavior must always be assessed in a client experiencing depression.

7. The nurse is preparing to care for a woman victimized by physical abuse. The nurse would plan to perform which action **first**?
   1 Support the woman, and facilitate access to a safe environment.
   2 Talk to the woman about how and why the abuser became provoked.
   3 Reinforce that dealing with the psychological aspects is of the highest priority.
   4 Establish firm timelines for the woman to make necessary changes in her life situation.

Level of Cognitive Ability: Applying
Client Needs: Safe and Effective Care Environment
Clinical Judgment/Cognitive Skills: Generate Solutions
Integrated Process: Caring
Content Area: Mental Health
Priority Concepts: Interpersonal Violence; Safety
Level of Nursing Student: Intermediate

ANSWER: 1

Rationale: The nurse must provide emotional support to the client and provide measures to ensure a safe environment. Option 2 fosters the notion that the client is at fault. In options 3 and 4, the nurse may be making unreasonable demands, which could cause further distress for the client.

Test-Taking Strategy: Apply the clinical judgment/cognitive skill, *generate solutions*. Note the strategic word, *first*. Use Maslow's Hierarchy of Needs theory to direct you to the correct option. Remember that if a physiological need does not exist in one of the options, then a safety need is the priority. Also, the correct option provides support to the client. **Review:** Care of the client victimized by **physical abuse**.

Tip for the Nursing Student: Physical abuse is a form of violence. In most states the nurse is required to report abuse to legal authorities if abuse is suspected or occurs in a child or older client. If abuse occurs, the priority is to treat any physical injuries sustained. Next it is important to provide support and a safe environment for the victim.

---

8. A client is scheduled for electroconvulsive therapy (ECT). The client says to the nurse, "I am so afraid that it will hurt and will make me worse off than I am." The nurse would make which **best** statement to the client?
   1 "Can you tell me what you understand about the procedure?"
   2 "Your fears are a sign that you really need this procedure."
   3 "Try not to worry. This is a well-known and easy procedure for the psychiatrist."
   4 "Those are very normal fears, but please be assured that everything will be okay."

Level of Cognitive Ability: Applying
Client Needs: Psychosocial Integrity
Clinical Judgment/Cognitive Skills: Take Action
Integrated Process: Caring
Content Area: Mental Health
Priority Concepts: Anxiety; Communication
Level of Nursing Student: Intermediate

ANSWER: 1

Rationale: The correct option is a therapeutic communication technique that explores the client's feelings, determines the level of client understanding about the procedure, and displays caring. Option 2 demeans the client and does not encourage further sharing by the client. Option 3 diminishes the client's feelings by directing attention away from the client and to the psychiatrist's importance. Option 4 does not address the client's fears and puts the client's feelings on hold.

Test-Taking Strategy: Apply the clinical judgment/cognitive skill, *take action*. Note the strategic word, *best*. Use therapeutic communication techniques, and remember to focus on the client's feelings and concerns. Option 1 is the only option that addresses the client's feelings, encourages client verbalization, and displays caring. **Review: Therapeutic communication techniques**.

Tip for the Nursing Student: ECT is a treatment in which a seizure is artificially induced in an anesthetized client by passing an electrical current through electrodes applied to the client's head. It is considered a safe and effective treatment for major depression.

9. A client with schizophrenia requires seclusion. The nurse plans care with the understanding that the determination for this treatment is made in which situation?
    1 For convenience of the health care staff
    2 When less restrictive methods are insufficient
    3 If a sedative is ineffective in calming the client down
    4 As a form of punishment to deter the client from continuing the behavior

Level of Cognitive Ability: Applying
Client Needs: Safe and Effective Care Environment
Clinical Judgment/Cognitive Skills: Generate Solutions
Integrated Process: Nursing Process/ Planning
Content Area: Mental Health
Priority Concepts: Caregiving; Safety
Level of Nursing Student: Intermediate

ANSWER: 2
Rationale: Seclusion or restraints require a written prescription from a primary health care provider and must be reviewed and renewed every 24 hours or per agency or state protocols. Seclusion would be used only when less restrictive methods (such as distraction or one-to-one supervision) are insufficient and the client still presents a risk for harm to self or others. This treatment must not be used for the convenience of the health care staff. A sedative is also a form of restraint (chemical) and would not be used without a primary health care provider's prescription. Seclusion would not be used as a form of punishment and can be considered a legal tort and violation of client rights if not used in the appropriate situation. Nursing measures include documenting the behavior leading to the restraint or seclusion; ensuring a prescription is in place for this treatment; ensuring the client in restraints or seclusion is protected from harm by having a staff member on one-to-one supervision within arm's length of the client; and assessing physical, safety, and comfort needs every 15 to 30 minutes, such as the need for food, fluids, range-of-motion exercises, and ambulation or the need to use the bathroom.

Test-Taking Strategy: Apply the clinical judgment/cognitive skill, *generate solutions.* Focus on the subject, indications for seclusion. Note that options 1 and 4 are comparable or alike options and indicate violation of client rights; this will assist in eliminating these options. Noting that option 3 is also a form of restraint will assist in eliminating this option. **Review:** Indications for **seclusion**.

Tip for the Nursing Student: Seclusion is a treatment measure in which the client is placed alone in a specially designed room that protects the client and allows for close supervision. In the process to maximize safety to the client and others, seclusion is the treatment of last resort. Physical restraints include any manual method or mechanical device, material, or equipment that inhibits free movement. Chemical restraints include the administration of medications for the specific purpose of inhibiting a specific behavior or movement. The important point to remember is that these treatment measures would be used as a last resort.

10. A mental health client is angry after an argument on the telephone with her son and tells the nurse about her conversation. Which statement by the nurse would be therapeutic?
    1 "You seem quite upset."
    2 "All mothers have arguments with their children."
    3 "You need to focus your energy on building your strength and getting better."
    4 "That is not very kind of your son. Does he not realize that you are trying to recuperate from surgery?"

ANSWER: 1
Rationale: The correct option provides an opportunity for the client to further share and discuss feelings. Option 2 is a stereotypical comment. Options 3 and 4 seem to console the client, but they indicate that the nurse has taken "a side" in the argument, which is nontherapeutic.

Test-Taking Strategy: Apply the clinical judgment/cognitive skill, *generate solutions.* Use therapeutic communication techniques. Remember to address the client's concerns or feelings and elicit further information from the client. This will direct you to the correct option. **Review: Therapeutic communication techniques.**

Level of Cognitive Ability: Applying
Client Needs: Psychosocial Integrity
Clinical Judgment/Cognitive Skills: Generate
Solutions
Integrated Process: Communication and
Documentation
Content Area: Mental Health
Priority Concepts: Anxiety; Communication
Level of Nursing Student: Beginning

Tip for the Nursing Student: Therapeutic communication techniques promote and encourage the client to communicate and share her or his feelings with the nurse. Nontherapeutic communication techniques block the communication process and are not methods that the nurse would use when caring for a client.

---

11. The mental health nurse is performing an admission interview with a depressed client who has suicidal ideation. After the interview, which intervention would the nurse carry out **first**?
    1 Develop a plan of activities for the client.
    2 Provide the client with diversional activities.
    3 Isolate the client from other clients in the nursing unit.
    4 Communicate the client's risk for suicide to all team members.

Level of Cognitive Ability: Applying
Client Needs: Safe and Effective Care
Environment
Clinical Judgment/Cognitive Skills: Take
Action
Integrated Process: Nursing Process/
Implementation
Content Area: Mental Health
Priority Concepts: Mood and Affect; Safety
Level of Nursing Student: Intermediate

ANSWER: 4
Rationale: The first priority intervention for the suicidal individual is to communicate the risk for suicide to all team members. The plan of activities (options 1 and 2) would take second priority. Client isolation is inappropriate. The client needs to be placed on 1:1 supervision if she or he is suicidal.

Test-Taking Strategy: Apply the clinical judgment/cognitive skill, *take action*. Note the strategic word, *first*. Eliminate options 1 and 2 first because they are comparable or alike options and relate to activities. From the remaining options, the priority item is communication to other members of the health care team, with the ultimate aim to increase client safety. **Review:** Care of the client with **suicidal ideation**.

Tip for the Nursing Student: Suicidal ideation means that the client is having thoughts about self-inflicted death. All suicidal behavior is serious and requires the nurse's immediate attention and highest-priority care.

---

12. A client has received electroconvulsive therapy (ECT) for the treatment of major depression. The nurse would implement which activity **first** in the posttreatment area when the client awakens?
    1 Discuss the treatment.
    2 Encourage the client to eat.
    3 Monitor the client's vital signs.
    4 Provide frequent reassurance to the client.

Level of Cognitive Ability: Applying
Client Needs: Physiological Integrity
Clinical Judgment/Cognitive Skills: Take
Action
Integrated Process: Nursing Process/
Implementation
Content Area: Mental Health
Priority Concepts: Caregiving; Perfusion
Level of Nursing Student: Intermediate

ANSWER: 3
Rationale: The nurse first monitors vital signs and then reviews the ECT treatment with the client. The nursing interventions outlined in options 1, 2, and 4 are also implemented but are not the first activity. In addition, the nurse would check for the return of a gag reflex before encouraging the client to eat.

Test-Taking Strategy: Apply the clinical judgment/cognitive skill, *take action*. Note the strategic word, *first*. Use the ABCs—airway, breathing, and circulation—to direct you to the correct option. **Review:** Care of the client receiving **ECT**.

Tip for the Nursing Student: Depression is a state of sadness or grief; it can range from mild and moderate states to severe states. ECT is an effective treatment for major depression in which a seizure is artificially induced in an anesthetized client by passing an electrical current through electrodes applied to the client's head. Because the client has been anesthetized and experienced an artificially induced seizure, monitoring vital signs is a priority.

13. The nurse is creating a plan of care for a client with mania and determines that the client is experiencing disturbed thoughts. Which activity related to disturbed thoughts would the nurse provide for the client **initially**?

1 Painting
2 Playing cards
3 Playing checkers
4 Playing a board game

Level of Cognitive Ability: Applying
Client Needs: Psychosocial Integrity
Clinical Judgment/Cognitive Skills: Generate Solutions
Integrated Process: Nursing Process/ Planning
Content Area: Mental Health
Priority Concepts: Caregiving; Cognition
Level of Nursing Student: Intermediate

ANSWER: 1

Rationale: When the client is manic, solitary activities requiring a short attention span or mild physical exertion activities, such as writing, painting, finger painting, woodworking, or walks with the staff, are best initially. Solitary activities minimize stimuli, and mild physical activities release tension constructively. When less manic, the client may join 1 or 2 other clients in quiet nonstimulating activities. Competitive games would be avoided because they can stimulate aggression and cause increased psychomotor activity.

Test-Taking Strategy: Apply the clinical judgment/cognitive skill, *generate solutions.* Focus on the strategic word, *initially.* Note that options 2, 3, and 4 are comparable or alike options in that they all involve activities with another individual. The correct option is the only solitary activity, which will minimize stimuli. **Review:** Care of the **manic client.**

Tip for the Nursing Student: Mania is a component of bipolar disorder and is characterized by an elevated, expansive, or irritable mood. The client lacks judgment in anticipating consequences and exhibits disturbed thought processes, pressured speech, flight of ideas, distractibility, inflated self-esteem, and hypersexuality.

---

14. A client who has been raped arrives at the emergency department. Which of these observations would be **most important** for the nurse to consider when planning the **immediate** care for the client?

1 The victim states that she "feels numb."
2 The victim states that she "feels as if it did not happen."
3 The victim states that she knows the rapist well; in fact, they had been dating for several weeks.
4 The victim states that the rapist knows where she lives and that "he will kill me if I tell anyone about the rape."

Level of Cognitive Ability: Analyzing
Client Needs: Safe and Effective Care Environment
Clinical Judgment/Cognitive Skills: Generate Solutions
Integrated Process: Nursing Process/ Planning
Content Area: Mental Health
Priority Concepts: Interpersonal Violence; Safety
Level of Nursing Student: Intermediate

ANSWER: 4

Rationale: The nurse's primary concern is to provide for safety. The priority statement by the victim is that the rapist will kill her. The victim who states that she *feels as if it did not happen* or that she *feels numb* is most likely in the denial stage, which can be a helpful defense mechanism for the client. The fact that the rapist and the victim knew each other is a common phenomenon; in many situations of rape, the victim does know the rapist.

Test-Taking Strategy: Apply the clinical judgment/cognitive skill, *generate solutions.* Note the strategic words, *most important* and *immediate.* Eliminate options 1 and 2 first because the client's statements are comparable or alike options. From the remaining options use Maslow's Hierarchy of Needs theory. The correct option indicates planning with a concern for safety. **Review:** Care of the **rape victim.**

Tip for the Nursing Student: Rape is the forced act of sexual intercourse with another person without that person's consent. Safety of the client is a primary concern. In addition, nonjudgmental listening and physical and psychological support are essential. Physical evidence may need to be obtained if the victim chooses to take legal action against the perpetrator.

15. A client says to the nurse, "Ever since my wife passed on, my life is empty and has no meaning." The nurse would make which appropriate nursing response?
  1 "Your life has no meaning?"
  2 "Most people who lose a loved one feel empty."
  3 "What would your children think if they knew how you felt?"
  4 "Let's talk about the positive things that you have in your life."

Level of Cognitive Ability: Applying
Client Needs: Psychosocial Integrity
Clinical Judgment/Cognitive Skills: Take Action
Integrated Process: Communication and Documentation
Content Area: Mental Health
Priority Concepts: Communication; Stress and Coping
Level of Nursing Student: Intermediate

ANSWER: 1
Rationale: In the correct option, the nurse uses the therapeutic technique of restating. In this technique, the nurse explores more thoroughly topics that are significant to the client. Option 2 generalizes and does not focus on the client. Option 3 focuses on the client's children rather than on the client's feelings. Option 4 avoids the client's feelings.

Test-Taking Strategy: Apply the clinical judgment/cognitive skill, *take action.* Use therapeutic communication techniques. Eliminate options 3 and 4 first because they are comparable or alike options and do not focus on the client's feelings. Next eliminate option 2 because it is a generalized statement and stereotypes the client. Option 1 uses the therapeutic technique of restating. **Review: Therapeutic communication techniques.**

Tip for the Nursing Student: Therapeutic communication techniques promote and encourage the client to communicate and share feelings with the nurse. Nontherapeutic communication techniques block the communication process and are not methods that the nurse would use when caring for a client.

---

16. The nurse is having a conversation with a client hospitalized in a mental health unit. The client says to the nurse, "I work in a factory doing piecework, and I am very competitive with the people with whom I work." The nurse would plan to make which appropriate response?
  1 "Do you find that your fellow employees are competitive also?"
  2 "When you are being paid by piecework, then you need to be competitive."
  3 "In other words, you seem to be saying that you try to do better than your fellow employees."
  4 "Why are you competitive? After all, you get paid based on the amount of work that you do, not your fellow employees."

Level of Cognitive Ability: Applying
Client Needs: Psychosocial Integrity
Clinical Judgment/Cognitive Skills: Generate Solutions
Integrated Process: Communication and Documentation
Content Area: Mental Health
Priority Concepts: Caregiving; Communication
Level of Nursing Student: Beginning

ANSWER: 3
Rationale: Option 3 uses the therapeutic technique of paraphrasing. In paraphrasing, the nurse restates in different words what the client has said to confirm an understanding of what has been said. Option 1 focuses on fellow employees and not the client. In option 2, the nurse agrees with the client. In option 4, the nurse uses the word *why*, which can make the client feel defensive and often implies criticism.

Test-Taking Strategy: Apply the clinical judgment/cognitive skill, *generate solutions.* Use therapeutic communication techniques. Eliminate option 1 first because it does not focus on the client. Next eliminate option 4 because the nurse uses the word *why*. From the remaining options, eliminate option 2 because the nurse agrees with the client. Additionally, the correct option uses the therapeutic technique of paraphrasing. **Review: Therapeutic communication techniques.**

Tip for the Nursing Student: Paraphrasing is a therapeutic communication technique that not only confirms an understanding of what the client said but also encourages the client to communicate and share feelings with the nurse.

17. A client receiving therapy at a mental health clinic says to the nurse, "When I have a stressful day at work and when my boss is 'on my case' all day, I go home and take my frustrations out on my children." The nurse would plan to make which appropriate response?
    1 "Let's talk about some other ways that you can handle your frustrations."
    2 "Why do you do this? Can you think of another way to take out your frustrations?"
    3 "Is there someplace that you can go after work to relieve your frustrations before going home?"
    4 "The only way to take out your frustrations is to join a health fitness center that provides equipment for weight lifting and boxing."

Level of Cognitive Ability: Applying
Client Needs: Psychosocial Integrity
Clinical Judgment/Cognitive Skills: Generate Solutions
Integrated Process: Communication and Documentation
Content Area: Mental Health
Priority Concepts: Communication; Stress and Coping
Level of Nursing Student: Beginning

ANSWER: 1
Rationale: The nursing response in option 1 provides the client the opportunity to problem-solve. Option 2 uses the word *why,* which can make the client feel defensive and often implies criticism. Option 3 avoids the fact that the client needs to deal with the issue, namely, taking frustrations out on the children. Option 4 is incorrect because physical activity is not the only way to relieve frustrations. In addition, this may not be appropriate for this client.

Test-Taking Strategy: Apply the clinical judgment/cognitive skill, *generate solutions.* Use therapeutic communication techniques. Eliminate option 2 because of the word *why.* Next eliminate option 4 because of the closed-ended word "only." From the remaining options, note that options 2 and 3 are comparable or alike options in that they both address other ways to deal with frustrations. Option 1 provides the client the opportunity to problem-solve. **Review: Therapeutic communication techniques.**

Tip for the Nursing Student: The nurse would involve the client in decision-making about the plan of care as much as possible. Involving the client in decision-making is a therapeutic action.

18. A client who is hospitalized in the mental health unit for treatment of depression says to the nurse, "Women always get put down. It is as if we are useless members of society." The nurse would plan to make which appropriate response?
    1 "Tell me how you feel as a woman."
    2 "Think about it. That is no longer true in today's society."
    3 "I never let anyone make me feel as though I am useless!"
    4 "Yes, that does happen to women, but it does not mean that women have to stand for that kind of treatment."

Level of Cognitive Ability: Applying
Client Needs: Psychosocial Integrity
Clinical Judgment/Cognitive Skills: Generate Solutions
Integrated Process: Communication and Documentation
Content Area: Mental Health
Priority Concepts: Mood and Affect; Communication
Level of Nursing Student: Beginning

ANSWER: 1
Rationale: In option 1, the nurse uses the therapeutic technique of focusing and encourages the client to verbalize and expand on her feelings. In option 2, the nurse disagrees with the client. In option 3, the nurse provides an opinion. In option 4, the nurse agrees with the client and then takes a forceful stance with regard to how the client should deal with these feelings.

Test-Taking Strategy: Apply the clinical judgment/cognitive skill, *generate solutions.* Use therapeutic communication techniques. Eliminate option 3 first because of the closed-ended word *never.* In addition, in this option the nurse provides an opinion, which is nontherapeutic. Next eliminate options 2 and 4. In option 2, the nurse disagrees with the client, and in option 4, the nurse agrees with the client. **Review: Therapeutic communication techniques.**

Tip for the Nursing Student: Depression is a state of sadness or grief and can range from mild and moderate states to severe states. The client with depression needs to be monitored closely for signs of potential self-harm.

19. The nurse employed in a mental health unit is meeting with a client for the first time. Which nursing statement would be **most appropriate** to initiate the conversation?

1 "Are you feeling sad?"
2 "What would you like to discuss?"
3 "Have you ever been admitted to a mental health facility?"
4 "Have psychiatric medications ever been prescribed for you?"

Level of Cognitive Ability: Applying
Client Needs: Psychosocial Integrity
Clinical Judgment/Cognitive Skills: Generate Solutions
Integrated Process: Communication and Documentation
Content Area: Mental Health
Priority Concepts: Caregiving; Communication
Level of Nursing Student: Intermediate

ANSWER: 2
Rationale: The nursing statement in option 2 is an open-ended question that encourages conversation because it requires more than a 1-word answer. In options 1, 3, and 4, the nurse attempts to obtain information from the client; however, these statements do not encourage conversation in that the client can respond with a *yes* or *no*.

Test-Taking Strategy: Apply the clinical judgment/cognitive skill, *generate solutions.* Note the strategic words, *most appropriate.* Use therapeutic communication techniques. Eliminate options 1, 3, and 4 because they are comparable or alike options and do not encourage conversation. **Review: Therapeutic communication techniques**.

Tip for the Nursing Student: The initial meeting of a client being admitted to the mental health unit is an important time to establish a therapeutic nurse–client relationship.

---

20. The emergency department nurse suspects that a client is a victim of physical abuse. The nurse would plan to make which appropriate statement to the client?

1 "If your partner is physically abusing you, you can get a restraining order."
2 "You have a huge bruise on your back. How often does your partner hit you?"
3 "That bruise looks very sore. I do not know how a person can do that to a woman."
4 "I sometimes see women who have been hurt by their partners. Did anyone hit you?"

Level of Cognitive Ability: Applying
Client Needs: Psychosocial Integrity
Clinical Judgment/Cognitive Skills: Generate Solutions
Integrated Process: Communication and Documentation
Content Area: Mental Health
Priority Concepts: Communication; Interpersonal Violence
Level of Nursing Student: Intermediate

ANSWER: 4
Rationale: Women must be asked in a caring and nonthreatening manner about violence in their lives. Options 1 and 2 are confrontational. Option 3 is a judgmental statement on the nurse's part. The nurse must avoid judgment of the victim or suspected victim's situation. It can take a great deal of time for a woman to admit that there is, in fact, abuse occurring, and the nurse must avoid becoming another controller in the woman's life. Only option 4 allows the client the option of rejecting or accepting further intervention because the nurse is making an indirect, general statement to the client.

Test-Taking Strategy: Apply the clinical judgment/cognitive skill, *generate solutions.* Use therapeutic communication techniques, and note that the client may be a victim of violence. Eliminate options 1 and 2 first because they are comparable or alike options and are both confrontational statements. Next eliminate option 3 because it is a judgmental statement. Also note that option 4 is a general statement. **Review: Therapeutic communication techniques**.

Tip for the Nursing Student: Physical abuse is a form of violence. If abuse occurs, the priority is to treat any physical injuries sustained. Next it is important to provide support and a safe environment for the victim. The nurse would use therapeutic communication techniques to communicate with the client because they promote and encourage the client to communicate and share feelings with the nurse.

21. Which statements made by the nurse indicate the use of a therapeutic communication technique? **Select all that apply.**
    1 "I would not worry about that."
    2 "You'll do just fine. You'll see."
    3 "What would you like to discuss?"
    4 "Can you describe your feelings?"
    5 "Can you tell me what the voices are saying?"
    6 "Let's not talk about that now, and let's focus on some other issues."

Level of Cognitive Ability: Applying
Client Needs: Psychosocial Integrity
Clinical Judgment/Cognitive Skills: Generate Solutions
Integrated Process: Communication and Documentation
Content Area: Mental Health
Priority Concepts: Caregiving; Communication
Level of Nursing Student: Beginning

ANSWER. 3, 4, 5
Rationale: The nursing statement "What would you like to discuss?" is therapeutic and an open-ended question that invites the client to share personal feelings. The nursing statements "Can you describe your feelings?" and "Can you tell me what the voices are saying?" are therapeutic and focused statements that are exploratory and will direct necessary nursing actions. The nursing statements "I would not worry about that" and "You'll do just fine. You'll see" are nontherapeutic and provide false reassurance. The statement "Let's not talk about that now, and let's focus on some other issues" avoids a client's feelings and concerns.

Test-Taking Strategy: Apply the clinical judgment/cognitive skill, *generate solutions.* Read each nursing statement and focus on the subject, use of therapeutic communication techniques. Recalling the therapeutic and nontherapeutic techniques will assist in answering the question. Also, remember that the priority is to address the client's feelings and encourage communication that will assist in directing necessary nursing actions. **Review: Therapeutic communication techniques.**

Tip for the Nursing Student: Therapeutic communication techniques promote and encourage the client to communicate and share feelings with the nurse. Nontherapeutic communication techniques block the communication process and are not methods that the nurse would use when caring for a client.

22. The primary health care provider prescribes aripiprazole for a client with a diagnosis of schizophrenia. Which intervention would the nurse take?
    1 Administer the medication only after meals.
    2 Inform the client to limit alcohol intake to 1 drink a day.
    3 Inform the client that the medication may cause sedation and needs to be taken at bedtime.
    4 Instruct the client to increase the usual exercise pattern threefold to help with medication absorption.

Level of Cognitive Ability: Applying
Client Needs: Physiological Integrity
Clinical Judgment/Cognitive Skills: Take Action
Integrated Process: Nursing Process/ Implementation
Content Area: Mental Health
Priority Concepts: Psychosis; Safety
Level of Nursing Student: Intermediate

ANSWER: 3
Rationale: Aripiprazole is an antipsychotic agent that may be referred to as a *dopamine system stabilizer (DSS).* Because antipsychotics cause sedation, bedtime dosing helps promote sleep while decreasing daytime drowsiness. Aripiprazole may be administered with or without food and is well absorbed both in the presence or absence of food. It is not necessary for the client to increase her or his usual exercise pattern to assist in absorption of the medication. Alcohol is avoided, not limited.

Test-Taking Strategy: Apply the clinical judgment/cognitive skill, *take action.* Noting that the client has schizophrenia will assist in determining that the medication is an antipsychotic. Eliminate option 1 because of the closed-ended word "only." Eliminate option 2 by recalling that alcohol intake is avoided, not limited. From the remaining options, eliminate option 4 because of the words *increase the usual exercise pattern threefold.* **Review: Aripiprazole.**

Tip for the Nursing Student: Schizophrenia is a psychotic disorder characterized by gross distortion of reality, disturbances of language and communication, withdrawal from social interactions, and disorganization and fragmentation of thoughts. Antipsychotic medication is administered to control the delusions and hallucinations that the client experiences.

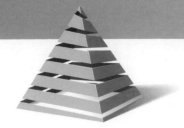

CHAPTER 16

Maternity Questions

1. The nurse is collecting data during an assessment and notes that the fundus feels soft and spongy. Which nursing actions are **most appropriate initially**? **Select all that apply.**
   1 Massage the fundus gently.
   2 Encourage the mother to ambulate.
   3 Notify the primary health care provider.
   4 Observe for increased vaginal bleeding or clots.
   5 Document fundal position, consistency, and height.

Level of Cognitive Ability: Analyzing
Client Needs: Physiological Integrity
Clinical Judgment/Cognitive Skills: Take Action
Integrated Process: Nursing Process/
   Implementation
Content Area: Maternity
Priority Concepts: Perfusion; Reproduction
Level of Nursing Student: Intermediate

ANSWER: 1, 4, 5
Rationale: If the uterus feels soft and spongy (boggy), it would be massaged gently, observing for increased vaginal bleeding or clots. Option 2 is inappropriate at this time and could be harmful. The nurse would document fundal position, consistency, and height and the need to perform fundal massage, along with the client's response to the intervention. Notifying the primary health care provider before beginning fundal massage is not appropriate.

Test-Taking Strategy: Apply the clinical judgment/cognitive skill, *take action*. Note the strategic words, *most appropriate initially*. Note the relationship of the data in the question (soft and spongy) and the data in the correct options. Also recall that actions need to be taken if the top of the uterus (fundus) is soft and spongy. **Review:** Nursing interventions related to **fundal assessment**.

Tip for the Nursing Student: The postpartum period is the time after delivery of a newborn. During this time, the nurse needs to check the new mother's fundus for firmness. If the fundus is soft and spongy (and not firm as it should be), the nurse would gently massage the fundus.

---

2. A client arrives at the prenatal clinic for her first prenatal assessment. She tells the nurse that the first day of her last menstrual period (LMP) was August 19, 2022. Using Naegele's rule, the nurse informs the client that the estimated date of delivery is which date?
   1 May 12, 2023
   2 May 26, 2023
   3 June 12, 2023
   4 June 26, 2023

Level of Cognitive Ability: Applying
Client Needs: Physiological Integrity
Clinical Judgment/Cognitive Skills: Recognize
   Cues

ANSWER: 2
Rationale: Accurate use of Naegele's rule requires that the woman have a regular 28-day menstrual cycle. Subtract 3 months from the first day of the LMP, add 7 days, and then add 1 year to that date if it is appropriate to change it to the next year. First day of the LMP is August 19, 2022; subtract 3 months: May 19, 2022; add 7 days: May 26, 2022; add 1 year: May 26, 2023.

Test-Taking Strategy: Apply the clinical judgment/cognitive skill, *recognize cues*. Focus on the subject, accurate use of this rule. Use Naegele's rule to answer this question, but use caution when following the steps to determine the estimated date of delivery. Read all options carefully, noting the dates and years in each before selecting an option. **Review: Naegele's rule**.

Tip for the Nursing Student: Naegele's rule is a method of determining the date of delivery for a client who is pregnant. Determining

Integrated Process: Nursing Process/
Assessment/Data Collection
Content Area: Maternity
Priority Concepts: Development; Reproduction
Level of Nursing Student: Intermediate

the date of delivery requires knowing the date of the LMP and then using the rule to determine the delivery date. This is a simple way to determine the date, and memorizing the rule will assist you in determining a client's delivery date.

---

3. The nurse is monitoring a client who is receiving magnesium sulfate for preeclampsia and is monitoring the client every 30 minutes. Which finding indicates a need to **immediately** contact the obstetrician?
   1 Urinary output of 20 mL
   2 Deep tendon reflexes of 2+
   3 Respirations of 10 breaths/minute
   4 Fetal heart rate (FHR) of 116 beats/minute

Level of Cognitive Ability: Analyzing
Client Needs: Physiological Integrity
Clinical Judgment/Cognitive Skills: Recognize Cues
Integrated Process: Nursing Process/
Assessment/Data Collection
Content Area: Maternity
Priority Concepts: Clinical Judgment;
Collaboration
Level of Nursing Student: Intermediate

ANSWER: 3
Rationale: Magnesium sulfate depresses the respiratory rate. If the rate is less than 12 breaths/minute, continuation of the medication needs to be reassessed. The acceptable criterion for urine output is at least 30 mL/hour. The amount of urine output identified in option 1 is adequate (20 mL of urine in 30 minutes). Deep tendon reflexes of 2+ are normal. The FHR is within normal limits for a resting fetus.

Test-Taking Strategy: Apply the clinical judgment/cognitive skill, *recognize cues*. Note the strategic word, *immediately*. Determine whether an abnormality exists. Select the option that indicates an abnormal finding that requires further intervention. Recalling the normal respiratory rate will direct you to option 3. **Review:** The findings in **preeclampsia**.

Tip for the Nursing Student: Preeclampsia is an abnormal condition of pregnancy characterized by the onset of acute hypertension after week 24 of pregnancy. One concern is that preeclampsia can progress to eclampsia (seizures). Preeclampsia may be treated with magnesium sulfate to prevent its progression to eclampsia. The nurse needs to monitor closely the client receiving this medication because of its many adverse effects and the risk of toxicity. One primary concern is that magnesium sulfate depresses respirations; therefore, the nurse monitors the client's respiratory status closely.

---

4. The nurse receives a report at the beginning of the shift about a client with an intrauterine fetal demise. When collecting data on assessment of the client, the nurse expects to note which finding?
   1 Intractable vomiting and dehydration
   2 Elevated blood pressure and proteinuria
   3 Uterine size greater than expected for gestational age
   4 Regression of pregnancy symptoms and absence of fetal heart tones

ANSWER: 4
Rationale: Symptoms of a fetal demise include decreased fetal movement, unchanged or decreased fundal height, and absent fetal heart tones. In addition, many symptoms of the pregnancy may diminish, such as breast size and tenderness. Option 1 is associated with hyperemesis gravidarum. Option 2 is associated with preeclampsia. Option 3 is unrelated to intrauterine fetal demise and can be associated with *a hydatidiform mole (molar pregnancy)*.

Test-Taking Strategy: Apply the clinical judgment/cognitive skill, *recognize cues*. Focus on the subject, intrauterine fetal demise. Note the relationship between the subject and option 4. Recalling that fetal demise means fetal death will direct you to the correct option. **Review:** The signs associated with **intrauterine fetal demise**.

Level of Cognitive Ability: Analyzing
Client Needs: Physiological Integrity
Clinical Judgment/Cognitive Skills: Recognize
Cues
Integrated Process: Nursing Process/
Assessment/Data Collection
Content Area: Maternity
Priority Concepts: Clinical Judgment;
Reproduction
Level of Nursing Student: Intermediate

Tip for the Nursing Student: Fetal demise refers to the intrauterine death of a fetus. If this occurs, fetal movement and heart tones would be absent. Hyperemesis gravidarum is an abnormal condition of pregnancy characterized by protracted vomiting, weight loss, and fluid and electrolyte imbalance. Preeclampsia is an abnormal condition of pregnancy characterized by the onset of acute hypertension after week 24 of pregnancy. The classic signs include hypertension and proteinuria (protein in the urine). *Hydatidiform mole* is a rare mass or growth that grows inside the uterus at the beginning of a pregnancy. It is a form of gestational trophoblastic disease.

---

5. Immediately after the delivery of a newborn, the nurse prepares to assist in the delivery of the placenta. What is the appropriate action to deliver the placenta?
   1 Pull on the umbilical cord.
   2 Instruct the mother to push during a uterine contraction.
   3 Place traction on the umbilical cord and pull on the placenta as it enters the vaginal canal.
   4 Separate the placenta from the uterine wall using the forceps, and then allow the placenta to deliver spontaneously.

Level of Cognitive Ability: Applying
Client Needs: Physiological Integrity
Clinical Judgment/Cognitive Skills: Take Action
Integrated Process: Nursing Process/
Implementation
Content Area: Maternity
Priority Concepts: Clinical Judgment; Safety
Level of Nursing Student: Intermediate

ANSWER: 2
Rationale: After the placenta separates, the mother is instructed to push during a uterine contraction. Pulling on the umbilical cord or placing traction on the umbilical cord may cause it to break, making the placenta harder to deliver. The placenta is not separated from the uterine wall using forceps. This may result in bleeding.

Test-Taking Strategy: Apply the clinical judgment/cognitive skill, *take action*. Focus on the subject, actions to assist in the delivery of a placenta. Eliminate option 1 because of the word *pull* and option 3 because of the word *traction*. From the remaining options, eliminate option 4 by recalling that the placenta is attached to the uterine wall and unnatural separation will result in bleeding. **Review:** The procedure for **placental delivery**.

Tip for the Nursing Student: The placenta is a fetal structure that provides nourishment to and removes wastes from the developing fetus. After the delivery of the baby, the placenta separates from the uterine wall and is delivered.

---

6. A client tells the nurse that she is really worried about knowing how to care for her firstborn child. The nurse would identify which **priority** problem for this client?
   1 Inability to cope
   2 Lack of knowledge
   3 Ineffective grieving
   4 Lowered self-esteem

Level of Cognitive Ability: Analyzing
Client Needs: Health Promotion and
Maintenance
Clinical Judgment/Cognitive Skills: Prioritize
Hypotheses

ANSWER: 2
Rationale: Lack of knowledge indicates a lack of information or psychomotor ability concerning a skill, condition, or treatment. This problem best describes the situation presented in the question. Inability to cope implies that the person is unable to manage stressors adequately. Ineffective grieving implies prolonged unresolved grief leading to detrimental activities. Lowered self-esteem represents temporary negative feelings about self in response to an event.

Test-Taking Strategy: Apply the clinical judgment/cognitive skill, *prioritize hypotheses*. Note the strategic word, *priority*. When a question asks to identify a priority client problem, focus on the data in the question. Option 2 will focus on the mother's concern about *knowing how to care for her firstborn child*. **Review: Psychosocial concerns of a new mother**.

Integrated Process: Nursing Process/
    Analysis
Content Area: Maternity
Priority Concepts: Anxiety; Family Dynamics
Level of Nursing Student: Intermediate

Tip for the Nursing Student: Teaching is an important nursing responsibility. It is common for a new mother to be concerned about how to care for her newborn. The nurse needs to alleviate fears and concerns by providing the mother with opportunities to care for the newborn after delivery while hospitalized.

---

7. The nurse is monitoring the status of a client in labor who is experiencing hypotonic uterine dysfunction. The nurse interprets that which findings are consistent with this type of dysfunctional labor? **Select all that apply.**
   1 Contractions weaken during the active stage of labor.
   2 Contractions become inefficient or stop during the active stage of labor.
   3 Contractions are painful and are ineffective in causing cervical dilation.
   4 The client is experiencing frequent contractions that are ineffective in causing effacement to progress.
   5 The client initially makes normal progress into the active stage of labor and then contractions weaken.

Level of Cognitive Ability: Analyzing
Client Needs: Physiological Integrity
Clinical Judgment/Cognitive Skills: Analyze
    Cues
Integrated Process: Nursing Process/
    Analysis
Content Area: Maternity
Priority Concepts: Clinical Judgment;
    Reproduction
Level of Nursing Student: Intermediate

ANSWER: 1, 2, 5
Rationale: In hypotonic uterine dysfunction the client initially makes normal progress into the active stage of labor and then contractions weaken, become inefficient, or stop. Options 3 and 4 are characteristic of hypertonic uterine dysfunction.

Test-Taking Strategy: Apply the clinical judgment/cognitive skill, *analyze cues.* Focus on the subject, characteristics of hypotonic uterine dysfunction. Noting that options 1, 2, and 5 are comparable or alike options and noting the word *hypotonic* in the question will direct you to the correct options. **Review:** Manifestations of **hypotonic uterine dysfunction**.

Tip for the Nursing Student: A contraction is a rhythmic tightening of the musculature of the upper uterus that begins as mild tightening and progresses to strong tightening late in labor. Contractions decrease the size of the uterus and push the fetus through the birth canal. Normal labor contractions are coordinated, involuntary, and intermittent.

---

8. A client has just experienced a precipitate labor. The nurse notes that the mother is lying quietly in bed and is avoiding physical contact with her newborn. What is the **most appropriate** nursing action?
   1 Request a psychiatric consult.
   2 Provide support to the mother.
   3 Contact the primary health care provider.
   4 Encourage the mother to breast-feed the infant.

Level of Cognitive Ability: Applying
Client Needs: Psychosocial Integrity
Clinical Judgment/Cognitive Skills: Take
    Action
Integrated Process: Caring
Content Area: Maternity

ANSWER: 2
Rationale: Precipitate labor is defined as labor that lasts less than 3 hours from the onset of contractions to the time of birth. After a precipitate labor, the mother may need help to process what has happened and time to assimilate it all. The mother may be exhausted, in pain, stunned by the rapid nature of the delivery, or simply following cultural norms. Providing support to the mother is the most appropriate and therapeutic action by the nurse. Options 1 and 3 do not enhance the therapeutic relationship. Option 4 is an appropriate nursing intervention, but the question does not indicate whether the mother is going to be breast-feeding.

Test-Taking Strategy: Apply the clinical judgment/cognitive skill, *take action.* Note the strategic words, *most appropriate.* Eliminate options 1 and 3 first because they are comparable or alike options. From the remaining options, note that no data indicate that the mother is going to breast-feed. This will direct you to the correct option. **Review:** Care of the client after **precipitate labor**.

Priority Concepts: Caregiving; Stress and
  Coping
Level of Nursing Student: Intermediate

Tip for the Nursing Student: The total duration of normal labor differs for women who have never given birth and for those who have previously given birth by the vaginal route. Normal labor consists of 4 stages. In the first stage, which normally lasts 6 to 10 hours (but can be longer), effacement and dilation occur. The second stage involves expulsion of the fetus and normally lasts 20 to 60 minutes. Stage 3 involves separation of the placenta and usually takes 5 to 30 minutes. Stage 4, which lasts 1 to 4 hours after delivery, is the time for physical recovery and newborn bonding.

---

9. A pregnant client experienced a uterine rupture with subsequent fetal death. After ensuring that the client is physiologically stable, the nurse would use which approach as the **first** step to support the client psychologically?
   1 Avoid talking about the dead fetus.
   2 Determine how the client perceived the event.
   3 Ask the client and husband about plans for future pregnancies.
   4 Suggest that family members see and hold the dead infant if they wish.

Level of Cognitive Ability: Applying
Client Needs: Psychosocial Integrity
Clinical Judgment/Cognitive Skills: Generate
  Solutions
Integrated Process: Caring
Content Area: Maternity
Priority Concepts: Caregiving; Stress and
  Coping
Level of Nursing Student: Intermediate

ANSWER: 2
Rationale: Because of anesthesia, anxiety, and the experience of a sudden catastrophic event, the client may well have experienced a decreased ability to take in and process information. The nurse would first assess the client's perception of the event before deciding how to intervene. Options 1 and 3 are unhelpful because they are nontherapeutic. Option 1 avoids the subject, and option 3 deals with a subject the client may not be ready to face. Option 4 may be helpful, but not as a first step.

Test-Taking Strategy: Apply the clinical judgment/cognitive skill, *generate solutions.* Note the strategic word, *first.* Use the steps of the nursing process, remembering that assessment/data collection comes first. This will direct you to the correct option. **Review:** Care of the mother psychosocially after a **fetal demise**.

Tip for the Nursing Student: Uterine rupture results when a tear in the wall of the uterus occurs because the uterine wall cannot stand the pressure placed against it from the growing fetus. Uterine rupture is a rare condition associated with previous uterine surgery, such as a cesarean birth or surgery to remove fibroids. If the placenta is involved, it often results in fetal demise.

---

10. A pregnant client with a suspected diagnosis of placenta previa arrives at the health care clinic for an examination. The nurse prepares the client for the examination and tells the client that which procedure will be deferred until the diagnosis is confirmed?
    1 Abdominal ultrasound
    2 Vital sign measurement
    3 Urine testing for glucose
    4 Vaginal speculum examination

Level of Cognitive Ability: Applying
Client Needs: Physiological Integrity
Clinical Judgment/Cognitive Skills: Take
  Action
Integrated Process: Nursing Process/
  Implementation

ANSWER: 4
Rationale: The placenta is implanted low in the uterus in placenta previa, and a vaginal speculum examination could cause disruption of the placenta and initiate severe hemorrhage. The abdominal ultrasound is used to confirm the diagnosis of placenta previa. There is no reason to defer urine testing or vital sign measurement.

Test-Taking Strategy: Apply the clinical judgment/cognitive skill, *take action.* Focus on the subject, care of the client with placenta previa. Note the word *deferred,* and focus on the client's suspected diagnosis. Recalling that in this condition the placenta is implanted low in the uterus and that the client is at risk for hemorrhage will direct you to the correct option. **Review:** Nursing care of the client with **placenta previa**.

Tip for the Nursing Student: The placenta is a fetal structure that provides nourishment to and removes wastes from the developing

Content Area: Maternity
Priority Concepts: Clinical Judgment; Safety
Level of Nursing Student: Intermediate

fetus. It is normally implanted in the upper uterine area. In placenta previa, the placenta is implanted low in the uterus near the cervix. Disruption of the placenta can cause severe hemorrhage and compromise fetal status. Therefore, any activity or procedure that could disrupt the placenta is avoided.

---

11. The nurse is collecting data on a client with placenta previa and would check which item **first**?
    1 The client's temperature
    2 The fetal heart rate (FHR)
    3 The client's compliance with activity limitations
    4 The client's understanding of the treatment for placenta previa

Level of Cognitive Ability: Analyzing
Client Needs: Physiological Integrity
Clinical Judgment/Cognitive Skills: Take Action
Integrated Process: Nursing Process/ Assessment/Data Collection
Content Area: Maternity
Priority Concepts: Clinical Judgment; Perfusion
Level of Nursing Student: Intermediate

ANSWER: 2
Rationale: A primary concern with placenta previa is fetal injury related to potentially decreased placental perfusion. Although all the options may be assessed, assessing the FHR is the priority and the item that needs to be checked first.

Test-Taking Strategy: Apply the clinical judgment/cognitive skill, *take action*. Note the strategic word, *first*, and that options 3 and 4 are comparable or alike options relating to treatment for placenta previa and therefore can be eliminated. Also use the ABCs—airway, breathing, and circulation—to direct you to option 2. **Review:** Care of the client with **placenta previa**.

Tip for the Nursing Student: Placenta previa is an abnormal condition in which the placenta is implanted low in the uterus near the cervix. A primary concern when a client has placenta previa is disruption of the placenta, leading to severe hemorrhage and a compromised fetal status. Both the mother and fetus are monitored closely. Any activity or procedure that could disrupt the placenta, such as a vaginal examination, is avoided.

---

12. The nurse is preparing to perform fundal massage on a client with uterine atony. How would the nurse perform this procedure?
    1 Place 1 hand just above the symphysis pubis and push on the uterus in a vertical direction.
    2 Place 1 hand just below the symphysis pubis and massage the fundus in a circular motion.
    3 Place 1 hand just below the symphysis pubis and massage the fundus in a horizontal motion.
    4 Place 1 hand just above the symphysis pubis and gently but firmly massage the fundus in a circular motion.

Level of Cognitive Ability: Applying
Client Needs: Physiological Integrity
Clinical Judgment/Cognitive Skills: Take Action
Integrated Process: Nursing Process/ Implementation
Content Area: Maternity
Priority Concepts: Perfusion; Safety
Level of Nursing Student: Intermediate

ANSWER: 4
Rationale: When performing fundal massage, 1 hand is placed just above the symphysis pubis to support the lower uterine segment while the fundus is gently but firmly massaged in a circular motion. Pushing on an uncontracted uterus could invert the uterus and cause massive hemorrhage.

Test-Taking Strategy: Apply the clinical judgment/cognitive skill, *take action*. Focus on the subject, the procedure to perform fundal massage. Eliminate option 1 first because of the word *push*, recalling that pushing on an uncontracted uterus could invert the uterus and cause massive hemorrhage. Next visualize the anatomy of the uterus. Eliminate options 2 and 3 because the hand is not placed below the symphysis pubis. **Review:** The procedure for **fundal massage**.

Tip for the Nursing Student: Uterine atony refers to a lack of uterine muscle tone and can result in bleeding. Bleeding occurs because the uterine muscle fibers fail to contract firmly around the blood vessels when the placenta separates. A soft or "boggy" feel on locating the uterine fundus is a manifestation of uterine atony. Fundal massage is performed to contract the uterus when uterine atony is present.

13. A pregnant client is seen in the prenatal clinic with morning sickness. The nurse would provide which instruction to the client regarding dietary measures?
    1 Eat 5 or 6 small meals per day.
    2 Gas-forming foods should be eaten only during the afternoon hours.
    3 A high-protein and high-fat snack should be eaten before getting out of bed.
    4 Fried foods should be eaten only during the afternoon and early evening hours.

Level of Cognitive Ability: Applying
Client Needs: Health Promotion and Maintenance
Clinical Judgment/Cognitive Skills: Take Action
Integrated Process: Teaching and Learning
Content Area: Maternity
Priority Concepts: Client Education; Nutrition
Level of Nursing Student: Intermediate

ANSWER: 1
Rationale: Morning sickness is common during the first trimester of pregnancy and is associated with increased levels of human chorionic gonadotropin (hCG) and changes in carbohydrate metabolism. It most often occurs on arising, although a few women experience it throughout the day. Several self-care measures can be implemented to prevent or alleviate morning sickness. These include avoiding an empty or overloaded stomach; eating a dry carbohydrate food item such as a dry cracker or toast before getting out of bed; eating 5 or 6 small meals per day; and avoiding fried, odorous, greasy, gas-forming, or spicy foods.

Test-Taking Strategy: Apply the clinical judgment/cognitive skill, *take action.* Focus on the subject, measures to prevent or alleviate morning sickness. Eliminate options 2 and 4 first because of the closed-ended word "only." From the remaining options eliminate option 3 because of the words *high-fat.* **Review:** Measures to prevent or alleviate **morning sickness**.

Tip for the Nursing Student: Morning sickness is nausea and vomiting that occur during pregnancy. It is called morning sickness because the symptoms are usually more acute in the morning (although it can occur at any time of the day). This is a common discomfort of pregnancy and is usually temporary.

14. A client in the third trimester of pregnancy seen in the clinic is experiencing urinary frequency. Which self-care measure would the nurse provide teaching on to the client?
    1 Perform Kegel exercises.
    2 Avoid fluid intake after 6:00 PM.
    3 Avoid emptying the bladder frequently.
    4 Sip on small amounts of fluids during the day, restricting intake to 1000 mL.

Level of Cognitive Ability: Applying
Client Needs: Health Promotion and Maintenance
Clinical Judgment/Cognitive Skills: Generate Solutions
Integrated Process: Teaching and Learning
Content Area: Maternity
Priority Concepts: Client Education; Elimination
Level of Nursing Student: Intermediate

ANSWER: 1
Rationale: Urinary frequency may occur in the first trimester and then again late in the third trimester because of the pressure placed on the bladder by the enlarged uterus. Self-care measures for urinary frequency include emptying the bladder frequently (every 2 hours), drinking at least 2000 mL of fluid per day, limiting fluid intake before bedtime (not avoiding fluid intake), performing Kegel exercises to strengthen the perineal muscles, and wearing a perineal pad. Options 2, 3, and 4 are incorrect and could lead to urinary stasis (option 3) or fluid volume deficit (options 2 and 4).

Test-Taking Strategy: Apply the clinical judgment/cognitive skill, *generate solutions.* Eliminate options 2 and 4 first because they are comparable or alike options and could lead to fluid volume deficit. Eliminate option 3 next because it does not make sense to avoid emptying the bladder frequently. This action could lead to urinary stasis and cause discomfort. **Review:** Measures that will assist with the discomfort of **urinary frequency**.

Tip for the Nursing Student: Urinary frequency is a common discomfort of pregnancy and usually occurs during the first trimester of pregnancy and near term. This is a temporary condition, and Kegel exercises help maintain bladder control. Kegel exercises involve contracting muscles around the vagina, holding tightly for 10 seconds, and then relaxing for 10 seconds. Thirty contraction–relaxation cycles should be done each day.

15. A client seen in the prenatal clinic is experiencing ankle edema. The nurse assesses the client and notes that the edema is nonpitting and the client's blood pressure is within normal limits. The nurse would provide which home care instruction to this client?
    1 Restrict fluid intake.
    2 Avoid exercising until the edema subsides.
    3 Rest periodically with the legs and hips elevated.
    4 Stop wearing the support stockings prescribed by the obstetrician.

Level of Cognitive Ability: Applying
Client Needs: Health Promotion and Maintenance
Clinical Judgment/Cognitive Skills: Generate Solutions
Integrated Process: Teaching and Learning
Content Area: Maternity
Priority Concepts: Client Education; Perfusion
Level of Nursing Student: Intermediate

ANSWER: 3
Rationale: Ankle edema is common in the third trimester of pregnancy and is caused by decreased venous return from the feet because of gravity. It is a minor discomfort, and as long as the edema is nonpitting and hypertension is not present, it is not a cause for concern. Self-care measures include resting periodically with the legs and hips elevated, wearing supportive stockings or hose as prescribed, drinking ample amounts of fluid, partaking in moderate exercise, and avoiding standing in 1 position or place for long periods.

Test-Taking Strategy: Apply the clinical judgment/cognitive skill, *generate solutions.* Focus on the subject, measures to relieve edema. Eliminate option 1 first because of the word *restrict.* Restricting fluids can be detrimental to the fetus. Next, eliminate option 4 because the nurse would not tell a client to ignore the obstetrician's prescription. From the remaining options, use principles related to the effects of gravity to direct you to the correct option. **Review:** The measures to alleviate ankle **edema.**

Tip for the Nursing Student: Edema refers to swelling from the accumulation of excess fluid in body tissues. Edema can occur during pregnancy because the weight of the uterus compresses the veins of the pelvis, delaying venous return. Edema of the feet and ankles is most noticeable at the end of the day. Dependent edema is not significant, but if edema of the face or hands occurs, the client needs to be further assessed for developing complications of pregnancy.

16. The nurse provides instructions to a prenatal client with heartburn about measures to alleviate the discomfort. Which statement by the client indicates a **need for further instruction**?
    1 "I need to lie down after eating."
    2 "I need to eat small, frequent meals."
    3 "I need to avoid fatty or spicy foods."
    4 "I need to drink about 2000 mL of fluid per day."

Level of Cognitive Ability: Evaluating
Client Needs: Health Promotion and Maintenance
Clinical Judgment/Cognitive Skills: Evaluate Outcomes
Integrated Process: Teaching and Learning
Content Area: Maternity
Priority Concepts: Client Education; Pain
Level of Nursing Student: Intermediate

ANSWER: 1
Rationale: Heartburn is associated with regurgitation of gastric acid contents into the esophagus. Self-care measures for heartburn include eating small, frequent meals; remaining upright for 30 minutes after eating; avoiding fatty or spicy foods; and drinking approximately 2000 mL of fluid per day.

Test-Taking Strategy: Apply the clinical judgment/cognitive skill, *evaluate outcomes.* Note the strategic words, *need for further instruction.* These words indicate a negative event query and the need to select the option that indicates an incorrect client statement. Recalling that heartburn is associated with regurgitation of gastric acid contents into the esophagus will direct you to the correct option. **Review:** Measures to relieve or prevent **heartburn.**

Tip for the Nursing Student: Heartburn is described as an acute burning sensation in the epigastric and sternal regions. During pregnancy it normally occurs as a result of diminished gastric motility, displacement of the stomach by the enlarging uterus, and relaxation of the lower esophageal sphincter.

17. The nurse is collecting data on a client who is at 38 weeks' gestation and notes that the fetal heart rate (FHR) is 174 beats/minute. Based on this finding, what is the **most appropriate** nursing action?
1 Document the finding.
2 Check the mother's heart rate.
3 Tell the client that the FHR is normal.
4 Notify the primary health care provider.

Level of Cognitive Ability: Applying
Client Needs: Physiological Integrity
Clinical Judgment/Cognitive Skills: Take Action
Integrated Process: Nursing Process/Implementation
Content Area: Maternity
Priority Concepts: Perfusion; Safety
Level of Nursing Student: Intermediate

ANSWER: **4**
Rationale: The FHR should be 110 to 160 beats/minute at term. Because the FHR is elevated from the normal range, the nurse would notify the primary health care provider. The FHR would be documented, but option 4 is the most appropriate action. Options 2 and 3 are inappropriate actions based on the data in the question.

Test-Taking Strategy: Apply the clinical judgment/cognitive skill, *take action*. Note the strategic words, *most appropriate*. Focus on the data in the question and note the FHR. Recalling that the normal FHR should be 110 to 160 beats/minute at term will direct you to the correct option. Remember that an abnormal finding noted in the pregnant client needs to be reported to the primary health care provider. **Review:** The normal **FHR**.

Tip for the Nursing Student: FHR monitoring is an important part of maternal assessment during pregnancy. The nurse usually uses a Doppler device to auscultate the FHR, which creates an electronic sound based on movements.

18. The nurse is monitoring a client in the fourth stage of labor and notes that the uterine fundus is firmly contracted and is midline at the level of the umbilicus. Based on this finding, what is the **most appropriate** nursing action?
1 Record the findings.
2 Massage the fundus.
3 Assist the mother to void.
4 Contact the primary health care provider.

Level of Cognitive Ability: Applying
Client Needs: Health Promotion and Maintenance
Clinical Judgment/Cognitive Skills: Take Action
Integrated Process: Nursing Process/Implementation
Content Area: Maternity
Priority Concepts: Clinical Judgment; Perfusion
Level of Nursing Student: Intermediate

ANSWER: **1**
Rationale: In the postpartum period the nurse checks for uterine atony and checks the consistency and location of the uterine fundus. The uterine fundus should be firmly contracted, at or near the level of the umbilicus, and midline. Therefore, the nurse would record the findings. Because the finding is normal, options 2, 3, and 4 are unnecessary. The nurse would massage the uterine fundus if it is soft and boggy. A full bladder may cause a displaced fundus and one that is above the level of the umbilicus. The primary health care provider needs to be contacted if the client experiences excessive bleeding.

Test-Taking Strategy: Apply the clinical judgment/cognitive skill, *take action*. Note the strategic words, *most appropriate*, and focus on the data in the question. Recalling the normal location and consistency of the fundus will direct you to the correct option. **Review:** The expected **uterine postpartum findings**.

Tip for the Nursing Student: Involution is a retrogressive change in the uterus to its nonpregnant size. In the fourth stage of labor (1 to 4 hours after delivery), the nurse monitors the location of the uterine fundus to determine whether involution is progressing normally. Immediately after delivery the fundus can be palpated midway between the symphysis pubis and the umbilicus. Within a few hours the fundus rises to the level of the umbilicus and should remain at this level for 24 hours. After 24 hours the fundus descends by approximately 1 cm/day.

19. The home care nurse is visiting a postpartum client. The nurse reviews the information in the client's medical record and collects data on the client. The nurse would suspect endometritis if which finding is noted?
1 Breast engorgement
2 Fever that began 3 days postpartum
3 Slightly elevated white blood cell count
4 Lochia rubra on the second day postpartum

Level of Cognitive Ability: Analyzing
Client Needs: Physiological Integrity
Clinical Judgment/Cognitive Skills: Recognize Cues
Integrated Process: Nursing Process/ Assessment/Data Collection
Content Area: Maternity
Priority Concepts: Clinical Judgment; Infection
Level of Nursing Student: Intermediate

ANSWER: **2**
Rationale: Fever on the third or fourth day postpartum should raise concerns about possible endometritis until proven otherwise. The woman with endometritis normally presents with a temperature over 100.4°F (38°C). Breast engorgement is a normal response and is not associated with endometritis. The white blood cell count of a postpartum woman is normally increased; thus, this method of detecting infection is not of great value in the postpartum period. Lochia rubra on the second day postpartum is a normal finding.

Test-Taking Strategy: Apply the clinical judgment/cognitive skill, *recognize cues.* Focus on the subject, suspected endometritis. Use medical terminology to recall that *-itis* indicates inflammation or infection. This will assist in eliminating options 1 and 4. From the remaining options, noting the word *slightly* in option 3 will assist in eliminating this option. Also note that options 1, 3, and 4 are comparable or alike options in that they are normal postpartum findings. **Review:** The signs of **endometritis**.

Tip for the Nursing Student: Endometritis is an inflammation of the endometrium or decidua and is usually caused by a bacterial infection. It occurs most frequently after childbirth or abortion and is associated with the use of an intrauterine device. Conservative treatment includes rest, antibiotics, pain medication, and adequate fluid intake.

---

20. A client in the second trimester of pregnancy is admitted to the maternity unit with a diagnosis of abruptio placentae. The nurse expects to note which clinical manifestation associated with this disorder?
1 Nontender uterus
2 Uterine hypertonicity
3 Painless vaginal bleeding
4 Soft, relaxed uterus with normal tone

Level of Cognitive Ability: Analyzing
Client Needs: Physiological Integrity
Clinical Judgment/Cognitive Skills: Recognize Cues
Integrated Process: Nursing Process/ Assessment/Data Collection
Content Area: Maternity
Priority Concepts: Pain; Perfusion
Level of Nursing Student: Intermediate

ANSWER: **2**
Rationale: In abruptio placentae, abdominal pain, uterine tenderness, and uterine hypertonicity are present. Uterine tenderness accompanies placental abruption, especially with a central abruption in which blood becomes trapped behind the placenta. The abdomen will feel hard and boardlike on palpation as the blood penetrates the myometrium and causes uterine irritability. Excessive uterine activity with poor relaxation between contractions is present. A nontender uterus; painless vaginal bleeding; and a soft, relaxed uterus with normal tone are signs of placenta previa.

Test-Taking Strategy: Apply the clinical judgment/cognitive skill, *recognize cues.* Eliminate options 1 and 3 first because they are comparable or alike options and indicate an absence of pain. From the remaining options note that option 2 indicates a sign opposite to the sign in option 4. This provides a clue that one of these options is the correct one. Recalling the signs of abruptio placentae will direct you to the correct option. **Review:** Signs of **abruptio placentae**.

Tip for the Nursing Student: In abruptio placentae the normally implanted placenta separates before the fetus is born. The major concerns for the mother are bleeding, shock, and clotting abnormalities. The major concerns for the fetus are blood loss, anoxia, preterm birth, and fetal death.

21. The nurse is collecting data on a client with severe preeclampsia. Which sign would indicate an improvement in the client's condition?

1 Headache is no longer present.
2 Blood pressure is 148/106 mm Hg.
3 Client complains of abdominal pain.
4 Blood urea nitrogen is 40 mg/dL (14.28 mmol/L).

Level of Cognitive Ability: Evaluating
Client Needs: Physiological Integrity
Clinical Judgment/Cognitive Skills: Evaluate Outcomes
Integrated Process: Nursing Process/ Evaluation
Content Area: Maternity
Priority Concepts: Clinical Judgment; Perfusion
Level of Nursing Student: Intermediate

ANSWER: 1
Rationale: Preeclampsia is considered mild when the diastolic blood pressure does not exceed 100 mm Hg and symptoms such as headache, visual disturbances, or abdominal pain are absent. In addition, signs of kidney or liver involvement are absent. An elevated blood urea nitrogen level indicates the presence of kidney damage as a result of preeclampsia.

Test-Taking Strategy: Apply the clinical judgment/cognitive skill, *evaluate outcomes.* Focus on the subject, an improvement in the client's condition, noting the words *severe preeclampsia* and *improvement in the client's condition.* Note the words *no longer present* in option 1. This is the only option that does not indicate severe preeclampsia. **Review:** The signs of mild and severe **preeclampsia** and the signs that indicate improvement.

Tip for the Nursing Student: Preeclampsia is an abnormal condition of pregnancy characterized by the onset of acute hypertension after week 24 of gestation. Manifestations include hypertension. If preeclampsia is untreated, it can lead to serious complications, such as premature separation of the placenta or eclampsia (seizures).

---

22. Artificial rupture of the membranes is done to induce labor in a client. After this procedure, what is the **immediate** nursing action?

1 Clean the client's perineal area.
2 Check the fetal heart rate (FHR).
3 Place the client in a comfortable position.
4 Tell the client that a wet feeling in the perineal area is normal and expected.

Level of Cognitive Ability: Analyzing
Client Needs: Physiological Integrity
Clinical Judgment/Cognitive Skills: Take Action
Integrated Process: Nursing Process/ Implementation
Content Area: Maternity
Priority Concepts: Clinical Judgment; Safety
Level of Nursing Student: Intermediate

ANSWER: 2
Rationale: Artificial rupture of the membranes may be done to augment or induce labor or to facilitate placement of internal monitors when fetal status indicates the need for some form of direct monitoring. Because the umbilical cord can prolapse when the membranes rupture, the FHR and fetal pattern need to be monitored immediately and for several minutes after the procedure to ascertain fetal well-being. Although options 1, 3, and 4 are appropriate, they are not the priority concern. In addition, in the preprocedure period (rather than postprocedure period), the client should be told that a wet feeling in the perineal area is normal and expected.

Test-Taking Strategy: Apply the clinical judgment/cognitive skill, *take action.* Note the strategic word, *immediate.* Use the ABCs—airway, breathing, and circulation—to direct you to the correct option. Also, use of the steps of the nursing process will direct you to option 2 because it is the only option that addresses assessment/ data collection. **Review:** Care of the client after **artificial rupture of the membranes**.

Tip for the Nursing Student: Artificial rupture of the membranes is also known as *amniotomy* and is done to stimulate labor. In this procedure, performed by the primary health care provider or nurse-midwife, a disposable plastic hook is inserted through the cervix to the amniotic membranes and a hole is made to allow the amniotic fluid to drain. Major risks associated with amniotomy include prolapse of the umbilical cord, infection, and abruptio placentae (abnormal separation of the placenta from the uterine wall).

23. A client in labor tells the nurse that she suddenly has a wet feeling in the vaginal area. The nurse quickly checks the client and notes a large amount of bright red blood. What is the **immediate** nursing action?
1 Notify the obstetrician.
2 Insert an intravenous catheter.
3 Prepare to perform a vaginal examination.
4 Prepare the client for an emergency cesarean birth.

Level of Cognitive Ability: Analyzing
Client Needs: Physiological Integrity
Clinical Judgment/Cognitive Skills: Take Action
Integrated Process: Nursing Process/ Implementation
Content Area: Maternity
Priority Concepts: Clinical Judgment; Perfusion
Level of Nursing Student: Intermediate

ANSWER: 1
Rationale: Vaginal bleeding (bright red, dark red, or in an amount in excess of that expected during normal cervical dilation) requires immediate notification of the obstetrician. This finding indicates an emergency situation and could have occurred as a result of placenta previa or placental separation. Although the nurse will prepare the client for an emergency cesarean delivery and insert an intravenous catheter, these are not the immediate actions. A vaginal examination is not performed on a pregnant client who is bleeding vaginally.

Test-Taking Strategy: Apply the clinical judgment/cognitive skill, *take action*. Note the strategic word, *immediate*, and focus on the data in the question. Noting the words *large amount of bright red blood* will direct you to the correct option. Remember that when an emergency situation is presented in the question, it is likely that the correct option will be to notify the obstetrician. **Review:** Care of the **pregnant client who is bleeding vaginally**.

Tip for the Nursing Student: Vaginal bleeding during pregnancy is always a concern. Two conditions that can cause vaginal bleeding are abruptio placentae and placenta previa. In abruptio placentae, the normally implanted placenta separates before the fetus is born. Placenta previa is an abnormal condition in which the placenta is implanted low in the uterus near the cervix.

24. While caring for a client in labor, the nurse suspects an umbilical cord prolapse. What is the **immediate** nursing action?
1 Set up for an emergency cesarean delivery.
2 Adjust the bed to Trendelenburg's position.
3 Encourage the woman to push with each contraction.
4 Calmly reassure the woman and her partner that all possible measures are being taken.

Level of Cognitive Ability: Applying
Client Needs: Physiological Integrity
Clinical Judgment/Cognitive Skills: Take Action
Integrated Process: Nursing Process/ Implementation
Content Area: Maternity
Priority Concepts: Clinical Judgment; Perfusion
Level of Nursing Student: Intermediate

ANSWER: 2
Rationale: Adjusting the bed into Trendelenburg's position (mattress flat, foot of bed elevated) uses gravity to reverse the direction of the pressure, keeping the fetal presenting part off the umbilical cord. In addition, the knee–chest or modified Sims' position can be used. Pushing with contractions is contraindicated because it will push the presenting part against the cord. Not all prolapsed cords require a cesarean delivery. The nurse would reassure the woman and her partner after placing the woman in Trendelenburg's position.

Test-Taking Strategy: Apply the clinical judgment/cognitive skill, *take action*. Note the strategic word, *immediate*, and visualize the situation. Using Maslow's Hierarchy of Needs theory, eliminate option 4 first because it does not address a physiological need. From the remaining options, select the option that addresses the physiological safety of the primary client (the fetus). Also remember that in a prioritizing question, if repositioning is indicated in one of the options, that may be the correct option. **Review:** Immediate interventions for **umbilical cord prolapse**.

Tip for the Nursing Student: A prolapsed umbilical cord refers to a condition in which the umbilical cord slips down after the amniotic membranes rupture, subjecting it to compression between the fetus and pelvis. This is a serious occurrence because it causes interruption in blood flow, and thus oxygenation, through the cord to the fetus and is potentially fatal.

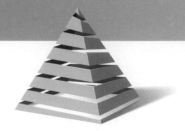

CHAPTER 17

Pediatric Questions

1. The nurse at a playground witnesses a child fall off a swing. The nurse rushes to the child and suspects that the child has a broken right leg. The nurse would take which **priority** action?
   1 Immobilize the leg.
   2 Remove the child's shoes.
   3 Tell the child that everything will be fine.
   4 Transport the child to the emergency department.

Level of Cognitive Ability: Applying
Client Needs: Physiological Integrity
Clinical Judgment/Cognitive Skills: Take Action
Integrated Process: Nursing Process/ Implementation
Content Area: Pediatrics
Priority Concepts: Clinical Judgment; Safety
Level of Nursing Student: Intermediate

ANSWER: 1
Rationale: When a fracture is suspected, the area is immobilized and splinted before the child is moved. Emergency help is called, and the nurse would remain with the child and provide realistic reassurance. Shoes are not removed because this action can cause increased trauma. Telling the child that everything will be fine is nontherapeutic.

Test-Taking Strategy: Apply the clinical judgment/cognitive skill, *take action*. Note the strategic word, *priority*. Focusing on the subject, a broken right leg, will direct you to the correct option. When a fracture is suspected, remember to immobilize and splint that area. **Review:** Care of the victim with a **fracture.**

Tip for the Nursing Student: A fracture is a break or disruption in a bone's continuity and generally occurs when traumatic or excessive force is placed on a bone. The signs and symptoms will vary, depending on the location, type, and cause of injury, but they generally include pain at the site of injury, immobility or decreased range of motion, deformity, and edema.

---

2. A newborn with a diagnosis of subdural hematoma is admitted to the newborn nursery. The nurse would perform which action to check for the major symptom associated with subdural hematoma?
   1 Monitor the urine for blood.
   2 Monitor the urinary output pattern.
   3 Test for contractures of the extremities.
   4 Test for equality of extremities when stimulating reflexes.

Level of Cognitive Ability: Analyzing
Client Needs: Physiological Integrity
Clinical Judgment/Cognitive Skills: Take Action
Integrated Process: Nursing Process/ Assessment/Data Collection
Content Area: Pediatrics
Priority Concepts: Clinical Judgment; Intracranial Regulation
Level of Nursing Student: Advanced

ANSWER: 4
Rationale: A subdural hematoma can cause pressure on a specific area of the cerebral tissue. If the newborn is actively bleeding, changes in the stimuli responses in the extremities on the opposite side of the body can occur. Options 1 and 2 are incorrect. Blood in the urine would indicate abdominal trauma and not be a result of the subdural hematoma. After delivery an infant is incontinent of urine. Option 3 is incorrect because contractures would not occur this soon after delivery.

Test-Taking Strategy: Apply the clinical judgment/cognitive skill, *take action*. Note the words *major symptom*. Eliminate options 1 and 2 first because they are comparable or alike options. Next focus on the infant's condition—subdural hematoma—and recall that this condition is a neurological disorder. Remember that the method of checking for complications and active bleeding into the cranial cavity would be a neurological assessment. Checking newborn reflexes is a neurological assessment. Although contractures of extremities could occur as residual effects, they would not occur immediately; therefore, eliminate option 3. **Review:** The signs of **subdural hematoma.**

Tip for the Nursing Student: A subdural hematoma is an accumulation of blood in the subdural space and is usually caused by an injury. It can be acute with rapid bleeding or subacute with the accumulation of blood occurring over a longer period. Because the accumulation of blood is in the cranial cavity, neurological assessment and monitoring for signs of increased intracranial pressure are priorities.

---

3. The nurse is reviewing the record of an infant admitted to the newborn nursery. The nurse notes that the primary health care provider has documented bladder exstrophy. On data collection, the nurse expects to note which finding?
   1 Undescended or hidden testes
   2 Urinary bladder on the outside of the body
   3 Opening of the urethral meatus on the ventral side of the glans penis
   4 Opening of the urethral meatus below the normal placement on the glans penis

Level of Cognitive Ability: Analyzing
Client Needs: Physiological Integrity
Clinical Judgment/Cognitive Skills: Recognize Cues
Integrated Process: Nursing Process/ Assessment/Data Collection
Content Area: Pediatrics
Priority Concepts: Clinical Judgment; Elimination
Level of Nursing Student: Advanced

ANSWER: 2
Rationale: Bladder exstrophy is a congenital anomaly characterized by the extrusion of the urinary bladder to the outside of the body through a defect in the lower abdominal wall. Option 1 describes cryptorchidism, option 3 describes epispadias, and option 4 describes hypospadias.

Test-Taking Strategy: Apply the clinical judgment/cognitive skill, *recognize cues.* Focus on the subject, findings associated with bladder exstrophy. Note the relationship between the prefix in the name of the disorder, *ex-*, and the word *outside* in option 2. In addition, note that options 3 and 4 are comparable or alike options and discuss the meatus. **Review: Bladder exstrophy.**

Tip for the Nursing Student: Bladder exstrophy is a congenital anomaly. In the newborn, the nurse would note the extrusion of the urinary bladder to the outside of the body. This occurs as a result of a defect in the lower abdominal wall. The nurse needs to institute measures as prescribed to protect the urinary bladder and prevent injury to the bladder mucosa.

---

4. The nurse notes that a child with Hirschsprung's disease who is scheduled for surgery has inadequate fluid volume. The nurse would plan to implement which intervention to stabilize the child's hydration status before surgery?
   1 Monitor daily weight.
   2 Monitor intake and output.
   3 Administer tap water enemas.
   4 Administer intravenous fluids and electrolytes.

Level of Cognitive Ability: Applying
Client Needs: Physiological Integrity
Clinical Judgment/Cognitive Skills: Generate Solutions
Integrated Process: Nursing Process/Planning
Content Area: Pediatrics
Priority Concepts: Clinical Judgment; Fluids and Electrolytes
Level of Nursing Student: Advanced

ANSWER: 4
Rationale: A child with inadequate fluid volume is stabilized with intravenous fluids and electrolytes before surgical management of the aganglionic portion of the bowel. Measurement of daily weight and intake and output assesses hydration status. Tap water enemas will alter the child's hydration status further.

Test-Taking Strategy: Apply the clinical judgment/cognitive skill, *generate solutions.* Focus on the subject, stabilizing the child's hydration status. Eliminate options 1 and 2 because they are assessments rather than interventions. Eliminate option 3 because it will cause a further decrease in fluid volume. The correct option addresses stabilization. **Review:** Care of the child with **Hirschsprung's disease.**

Tip for the Nursing Student: Hirschsprung's disease is also known as *congenital aganglionosis* or *megacolon* and is the result of an absence of ganglion cells in the rectum and, to varying degrees, upward in the colon. Constipation, signs of bowel obstruction, abdominal pain and distention, vomiting, and failure to thrive are manifestations.

5. The nurse provides home care instructions to the parents of a toddler newly diagnosed with hemophilia. Which statement by the parents indicates a **need for further instruction?**
   1 "We need to pad crib rails and table corners."
   2 "We need to obtain a medical identification bracelet for our child."
   3 "We need to administer aspirin to our child if any signs of discomfort are noted."
   4 "We need to have our child use a small, soft-bristled toothbrush for dental hygiene."

Level of Cognitive Ability: Evaluating
Client Needs: Safe and Effective Care Environment
Clinical Judgment/Cognitive Skills: Evaluate Outcomes
Integrated Process: Teaching and Learning
Content Area: Pediatrics
Priority Concepts: Perfusion; Safety
Level of Nursing Student: Intermediate

ANSWER: 3
Rationale: In the child with hemophilia, bleeding is a priority concern. Therefore, measures are implemented to prevent this occurrence. The environment needs to be made as safe as possible, and the parents are instructed to pad crib side rails and table corners to prevent injury. The child needs to wear a medical identification bracelet to alert others of the disorder. The parents are instructed about dental hygiene measures, such as using a small, soft-bristled toothbrush. Neither aspirin nor aspirin-containing compounds would be used, primarily because of their antiplatelet properties; their use can result in bleeding. Acetaminophen can be used for discomfort if needed.

Test-Taking Strategy: Apply the clinical judgment/cognitive skill, *evaluate outcomes.* Note the strategic words, *need for further instruction.* These words indicate a negative event query and the need to find the option that indicates an incorrect parental statement. Recalling that bleeding is the priority concern and that aspirin has antiplatelet properties will direct you to the correct option. **Review:** Discharge teaching points for a child with **hemophilia.**

Tip for the Nursing Student: Hemophilia is a hereditary bleeding disorder characterized by a deficiency of 1 of the factors necessary for the coagulation of blood. The severity of the disorder varies with the extent of the deficiency. Nursing care focuses on preventing bleeding and providing a safe environment.

6. The nurse is preparing to care for a pediatric client with an intravenous solution infusing. The nurse would ensure that which item is in place to prevent fluid overload in this client?
   1 Armboard
   2 Infusion pump
   3 Macrodrip infusion set
   4 Large-bore intravenous catheter

Level of Cognitive Ability: Applying
Client Needs: Safe and Effective Care Environment
Clinical Judgment/Cognitive Skills: Generate Solutions
Integrated Process: Nursing Process/ Planning
Content Area: Pediatrics
Priority Concepts: Fluids and Electrolytes; Safety
Level of Nursing Student: Intermediate

ANSWER: 2
Rationale: The most effective means of preventing irregularities in volume infusion for the pediatric client is the use of an infusion pump. This prevents both overhydration and underhydration. An armboard may be helpful in certain instances to minimize movement of the extremity with the catheter, but it is not an effective means for regulating intravenous flow. A small-bore catheter and a microdrip infusion set, rather than a macrodrip set, are used in the pediatric client.

Test-Taking Strategy: Apply the clinical judgment/cognitive skill, *generate solutions.* Focus on the subject, preventing fluid overload. The only item in the options that will accomplish this is an infusion pump. **Review:** Care of the **pediatric client** receiving an **intravenous infusion.**

Tip for the Nursing Student: When a child (or adult) is receiving fluids by the intravenous route, the nurse needs to monitor the client and infusion closely to ensure that the fluid is infusing at the prescribed rate. If the fluid infuses too rapidly, serious complications can occur from the excess fluid. An infusion pump, which controls the amount of fluid infusing, needs to be used to administer intravenous fluids to a pediatric client.

7. A mother tells the clinic nurse that she does not want her child to receive any immunizations because she has heard that they cause serious illnesses. The nurse would make which appropriate statement to the mother?

1 "Are you afraid your child is going to die from the injection?"

2 "Why are you afraid? Children are immunized every day without a problem."

3 "There will be a slight discomfort at the time of the injection, but that is all that will happen."

4 "I can see you are very concerned about your child. What do you think might happen after an immunization is given?"

Level of Cognitive Ability: Applying
Client Needs: Psychosocial Integrity
Clinical Judgment/Cognitive Skills: Generate Solutions
Integrated Process: Caring
Content Area: Pediatrics
Priority Concepts: Anxiety; Immunity
Level of Nursing Student: Intermediate

ANSWER: 4
Rationale: The correct option acknowledges the mother's concern, which provides an opportunity for the mother to respond to the nurse's open-ended question. Options 1, 2, and 3 are nontherapeutic. Option 1 attempts to verify an assumption not supported in the question. Option 2 can make the mother feel defensive, devalues the mother's feelings, and requires an explanation from the mother. Option 3 provides false reassurance.

Test-Taking Strategy: Apply the clinical judgment/cognitive skill, *generate solutions.* Use therapeutic communication techniques. The correct option demonstrates empathy and helps the mother focus on specific fears so that the nurse can clarify information. Remember to focus on the client's feelings. **Review: Therapeutic communication techniques.**

Tip for the Nursing Student: An immunization is a procedure in which resistance to an infectious disease is induced. A schedule of various types of immunizations needs to be followed to prevent infectious childhood diseases. In addition, all states require immunizations for children enrolled in licensed child care programs and school (with few exceptions).

---

8. A child with hemophilia is brought into the emergency department after being hit on the neck with a baseball. The nurse would **immediately** check the child for which finding?

1 Headache
2 Slurred speech
3 Airway obstruction
4 Spontaneous hematuria

Level of Cognitive Ability: Analyzing
Client Needs: Physiological Integrity
Clinical Judgment/Cognitive Skills: Take Action
Integrated Process: Nursing Process/ Assessment/Data Collection
Content Area: Pediatrics
Priority Concepts: Gas Exchange; Perfusion
Level of Nursing Student: Intermediate

ANSWER: 3
Rationale: Trauma to the neck may cause bleeding into the tissues of the neck, which may compromise the airway. Although headache and slurred speech are associated with head trauma, from the options provided, they are not the priorities in this situation. Hematuria is a symptom of hemophilia, although it is not associated with neck injury.

Test-Taking Strategy: Apply the clinical judgment/cognitive skill, *take action.* Note the strategic word, *immediately.* Use the ABCs— airway, breathing, and circulation. Airway assessment is always a first priority. This directs you to the correct option. **Review: Care of the child with hemophilia.**

Tip for the Nursing Student: Hemophilia is a hereditary bleeding disorder characterized by a deficiency of 1 of the factors necessary for the coagulation of blood. The severity of the disorder varies with the extent of the deficiency. Bleeding is always a concern if the child is injured.

---

9. A 4-year-old child is admitted to the hospital for surgery. The nurse would ask the parents which **priority** question to identify the adequacy of support for the child's psychosocial needs?

ANSWER: 3
Rationale: Separation from family is the most stressful aspect of hospitalization in young children. A primary goal is to prevent separation from family in children under the age of 5 years. Identifying support and the ability of family members to stay with the child takes priority over favorite toys or diversional activities. Options 2 and 4 relate to physiological needs.

1 "What are your child's favorite toys?"
2 "What signs and symptoms has your child been having?"
3 "Will a family member be able to stay with the child most of the time?"
4 "How much do you know about the surgery and its expected outcome?"

Level of Cognitive Ability: Analyzing
Client Needs: Psychosocial Integrity
Clinical Judgment/Cognitive Skills: Take Action
Integrated Process: Nursing Process/ Assessment/Data Collection
Content Area: Pediatrics
Priority Concepts: Anxiety; Stress and Coping
Level of Nursing Student: Intermediate

Test-Taking Strategy: Apply the clinical judgment/cognitive skill, *take action*. Note the strategic word, *priority*. Focus on the subject, adequacy of support and the child's psychosocial needs. Options 2 and 4 relate to physiological needs, so eliminate these options. From the remaining options, use Maslow's Hierarchy of Needs theory to select the security issue instead of the diversional activity. **Review:** Psychosocial needs of a **hospitalized toddler.**

Tip for the Nursing Student: Hospitalization can be a stressful experience for the child, who can experience separation anxiety. How a child reacts to the experience depends on a number of factors, including age, cognitive development, preparation for the experience, coping skills, cultural influences, and previous experience with the health care system.

---

10. The nurse is assessing a child who has just returned from surgery in a hip spica cast. Which outcome is the **priority**?
    1 The hips are adducted.
    2 Circulation is adequate.
    3 The child is on the right side.
    4 The head of the bed is elevated.

Level of Cognitive Ability: Evaluating
Client Needs: Physiological Integrity
Clinical Judgment/Cognitive Skills: Evaluate Outcomes
Integrated Process: Nursing Process/ Evaluation
Content Area: Pediatrics
Priority Concepts: Clinical Judgment; Perfusion
Level of Nursing Student: Intermediate

ANSWER: 2
Rationale: The priority concern during the first few hours after a cast is applied is swelling, which may cause the cast to act as a tourniquet and constrict circulation. Therefore, circulatory assessment is a high priority. The hip spica cast immobilizes the hip and knee. Turning the child side to side at least every 2 hours is important because it allows the body cast to dry evenly and prevents complications related to immobility; however, it is not a higher priority than checking circulation. Elevating the head of a bed of a child in a hip spica cast is not recommended, as it causes discomfort.

Test-Taking Strategy: Apply the clinical judgment/cognitive skill, *evaluate outcomes*. Note the strategic word, *priority*. Use the ABCs— airway, breathing, and circulation. The correct option addresses circulation. **Review:** Care of the child in a **hip spica cast.**

Tip for the Nursing Student: A hip spica cast is an orthopedic cast that is applied to immobilize part or all of the body trunk and part or all of the lower extremities. It is used to treat various fractures, such as fractures of the hip or femur, and to correct a hip deformity. It may be used to treat developmental dysplasia of the hip, a condition in which the head of the femur is improperly seated in the acetabulum of the pelvis.

---

11. The parents of a newborn diagnosed with esophageal atresia ask the nurse to explain the diagnosis. What would the nurse plan to tell the parents regarding this condition?
    1 Gastric contents regurgitate back into the esophagus.
    2 The esophagus terminates before it reaches the stomach.
    3 A portion of the stomach protrudes through part of the diaphragm.
    4 Abdominal contents herniate through an opening of the diaphragm.

ANSWER: 2
Rationale: Esophageal atresia and tracheoesophageal fistula (TEF) are congenital malformations in which the esophagus terminates before it reaches the stomach and/or a fistula is present that forms an unnatural connection with the trachea. Option 1 describes gastroesophageal reflux. Option 3 describes a hiatal hernia. Option 4 describes a congenital diaphragmatic hernia.

Test-Taking Strategy: Apply the clinical judgment/cognitive skill, *generate solutions*. Focus on the subject and diagnosis, esophageal atresia. Note the relationship between the word *atresia* and the correct option. **Review:** The characteristics of **esophageal atresia.**

Level of Cognitive Ability: Applying
Client Needs: Physiological Integrity
Clinical Judgment/Cognitive Skills: Generate
  Solutions
Integrated Process: Nursing Process/Planning
Content Area: Pediatrics
Priority Concepts: Client Education; Tissue
  Integrity
Level of Nursing Student: Intermediate

Tip for the Nursing Student: Esophageal atresia is a congenital malformation in which the esophagus terminates before it reaches the stomach. It can cause respiratory distress secondary to the aspiration of saliva and any oral fluids that may be given to the newborn. Some manifestations of the disorder include excessive oral secretions, abdominal distention, and vomiting. Surgical repair will need to be done to correct the condition.

---

12. A mother brings her child to the emergency department because the child said that dirt flew into their eye during softball practice. The nurse would plan to assist with which action **first?**
    1 Assess vision.
    2 Remove the dirt.
    3 Place ice on the eye.
    4 Irrigate the eye with sterile saline.

Level of Cognitive Ability: Applying
Client Needs: Physiological Integrity
Clinical Judgment/Cognitive Skills: Generate
  Solutions
Integrated Process: Nursing Process/
  Planning
Content Area: Pediatrics
Priority Concepts: Sensory Perception; Tissue
  Integrity
Level of Nursing Student: Advanced

ANSWER: 1
Rationale: If a surface foreign body injury occurs to the eye, the nurse would first assess visual acuity. The eye will then be assessed for corneal abrasions, followed by irrigating the eye with sterile normal saline to gently remove the particles. There is no reason to place ice on the eye. Placing ice on the eye would be done if the client sustained an eye contusion.

Test-Taking Strategy: Apply the clinical judgment/cognitive skill, *generate solutions.* Note the strategic word, *first,* and use the steps of the nursing process. The correct option is the only option that relates to assessment/data collection. Options 2, 3, and 4 relate to implementation. **Review:** Content related to initial treatment of various **eye injuries**.

Tip for the Nursing Student: Interventions to treat an eye injury are based on the type of injury that occurred. If a contusion (blow) to the eye occurred, the nurse would immediately place ice on the eye. If a chemical substance splashed into the eye, the immediate intervention is to flush (irrigate) the eye. If dirt flew into the eye, the nurse would assess vision and check for the presence of the dirt substances and corneal abrasions before irrigating the eye.

---

13. The nurse is monitoring a child with increased intracranial pressure who has been exhibiting decorticate posturing. On data collection, the nurse notes extension of the upper and lower extremities with internal rotation of the upper arms, wrists, knees, and feet. How would the nurse interpret the child's condition?
    1 Is unchanged
    2 Has improved
    3 Indicates decreased intracranial pressure
    4 Indicates a deterioration in neurological function

Level of Cognitive Ability: Analyzing
Client Needs: Physiological Integrity
Clinical Judgment/Cognitive Skills: Analyze
  Cues

ANSWER: 4
Rationale: In decorticate posturing the nurse would note flexion of the upper extremities and extension of the lower extremities. In decerebrate posturing the nurse would note extension of the upper and lower extremities with internal rotation of the upper arms, wrists, knees, and feet. The progression from decorticate to decerebrate posturing usually indicates deteriorating neurological function and warrants primary health care provider notification. Options 1, 2, and 3 are inaccurate interpretations.

Test-Taking Strategy: Apply the clinical judgment/cognitive skill, *analyze cues.* Focus on the data in the question and determine whether an abnormality exists. Eliminate options 2 and 3 first because they are comparable or alike options. From the remaining options, recalling the significance of decerebrate posturing will direct you to the correct option. **Review:** The significance of **posturing.**

Integrated Process: Nursing Process/Analysis
Content Area: Pediatrics
Priority Concepts: Clinical Judgment;
Intracranial Regulation
Level of Nursing Student: Advanced

Tip for the Nursing Student: Posture is the position of the body and is determined and maintained by coordination of the muscles that move the limbs and a sense of balance. Abnormal postures occur in neurological disorders, such as head injuries, and in conditions that cause increased intracranial pressure. These types of posturing include decorticate, decerebrate, and flaccid.

---

14. The nurse is reviewing the assessment findings and laboratory results of a child diagnosed with new-onset glomerulonephritis. Which finding would the nurse **most likely** expect to note?
    1 Hypotension
    2 Tea-colored urine
    3 Low serum potassium
    4 Elevated creatinine levels

Level of Cognitive Ability: Analyzing
Client Needs: Physiological Integrity
Clinical Judgment/Cognitive Skills: Recognize Cues
Integrated Process: Nursing Process/ Assessment/Data Collection
Content Area: Pediatrics
Priority Concepts: Elimination; Inflammation
Level of Nursing Student: Intermediate

ANSWER: 2
Rationale: Gross hematuria resulting in dark brown or smoky, tea-colored urine is a classic finding in glomerulonephritis. Hypertension is also a common finding in glomerulonephritis. Blood urea nitrogen levels and creatinine levels are elevated only when there is an 80% decrease in glomerular filtration rate and renal insufficiency is severe. A high serum potassium level results from inadequate glomerular filtration.

Test-Taking Strategy: Apply the clinical judgment/cognitive skill, *recognize cues*. Note that the child is experiencing a renal disorder, and note the words *new-onset* and the strategic words, *most likely*. Recalling that the creatinine level is elevated only when there is an 80% decrease in glomerular filtration rate will assist in eliminating option 4. Next eliminate options 1 and 3, knowing that hypertension, rather than hypotension, and hyperkalemia, rather than hypokalemia, will occur in this renal disorder. **Review:** The clinical manifestations associated with **glomerulonephritis.**

Tip for the Nursing Student: Glomerulonephritis is a kidney disorder characterized by an inflammatory injury in the glomerulus. It is characterized by proteinuria, hematuria, decreased urine production, and edema (swelling). Acute poststreptococcal glomerulonephritis is the most common type and occurs as an immune reaction to a group A beta-hemolytic streptococcal infection of the throat.

---

15. A child newly diagnosed with type 1 diabetes mellitus who is receiving insulin suddenly experiences signs of a hypoglycemic reaction. Which item would the nurse give to the child **immediately?**
    1 1 cup of diet cola
    2 8 oz of skim milk
    3 ½ teaspoon of sugar
    4 ½ teaspoon of honey

Level of Cognitive Ability: Applying
Client Needs: Physiological Integrity
Clinical Judgment/Cognitive Skills: Take Action
Integrated Process: Nursing Process/ Implementation
Content Area: Pediatrics
Priority Concepts: Clinical Judgment; Glucose Regulation
Level of Nursing Student: Intermediate

ANSWER: 2
Rationale: Hypoglycemia is immediately treated with 15 g of carbohydrate. Glucose tablets or glucose gel may be administered. Other items used to treat hypoglycemia include 8 oz of skim milk, ½ cup of fruit juice, ½ cup of regular (nondiet) soft drink, 6 to 10 hard candies, 4 cubes or 4 teaspoons of sugar, 6 saltines, 3 graham crackers, or 1 tablespoon of honey or syrup. The items in options 1, 3, and 4 would not adequately treat hypoglycemia.

Test-Taking Strategy: Apply the clinical judgment/cognitive skill, *take action*. Note the strategic word, *immediately*. Eliminate options 3 and 4 first because they are comparable or alike options. From the remaining options, select option 2 because a diet cola does not contain the amount of carbohydrate needed to treat hypoglycemia. **Review:** The treatment measures for **hypoglycemia.**

Tip for the Nursing Student: Diabetes mellitus is a disorder of carbohydrate, fat, and protein metabolism that is primarily the result of a deficiency or complete lack of insulin secretion by the beta cells of the pancreas or resistance to insulin. Hypoglycemia (a low blood glucose level) is a complication and is characterized by symptoms such as weakness, headache, hunger, and visual disturbances. It is immediately treated with 15 g of carbohydrate. It is important to recognize the signs and symptoms of hypoglycemia and how to treat it.

16. The clinic nurse has provided instructions to the mother of a child with a urinary tract infection. Which statements by the mother indicate a **need for further instruction? Select all that apply.**
    - ☐ 1 "I need to increase my child's fluid intake."
    - ☐ 2 "I need to not use bubble baths with my child."
    - ☐ 3 "I need to wipe my child from front to back after urination or a bowel movement."
    - ☐ 4 "I should encourage my child to hold the urine and to urinate only four times each day."
    - ☐ 5 "I need to administer the antibiotics to my child until urinary tract infection symptoms disappear."

Level of Cognitive Ability: Evaluating
Client Needs: Physiological Integrity
Clinical Judgment/Cognitive Skills: Evaluate Outcomes
Integrated Process: Teaching and Learning
Content Area: Pediatrics
Priority Concepts: Client Education; Infection
Level of Nursing Student: Intermediate

ANSWER: 4, 5
Rationale: Fluid intake, including water, needs to be encouraged. Bubble baths are avoided secondary to possible urethral irritation. The parents need to be taught to wipe the child from front to back after urination or a bowel movement to avoid moving bacteria from the anus to the urethra. The child needs to be encouraged to avoid holding urine and to urinate at least every 2 to 3 hours and should be told that the bladder should be emptied with each void to avoid residual urine (have child sit for a full minute or two). Additionally, the full course of prescribed antibiotics need to be taken to prevent recurrence and emergence of resistant organisms.

Test-Taking Strategy: Apply the clinical judgment/cognitive skill, *evaluate outcomes.* Note the strategic words, *need for further instruction.* These words indicate a negative event query and the need to look for the incorrect statement. Careful reading of the options and applying principles related to prevention of urinary tract infections will direct you to options 4 and 5 as incorrect actions. Also, note the closed-ended word "only" in option 4. **Review:** Client instructions related to a **urinary tract infection.**

Tip for the Nursing Student: A urinary tract infection is an infection of one or more structures in the urinary system. The infection is usually characterized by urinary frequency, burning pain with urinating, fever, back pain, and possible blood or pus in the urine. The symptoms differ if infection is in the kidneys or in the bladder only. A sterile urine specimen is collected to check for the bacteria causing the infection and to determine treatment.

---

17. The nurse is monitoring a newborn of a mother with diabetes mellitus. The nurse recognizes that the newborn is at risk for which complication?
    1 Hypercalcemia
    2 Hyperglycemia
    3 Hypobilirubinemia
    4 Respiratory distress syndrome

Level of Cognitive Ability: Analyzing
Client Needs: Physiological Integrity
Clinical Judgment/Cognitive Skills: Analyze Cues
Integrated Process: Nursing Process/Analysis
Content Area: Pediatrics
Priority Concepts: Clinical Judgment; Glucose Regulation
Level of Nursing Student: Advanced

ANSWER: 4
Rationale: The major neonatal complications of preexisting diabetes mellitus in the mother are hypoglycemia, hypocalcemia, hypomagnesemia, hyperbilirubinemia, and polycythemia. Congenital anomalies, macrosomia, birth trauma, perinatal asphyxia, respiratory distress syndrome, and cardiomyopathy are also problems that can occur in newborns of a diabetic mother.

Test-Taking Strategy: Apply the clinical judgment/cognitive skill, *analyze cues.* Note the subject, complications in the newborn of a mother with diabetes mellitus. Focusing on the mother's diagnosis will assist in eliminating option 2. From the remaining options, it is necessary to know these complications. **Review:** The complications associated with the newborn of the mother with **diabetes mellitus.**

Tip for the Nursing Student: It is important to know the effects of maternal diabetes on the newborn. Respiratory distress syndrome is an acute lung disease caused by a deficiency of pulmonary surfactant. Fetal hyperinsulinemia retards cortisol production, which is necessary for surfactant production. It is characterized by airless alveoli, inelastic lungs, a respiration rate greater than 60 breaths/minute, nasal flaring, retractions, grunting, and edema.

18. An adolescent client who underwent emergency surgery for a ruptured appendix refuses to allow the nurse to change the abdominal dressing, saying, "Go away. There is nothing wrong with this dressing." Which nursing response would be **best**?

1 "Please do not be upset with me. I am just doing my job."

2 "I promise to do this really quickly, and then I will leave you alone."

3 "You can refuse the dressing change at this time, but your friends cannot visit you until it is done."

4 "I will draw the curtain and expose just the area on your abdomen that is needed. Can I go ahead with that?"

Level of Cognitive Ability: Applying
Client Needs: Health Promotion and Maintenance
Clinical Judgment/Cognitive Skills: Take Action
Integrated Process: Communication and Documentation
Content Area: Pediatrics
Priority Concepts: Clinical Judgment; Development
Level of Nursing Student: Intermediate

ANSWER: 4
Rationale: The primary developmental need of the hospitalized adolescent is maintenance of privacy, modesty, and control. The correct option strives to meet these needs. Options 1 and 2 do not address the client's concerns, and option 3 contains a threat.

Test-Taking Strategy: Apply the clinical judgment/cognitive skill, *take action*. Note the strategic word, *best*, and the words *adolescent client*. Think about the developmental needs of the adolescent when answering this question. Also use therapeutic communication techniques. The correct option is the only one that focuses on the client's feelings and needs. **Review: Therapeutic communication techniques** and psychosocial needs of the **adolescent**.

Tip for the Nursing Student: Adolescence is a time of transition from childhood to adulthood and is characterized by biological and psychological changes, including the appearance of secondary sex characteristics. The adolescent is very aware of the body changes that are taking place, and the nurse needs to respect the adolescent's need for body privacy.

---

19 The nurse is caring for a child who sustained a head injury from a fall. The nurse would perform which actions in the care of the child? **Select all that apply.**

☐ **1** Restrict oral fluid intake.

☐ **2** Elevate the head of the bed.

☐ **3** Perform neurological assessments.

☐ **4** Encourage coughing and deep breathing.

☐ **5** Place the child in a flat position during sleep.

Level of Cognitive Ability: Analyzing
Client Needs: Physiological Integrity
Clinical Judgment/Cognitive Skills: Take Action
Integrated Process: Nursing Process/ Implementation
Content Area: Pediatrics
Priority Concepts: Clinical Judgment; Intracranial Regulation
Level of Nursing Student: Advanced

ANSWER: 1, 2, 3
Rationale: A child with a head injury is at risk for increased intracranial pressure (ICP). Fluids may be restricted to reduce the chance of fluid overload and resultant increased ICP. Elevating the head of the bed decreases fluid retention in cerebral tissue and promotes drainage. Neurological assessments need to be performed to monitor for increased ICP. The Valsalva maneuver associated with coughing acutely elevates ICP. Additionally, the flat position can elevate ICP and needs to be avoided.

Test-Taking Strategy: Apply the clinical judgment/cognitive skill, *take action*. Note the subject, nursing actions in the care of the child with a head injury. Recall that a head injury places the child at risk for increased ICP. From this point, identify the options that would cause an increase in the ICP; this will assist in answering correctly. **Review:** Care of the child who sustained a **head injury.**

Tip for the Nursing Student: A head injury results from trauma to the head from any mechanical force to the scalp, skull, meninges, or brain. A primary concern when a child sustains a head injury is resultant pressure in the brain from swelling. This is known as increased ICP. If this occurs, structures within the cranium are compressed, which can result in serious neurological complications.

CHAPTER 18

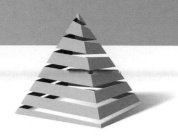

Pharmacology Questions

1. The nurse is instructing a client about quinapril hydrochloride. The nurse would make which statement to the client?
   1 To take the medication with food only
   2 To rise slowly from a lying to a sitting position
   3 To discontinue the medication if nausea occurs
   4 That a therapeutic effect will be seen immediately

Level of Cognitive Ability: Applying
Client Needs: Physiological Integrity
Clinical Judgment/Cognitive Skills: Take Action
Integrated Process: Teaching and Learning
Content Area: Pharmacology
Priority Concepts: Clinical Judgment; Safety
Level of Nursing Student: Intermediate

ANSWER: 2

Rationale: Quinapril hydrochloride is an angiotensin-converting enzyme (ACE) inhibitor used in the treatment of hypertension. The client should be instructed to rise slowly from a lying to a sitting position and to permit the legs to dangle from the bed momentarily before standing to reduce the hypotensive effect. The medication may be given without regard to food. The client needs to be instructed to drink a noncaffeinated carbonated beverage and eat crackers or dry toast if nauseated. A full therapeutic effect may occur in 1 to 2 weeks.

Test-Taking Strategy: Apply the clinical judgment/cognitive skill, *take action.* Eliminate option 1 because of the closed-ended word "only" and option 4 because of the word *immediately.* Next focus on the name of the medication and recall that most ACE inhibitor medication names end with the letters *-pril* and that these medications are used to treat hypertension. This will direct you to the correct option. **Review: Quinapril hydrochloride.**

Tip for the Nursing Student: Hypertension refers to an elevated blood pressure and is a known cardiovascular risk factor. ACE inhibitor medications are one class of medications used to treat hypertension. Because medication used to treat hypertension lowers the blood pressure, light-headedness and dizziness can occur. Therefore, it is important for the nurse to teach the client safety measures.

---

2. The nurse notes that a client is receiving ganciclovir sodium. The nurse suspects that the client is receiving this medication for the treatment of which disorder?
   1 Pancreatitis
   2 Urolithiasis
   3 Nephrotic syndrome
   4 Cytomegalovirus (CMV) retinitis

Level of Cognitive Ability: Analyzing
Client Needs: Physiological Integrity
Clinical Judgment/Cognitive Skills: Analyze Cues
Integrated Process: Nursing Process/ Analysis
Content Area: Pharmacology

ANSWER: 4

Rationale: Ganciclovir sodium is an antiviral medication used to treat CMV retinitis in immunocompromised clients and CMV gastrointestinal infections and pneumonitis; it is also used to prevent CMV disease in transplant clients. It is not used to treat pancreatitis, urolithiasis, or nephrotic syndrome.

Test-Taking Strategy: Apply the clinical judgment/cognitive skill, *analyze cues.* Note the subject, the intended effect of ganciclovir sodium. Focus on the name of the medication. Recalling that most names for antiviral medications contain the letters *vir* will direct you to the correct option. **Review: Ganciclovir sodium.**

Tip for the Nursing Student: CMV retinitis is an infection of the retina caused by a herpes type of virus. Pancreatitis is an inflammatory condition of the pancreas that can be acute or chronic. Urolithiasis

Priority Concepts: Clinical Judgment; Infection
Level of Nursing Student: Intermediate

refers to the presence of calculi (stones) in the urinary system. Nephrotic syndrome is an abnormal condition of the kidney characterized by marked proteinuria, hypoalbuminemia, and edema.

---

3. The nurse is teaching a client how to mix regular insulin (Humulin R) and isophane (Humulin N) insulin in the same syringe. Which instruction would be included?
    1 Draw up Humulin R first into the syringe.
    2 Take all air out of the bottle before mixing.
    3 Shake the Humulin N bottle before mixing.
    4 Keep both bottles stored in the refrigerator for 1 month.

Level of Cognitive Ability: Applying
Client Needs: Physiological Integrity
Clinical Judgment/Cognitive Skills: Generate Solutions
Integrated Process: Teaching and Learning
Content Area: Pharmacology
Priority Concepts: Client Education; Safety
Level of Nursing Student: Intermediate

ANSWER: **1**
Rationale: Before mixing different types of insulin, the bottle should be rotated for at least 1 minute between both hands. This resuspends the insulin and helps warm the medication. The nurse should not shake the bottles. Shaking causes foaming and bubbles to form, which may trap particles of insulin and alter the dosage. Insulin may be maintained at room temperature. Additional bottles of insulin should be stored in the refrigerator for future use. Humulin R is drawn up before Humulin N so the intermediate-acting insulin does not contaminate the regular insulin vial. Air does not need to be removed from the insulin bottle.

Test-Taking Strategy: Apply the clinical judgment/cognitive skill, *generate solutions*. Note the subject, the procedure for mixing Humulin R and Humulin N in the same syringe. Visualize the procedure as you carefully read each option. When answering questions that relate to mixing insulin, remember the letters *RN*—draw Humulin R into the syringe before Humulin N. **Review:** The procedures for administering **insulin**.

Tip for the Nursing Student: Insulin is a medication used to treat diabetes mellitus, a disorder of fat, carbohydrate, and protein metabolism. Humulin R is a short-acting insulin, and Humulin N is an intermediate-acting insulin. When both types of insulin are prescribed, they can be mixed together in one syringe so that only one injection is necessary.

---

4. A client has been taking lansoprazole. The nurse would monitor the client for the relief of which symptom?
    1 Diarrhea
    2 Heartburn
    3 Flatulence
    4 Constipation

Level of Cognitive Ability: Evaluating
Client Needs: Physiological Integrity
Clinical Judgment/Cognitive Skills: Evaluate Outcomes
Integrated Process: Nursing Process/ Evaluation
Content Area: Pharmacology
Priority Concepts: Clinical Judgment; Pain
Level of Nursing Student: Intermediate

ANSWER: **2**
Rationale: Lansoprazole is a gastric pump inhibitor (proton pump inhibitor). Its intended effect is relief of gastric irritation pain, often referred to as *heartburn*. The medication does not improve diarrhea, flatulence, or constipation.

Test-Taking Strategy: Apply the clinical judgment/cognitive skill, *evaluate outcomes*. Note the subject, intended effect of lansoprazole. Focus on the words *relief of*. Note the name of the medication, and recall that most proton pump inhibitor medication names end with the letters *-zole*. This will direct you to the correct option. **Review: Lansoprazole.**

Tip for the Nursing Student: Heartburn is a painful burning sensation in the esophagus. It is usually caused by the reflux of gastric acid into the esophagus. Proton pump inhibitors are one type of medication used to treat heartburn.

5. A client is taking amiloride hydrochloride daily. The nurse would tell the client to take the dose at what time?
   1 At bedtime
   2 On an empty stomach
   3 Between lunch and dinner
   4 In the morning with breakfast

Level of Cognitive Ability: Applying
Client Needs: Physiological Integrity
Clinical Judgment/Cognitive Skills: Generate Solutions
Integrated Process: Teaching and Learning
Content Area: Pharmacology
Priority Concepts: Client Education; Fluids and Electrolytes
Level of Nursing Student: Intermediate

ANSWER: 4
Rationale: Amiloride hydrochloride is a potassium-sparing diuretic used to treat edema or hypertension. A daily dose should be taken in the morning to avoid nocturia. The dose should be taken with food to increase bioavailability.

Test-Taking Strategy: Apply the clinical judgment/cognitive skill, *generate solutions.* Eliminate options 1, 2, and 3 because they are comparable or alike options in that they all indicate taking the medication dose without food. **Review: Amiloride hydrochloride.**

Tip for the Nursing Student: Edema is the abnormal accumulation of fluid in body tissues. Hypertension refers to an elevated blood pressure and is a known cardiovascular risk factor. Potassium-sparing diuretics are one class of medications used to treat edema or hypertension. Only a few medications are potassium sparing, and amiloride is one of them. A concern with potassium-sparing diuretics is that the client retains potassium, which can lead to hyperkalemia (a high potassium level). Therefore, the nurse monitors the client for signs of hyperkalemia.

6. The nurse is caring for a client with a diagnosis of rheumatoid arthritis who is receiving aspirin 5 g orally daily. The nurse recognizes which finding as an adverse effect related to the medication?
   1 Tinnitus
   2 Joint pain
   3 Urinary retention
   4 Difficulty voiding

Level of Cognitive Ability: Analyzing
Client Needs: Physiological Integrity
Clinical Judgment/Cognitive Skills: Recognize Cues
Integrated Process: Nursing Process/Assessment/Data Collection
Content Area: Pharmacology
Priority Concepts: Safety; Sensory Perception
Level of Nursing Student: Intermediate

ANSWER: 1
Rationale: Aspirin is a nonsteroidal anti-inflammatory medication. Adverse effects include gastrointestinal bleeding or gastric mucosal lesions, ringing in the ears (tinnitus), or generalized pruritus. Headache, dizziness, flushing, tachycardia, hyperventilation, sweating, and thirst are also adverse effects. Options 2, 3, and 4 are not adverse effects. In addition, aspirin is administered to the client with rheumatoid arthritis to relieve joint pain.

Test-Taking Strategy: Apply the clinical judgment/cognitive skill, *recognize cues.* Focus on the subject, an adverse effect of aspirin. Eliminate options 3 and 4 first because they are comparable or alike options. Next eliminate option 2 because aspirin is administered to relieve joint pain. Last, remembering that aspirin can cause gastrointestinal disturbances and ototoxicity will direct you to the correct option. **Review: Aspirin.**

Tip for the Nursing Student: Arthritis is an inflammatory condition of the joints characterized by pain, swelling, heat, redness, and limitation of movement. It can affect the client's ability to perform activities of daily living and result in debilitation. Arthritis can occur in childhood or adulthood. Large doses of aspirin may be administered to alleviate the joint pain. However, aspirin can cause gastrointestinal bleeding, ringing in the ears (tinnitus), or generalized pruritus.

7. The nurse is creating a plan of care for a client who is receiving meperidine hydrochloride for pain. The nurse would include in the plan to monitor for which adverse effect of this medication?

ANSWER: 4
Rationale: Frequent side effects of this medication include sedation, decreased blood pressure, diaphoresis, flushed face, dizziness, nausea, vomiting, and constipation. Adverse effects include respiratory depression; skeletal muscle flaccidity; cold and clammy skin; cyanosis; and extreme somnolence progressing to seizures, stupor, and coma.

1 Nausea
2 Sedation
3 Flushed face
4 Skeletal muscle flaccidity

Level of Cognitive Ability: Creating
Client Needs: Physiological Integrity
Clinical Judgment/Cognitive Skills: Generate Solutions
Integrated Process: Nursing Process/Planning
Content Area: Pharmacology
Priority Concepts: Pain; Safety
Level of Nursing Student: Intermediate

Test-Taking Strategy: Apply the clinical judgment/cognitive skill, *generate solutions*. Focus on the subject, an adverse effect, and recall that meperidine hydrochloride is an opioid analgesic. Recalling that an adverse effect is more severe than a side effect and is always an undesirable effect will direct you to the correct option. **Review:** The adverse effects of **meperidine hydrochloride**.

Tip for the Nursing Student: Meperidine hydrochloride is an opioid analgesic that has been used to alleviate pain in many types of disorders. This medication is not prescribed as frequently as it has been in the past because a metabolite of meperidine can be toxic, and the buildup of toxin in the blood can cause seizures and other mental status changes such as acute confusion. The nurse would monitor the client who is receiving this medication closely. Because meperidine hydrochloride is an opioid analgesic, it may cause skeletal muscle flaccidity, which can place the client at risk for injury. Another critical adverse effect of opioid analgesics is respiratory depression, so assessment of respiratory status is an important part of your nursing interventions.

---

8. Theophylline is prescribed for a client with bronchial asthma. The nurse provides dietary instructions to the client and would tell the client to avoid consuming which item?
    1 Iced tea
    2 Lemonade
    3 Orange juice
    4 Tomato juice

Level of Cognitive Ability: Applying
Client Needs: Physiological Integrity
Clinical Judgment/Cognitive Skills: Generate Solutions
Integrated Process: Teaching and Learning
Content Area: Pharmacology
Priority Concepts: Client Education; Gas Exchange
Level of Nursing Student: Intermediate

ANSWER: 1
Rationale: The client is instructed to avoid the use of products that contain caffeine, such as cola, coffee, tea, and chocolate, because caffeine could lead to an increased incidence of cardiovascular and central nervous system side/adverse effects of the medication. The items in options 2, 3, and 4 are acceptable to consume.

Test-Taking Strategy: Apply the clinical judgment/cognitive skill, *generate solutions*. Recall that medication names that end with the letters *-line* are xanthine bronchodilators and that these medications can cause cardiovascular and central nervous system side/adverse effects. Also, eliminate options 2, 3, and 4 because they are comparable or alike options in that they are fruit drinks. **Review:** The items to be avoided by a client taking a **xanthine bronchodilator**.

Tip for the Nursing Student: Theophylline is a xanthine bronchodilator that dilates bronchial airways and pulmonary blood vessels and is used to treat respiratory disorders, such as bronchial asthma, bronchitis, emphysema, chronic obstructive pulmonary disease, or bronchospasm. An important point to remember is that these medications can cause cardiovascular and central nervous system side/adverse effects, particularly if taken with caffeine-containing products. Therefore, an important teaching point is to tell the client to avoid caffeine-containing products. In addition, another important intervention is to monitor the client for changes in the cardiovascular or central nervous system.

---

9. The nurse is providing instructions to a client about lithium carbonate, which has been prescribed for acute mania. The nurse would provide which information to the client?

ANSWER: 4
Rationale: Because therapeutic and toxic dosage ranges are so close, lithium blood levels must be monitored closely (every 3 or 4 days at the initiation of therapy and then every 1 to 2 months). The client needs to be instructed to notify the primary health care provider if excessive diarrhea, vomiting, blurred vision, or other signs

1 Foods that contain salt need to be avoided.

2 Medication blood levels need to be checked yearly.

3 Vomiting and diarrhea are expected effects of the medication.

4 Blurred vision needs to be reported to the primary health care provider.

Level of Cognitive Ability: Applying
Client Needs: Physiological Integrity
Clinical Judgment/Cognitive Skills: Generate Solutions
Integrated Process: Teaching and Learning
Content Area: Pharmacology
Priority Concepts: Client Education; Safety
Level of Nursing Student: Intermediate

of toxicity occur. A normal diet and normal salt and fluid intake (1500 to 2500 mL per day of fluid) needs to be maintained because lithium decreases sodium reabsorption in the renal tubules, which could cause sodium depletion. A low sodium intake causes an increase in lithium retention and could lead to toxicity.

Test-Taking Strategy: Apply the clinical judgment/cognitive skill, *generate solutions.* Focus on the subject, client instructions regarding lithium carbonate. Recall the action of this medication and that toxicity is a concern with its use. This will direct you to the correct option. Also eliminate options 1, 2, and 3 because of the words *avoided, yearly,* and *are expected,* respectively, in these options. **Review:** The client teaching points related to the administration of **lithium carbonate**.

Tip for the Nursing Student: Lithium carbonate is an antimanic and antidepressant medication used to treat the manic phase of bipolar disease, which is a manic-depressive disorder. A primary concern when administering this medication is the risk for toxicity. Therefore, monitoring blood levels for toxicity is important. For long-term control, a therapeutic maintenance serum lithium level ranges between approximately 0.8 and 1.2 mEq/L (0.8 and 1.2 mmol/L). The client is taught about the importance of monitoring follow-up blood levels, diet and fluid requirements, and the signs and symptoms of toxicity.

---

10. Allopurinol has been prescribed for a client with gout, and the nurse provides instructions to the client about the medication. The nurse would tell the client that this medication has been prescribed to perform which therapeutic action?

1 Relieve pain

2 Maintain dilute urine

3 Reduce the uric acid level in the body

4 Reduce the need to consume large amounts of fluid

Level of Cognitive Ability: Applying
Client Needs: Physiological Integrity
Clinical Judgment/Cognitive Skills: Generate Solutions
Integrated Process: Teaching and Learning
Content Area: Pharmacology
Priority Concepts: Cellular Regulation; Client Education
Level of Nursing Student: Intermediate

ANSWER: 3

Rationale: Allopurinol is used in the treatment of gout to reduce uric acid production. Options 1, 2, and 4 are not actions of the medication. Clients taking allopurinol are encouraged to drink at least 10 to 12 (8-ounce) glasses of water per day to aid in uric acid excretion. Although the urine may become dilute as a result of increased fluid intake, dilute urine is not an action of the medication. This medication does not relieve pain.

Test-Taking Strategy: Apply the clinical judgment/cognitive skill, *generate solutions.* Focus on the subject, the therapeutic action of allopurinol. Note that the question identifies the client's diagnosis. Recalling the pathophysiology associated with gout will direct you to option 3. **Review:** The action of **allopurinol**.

Tip for the Nursing Student: Gout is a disease associated with an inborn error of metabolism that increases the production of or interferes with the excretion of uric acid. The excess uric acid is converted to urate crystals and deposits in joints and other tissues. The great toe is a common site for the accumulation of urate crystals. This condition can cause exceedingly painful swelling of the joint. Medication to reduce uric acid production is an important component of treatment. It is important to remind clients who take allopurinol that periodic liver function testing is needed because the medication can be hepatotoxic.

11. A client with bulimia nervosa was started on fluoxetine hydrochloride 10 mg daily 3 days ago. The client calls the clinic and reports experiencing nausea after taking the medication and wants to stop taking it. What would the nurse instruct the client to do?
   1 Take the medication with milk.
   2 Contact the primary health care provider.
   3 Lie down for 30 minutes after taking the medication.
   4 Decrease the medication dose until a different medication can be prescribed.

Level of Cognitive Ability: Applying
Client Needs: Physiological Integrity
Clinical Judgment/Cognitive Skills: Generate Solutions
Integrated Process: Teaching and Learning
Content Area: Pharmacology
Priority Concepts: Adherence; Client Education
Level of Nursing Student: Intermediate

ANSWER: 1
Rationale: Fluoxetine hydrochloride is an antidepressant, antiobsessional agent, and antibulimic. The client who experiences gastrointestinal distress needs to be instructed to take the medication with food or milk. Although nausea may be a sign of toxicity (overdosage), this client has been taking the medication for only 3 days, and overdosage is unlikely to occur in this short period. Therefore, it is unnecessary to contact the primary health care provider. Lying down for 30 minutes after taking the medication is not the best measure to alleviate the client's complaint. The nurse would not instruct a client to alter a medication dose or stop a medication.

Test-Taking Strategy: Apply the clinical judgment/cognitive skill, *generate solutions.* Note the subject, client instructions regarding fluoxetine hydrochloride. Eliminate option 4 using general guidelines related to medication administration. Focus on the data in the question, and note that the client has been taking the medication for 3 days. This will assist in directing you to the correct option. **Review: Fluoxetine hydrochloride.**

Tip for the Nursing Student: Bulimia nervosa is an eating disorder that is characterized by craving for food, often resulting in episodes of continuous eating followed by purging, depression, and self-deprivation. Treatment consists of measures to improve nourishment and therapy to overcome the underlying emotional conflicts leading to the disorder.

---

12. The nurse is caring for a client with a diagnosis of venous thrombosis in the left lower leg who is receiving heparin sodium by continuous intravenous (IV) infusion. The nurse would monitor the client for which manifestation indicating an adverse effect of this therapy?
   1 Nausea
   2 Dark urine
   3 Left calf tenderness
   4 Increased blood pressure

Level of Cognitive Ability: Analyzing
Client Needs: Physiological Integrity
Clinical Judgment/Cognitive Skills: Recognize Cues
Integrated Process: Nursing Process/ Assessment/Data Collection
Content Area: Pharmacology
Priority Concepts: Clinical Judgment; Perfusion
Level of Nursing Student: Advanced

ANSWER: 2
Rationale: The client who receives heparin sodium is at risk for bleeding. The nurse monitors for signs of bleeding, which include bleeding from the gums, ecchymoses on the skin, red or dark urine, black or red stools, and body fluids that test positive for occult blood. Tenderness is likely to be noted in the area of the thrombosis. Nausea and increased blood pressure are not signs of an adverse effect of the medication.

Test-Taking Strategy: Apply the clinical judgment/cognitive skill, *recognize cues.* Note the subject, an adverse effect. Focus on the name of the medication and the client's diagnosis. Recalling the manifestations of venous thrombosis will assist in eliminating option 3. Next, recalling that this medication is an anticoagulant will direct you to option 2. **Review: Heparin sodium.**

Tip for the Nursing Student: Venous thrombosis is also known as *phlebothrombosis* and is an abnormal condition in which a clot forms within a vein. It is usually caused by hemostasis, hypercoagulability, or occlusion. A concern with this disorder is that the clot will break free from the vein and travel to the lungs, causing a pulmonary embolus, which can be life threatening. Therefore, heparin sodium is administered to prevent further extension of the existing clot or new clot formation.

13. A postoperative client has a prescription to begin short-term therapy with enoxaparin. The nurse would plan to explain to the client that this medication is being prescribed for which therapeutic action?
1 Prevent pain
2 Relieve back spasms
3 Increase energy levels
4 Reduce the risk of deep vein thrombosis

Level of Cognitive Ability: Applying
Client Needs: Physiological Integrity
Clinical Judgment/Cognitive Skills: Generate Solutions
Integrated Process: Nursing Process/ Planning
Content Area: Pharmacology
Priority Concepts: Client Education; Perfusion
Level of Nursing Student: Intermediate

ANSWER: 4
Rationale: Enoxaparin is an anticoagulant that is administered to prevent deep vein thrombosis and thromboembolism in selected clients, such as postoperative clients after hip or knee replacement therapy. It is not used to prevent pain, relieve back spasms, or increase energy levels.

Test-Taking Strategy: Apply the clinical judgment/cognitive skill, *generate solutions*. Focus on the subject, an intended medication effect. Noting the word *postoperative* in the question will assist in eliminating options 2 and 3. From the remaining options, recalling that this medication is an anticoagulant will direct you to the correct option. **Review:** Intended effects of **enoxaparin**.

Tip for the Nursing Student: Deep vein thrombosis is a disorder involving a thrombus in one of the deep veins in the body. Thromboembolism is a condition in which a blood vessel is obstructed by a clot carried in the bloodstream from its site of formation. These are potentially life-threatening disorders, and treatment may include bed rest and the use of anticoagulant medications. Enoxaparin is a medication that will prevent deep vein thrombosis and thromboembolism and is prescribed for clients at risk for the development of these disorders.

---

14. The clinic nurse notes that a client is taking metoprolol. The nurse would perform which assessment to determine medication **effectiveness?**
1 Take the client's temperature.
2 Take the client's blood pressure.
3 Check the client's peripheral pulses.
4 Check the client's eyes for peripheral vision.

Level of Cognitive Ability: Evaluating
Client Needs: Physiological Integrity
Clinical Judgment/Cognitive Skills: Evaluate Outcomes
Integrated Process: Nursing Process/ Assessment/Data Collection
Content Area: Pharmacology
Priority Concepts: Clinical Judgment; Evidence
Level of Nursing Student: Intermediate

ANSWER: 2
Rationale: Metoprolol is a beta blocker that is used to treat mild-to moderate hypertension. Therefore, to determine medication effectiveness, the nurse would monitor the client's blood pressure. Options 1, 3, and 4 are unrelated to the medication's effectiveness.

Test-Taking Strategy: Apply the clinical judgment/cognitive skill, *evaluate outcomes*. Note the strategic word, *effectiveness*. Also, note the subject, assessment findings to determine medication effectiveness. Recalling that medication names that end with the letters -*lol* are beta blockers and that beta blockers are used to treat hypertension will direct you to the correct option. **Review:** Intended effects of **metoprolol**.

Tip for the Nursing Student: Metoprolol is a medication that is primarily used to treat hypertension. A priority nursing intervention when a medication with antihypertensive effects is administered is to monitor the client's blood pressure. Additional important interventions include client teaching related to safety because of the hypotensive effects of the medication. One important point to teach the client is to rise slowly from a lying to sitting position and to permit the legs to dangle from the bed momentarily before standing.

---

15. Betaxolol eye drops have been prescribed for a client for the treatment of glaucoma. The nurse would tell the client that it is important to return to the clinic for assessment of the presence of which condition?

ANSWER: 1
Rationale: Betaxolol is an antiglaucoma medication and a beta blocker. Systemic effects of the medication include hypotension manifested as dizziness, nausea, diaphoresis, headache, fatigue, constipation, and diarrhea. Nursing interventions include monitoring the blood pressure for hypotension and assessing the pulse for

1 Hypotension
2 Hyperglycemia
3 The presence of Trousseau's sign
4 The presence of redness and warmth in the calf area

Level of Cognitive Ability: Applying
Client Needs: Physiological Integrity
Clinical Judgment/Cognitive Skills: Generate Solutions
Integrated Process: Teaching and Learning
Content Area: Pharmacology
Priority Concepts: Client Education; Safety
Level of Nursing Student: Intermediate

strength, weakness, irregularities, and bradycardia. This medication may mask the symptoms of hypoglycemia and prolong the hypoglycemic effect in the client taking insulin or oral hypoglycemics. The presence of Trousseau's sign is unrelated to the use of this medication. A positive Trousseau's sign indicates a calcium imbalance. Redness and warmth in the calf area may be indicative of deep vein thrombosis; however, this assessment is not specifically related to this medication.

Test-Taking Strategy: Apply the clinical judgment/cognitive skill, *generate solutions.* Remember that beta-blocker medication names end with the letters *-lol*, and recall that beta blockers are used to treat hypertension. Also use the ABCs—airway, breathing, and circulation—to direct you to the correct option. **Review: Betaxolol.**

Tip for the Nursing Student: Glaucoma is an abnormal eye disorder characterized by elevated pressure within the eye. It is caused by the obstruction of the outflow of aqueous humor. If untreated, it will result in complete and permanent blindness. Medication therapy is extremely important to keep the intraocular pressure within the normal range of 10 to 21 mm Hg, and the client needs to be instructed about the importance of the medication.

---

16. Bupropion is prescribed for a client to treat an anxiety disorder. The nurse would tell the client that which is a common side effect of the medication?
    1 Diarrhea
    2 Dry mouth
    3 Sleepiness
    4 Slowed pulse rate

Level of Cognitive Ability: Applying
Client Needs: Physiological Integrity
Clinical Judgment/Cognitive Skills: Generate Solutions
Integrated Process: Teaching and Learning
Content Area: Pharmacology
Priority Concepts: Adherence; Client Education
Level of Nursing Student: Intermediate

ANSWER: 2
Rationale: Bupropion is an antianxiety medication. Common side effects include agitation, headache, dry mouth, constipation, gastrointestinal upset, dizziness, tremors, insomnia, blurred vision, and tachycardia. Options 1, 3, and 4 are not side effects of this medication.

Test-Taking Strategy: Apply the clinical judgment/cognitive skill, *generate solutions.* Focus on the subject, a common side effect of bupropion. Noting the words *to treat an anxiety disorder* will assist in determining that the medication is an antianxiety medication. Recall that dry mouth can occur with the use of some antianxiety medications. **Review: The side effects of bupropion.**

Tip for the Nursing Student: Anxiety is the anticipation of danger or dread accompanied by restlessness, tension, tachycardia, and breathing difficulty. In an anxiety disorder, the anxiety the client experiences can range from a mild to a severe state.

---

17. The nurse is caring for a client with systemic candidiasis who is receiving amphotericin B intravenously (IV). The nurse would perform which action during administration of the medication to monitor for an adverse effect?
    1 Monitor urinary output.
    2 Check peripheral pulses.
    3 Monitor for hypothermia.
    4 Check the neurological status.

ANSWER: 1
Rationale: Amphotericin B is an antifungal medication and can cause toxicity, which during administration can produce symptoms such as chills, fever, headache, vomiting, and impaired renal function. The medication is also very irritating to the IV site, commonly causing thrombophlebitis. The nurse administering this medication watches for signs of these problems. Options 2, 3, and 4 are not specifically related to the administration of this medication.

Test-Taking Strategy: Apply the clinical judgment/cognitive skill, *take action.* Note the subject, an adverse effect. Recalling that nephrotoxicity can occur with the use of this medication will direct you to the correct option. **Review: The adverse effects of amphotericin B.**

Level of Cognitive Ability: Analyzing
Client Needs: Physiological Integrity
Clinical Judgment/Cognitive Skills: Take Action
Integrated Process: Nursing Process/
   Implementation
Content Area: Pharmacology
Priority Concepts: Clinical Judgment; Safety
Level of Nursing Student: Advanced

Tip for the Nursing Student: Candidiasis is an infection caused by a species of *Candida*, usually *Candida albicans*. It usually occurs in a local area, such as the oral cavity, but can also occur in other areas. Treatment includes oral or topical administration of antifungal medication if candidiasis occurs locally. If it becomes a systemic infection, IV antifungal medications are prescribed. One adverse effect of antifungal medications administered by IV is nephrotoxicity (destruction to the kidney cells)

---

18. The nurse is reviewing the laboratory results of a client receiving intravenous (IV) chemotherapy. The nurse would initiate neutropenic precautions if which laboratory result is noted?
    1 Clotting time of 10 minutes
    2 Ammonia level of 10 mcg/dL (6 mcmol/L)
    3 Platelet count of 100,000 mm³ (100 × 10⁹/L)
    4 White blood cell (WBC) count of 2000 mm³ (2.0 × 10⁹/L)

Level of Cognitive Ability: Applying
Client Needs: Safe and Effective Care
   Environment
Clinical Judgment/Cognitive Skills: Take
   Action
Integrated Process: Nursing Process/
   Implementation
Content Area: Pharmacology
Priority Concepts: Immunity; Safety
Level of Nursing Student: Intermediate

ANSWER: 4
Rationale: The normal WBC count is 5000 to 10,000 mm³ (5 to 10 × 10⁹/L). When the WBC count drops, neutropenic precautions need to be implemented. These include protective isolation measures to protect the client from infection. Bleeding precautions need to be initiated when the platelet count drops. Bleeding precautions include avoiding all trauma, such as rectal temperatures or injections. The normal clotting time is 8 to 15 minutes. The normal ammonia value is 10 to 80 mcg/dL (6 to 47 mcmol/L). The normal platelet count is 150,000 to 450,000 mm³ (150 to 450 × 10⁹/L).

Test-Taking Strategy: Apply the clinical judgment/cognitive skill, *take action.* Eliminate options 1 and 2 first because they are comparable or alike options and identify normal laboratory values. To select between the remaining options, note that the client is receiving chemotherapy and focus on the words *neutropenic precautions.* Correlate a low WBC count with the need for neutropenic precautions and a low platelet count with the need for bleeding precautions. **Review:** The interventions associated with caring for the client receiving **chemotherapy.**

Tip for the Nursing Student: Neutropenia is an abnormal decrease in the number of neutrophils in the blood. This can occur in conditions such as acute leukemia, infection, and chronic splenomegaly and in the client receiving chemotherapy because chemotherapy destroys normal cells in addition to cancer cells. When neutropenia occurs, the client is at risk for developing an infection, and the nurse needs to implement measures to protect the client from infection, such as strict hand washing, wearing protective clothing when caring for the client, and keeping fresh fruits and flowers and standing water out of the client's room because these items harbor bacteria. The nurse should also restrict visits with the client from anyone who is ill.

---

19. The nurse is providing instructions to a client who is taking codeine sulfate. What instruction would the nurse provide to the client?
    1 Decrease fluid intake.
    2 Change positions slowly.
    3 Maintain a low-fiber diet.
    4 Limit the intake of alcoholic beverages.

Level of Cognitive Ability: Applying
Client Needs: Physiological Integrity

ANSWER: 2
Rationale: Codeine sulfate is an opioid analgesic. The medication can cause constipation, and the client is instructed to increase fluid intake and maintain a high-fiber diet. Alcohol intake is avoided, not limited. The medication can cause drowsiness, light-headedness, and hypotension, and the client is instructed to change positions slowly to prevent orthostatic hypotension.

Test-Taking Strategy: Apply the clinical judgment/cognitive skill, *generate solutions.* Focus on the subject, client instructions related to codeine sulfate. Eliminate option 4 first, using general pharmacology guidelines and recalling that alcohol is avoided, not limited.

Clinical Judgment/Cognitive Skills: Generate Solutions
Integrated Process: Teaching and Learning
Content Area: Pharmacology
Priority Concepts: Client Education; Pain
Level of Nursing Student: Intermediate

From the remaining options, recalling that codeine sulfate can cause constipation will eliminate options 1 and 3. **Review:** Nursing measures related to the administration of **codeine sulfate**.

Tip for the Nursing Student: Codeine sulfate is an opioid analgesic that is used primarily to treat pain. Opioid analgesics can cause many side effects, including drowsiness, light-headedness, and hypotension. Therefore, client safety is a concern with the use of opioid analgesics. Nursing interventions with the use of opioid analgesics focus on implementing measures that protect the client from injury and teaching the client measures to prevent injury.

---

20. A client is receiving diazepam to treat painful muscle spasms. The nurse would monitor the client for which frequent side effect of the medication?
    1 Ataxia
    2 Diarrhea
    3 Nervousness
    4 Hypertension

Level of Cognitive Ability: Analyzing
Client Needs: Physiological Integrity
Clinical Judgment/Cognitive Skills: Recognize Cues
Integrated Process: Nursing Process/ Assessment/Data Collection
Content Area: Pharmacology
Priority Concepts: Clinical Judgment; Safety
Level of Nursing Student: Intermediate

ANSWER: 1
Rationale: Diazepam is a centrally acting skeletal muscle relaxant. Incoordination (ataxia), fatigue, and drowsiness are frequent side effects. Occasional side effects include slurred speech, orthostatic hypotension, headache, hypoactivity, constipation, nausea, and blurred vision.

Test-Taking Strategy: Apply the clinical judgment/cognitive skill, *recognize cues.* Focus on the subject, a frequent side effect of diazepam. Note the name of the medication. Recalling that some benzodiazepine medication names end with the letters *-pam* will assist in answering the question. Also noting that the medication is used for muscle spasms will direct you to think that this medication relaxes muscles. The correct option is the only one that directly relates to this medication action. **Review:** The action and side effects of **diazepam**.

Tip for the Nursing Student: Muscle spasms are involuntary contractions or twitching that occurs in a muscle. These can be quite painful for the client, and one component of therapy is to treat the spasms with a centrally acting skeletal muscle relaxant. Because the medication is centrally acting, it can cause incoordination. This places the client at risk for injury, so nursing interventions focus on implementing measures to protect the client from injury.

---

21. The nurse is preparing to administer medications to a hospitalized client and notes that the client takes levothyroxine daily. The nurse suspects that the client has a history of which condition?
    1 Hypotension
    2 Hypertension
    3 Hypothyroidism
    4 Hyperthyroidism

Level of Cognitive Ability: Analyzing
Client Needs: Physiological Integrity
Clinical Judgment/Cognitive Skills: Recognize Cues
Integrated Process: Nursing Process/ Assessment/Data Collection
Content Area: Pharmacology

ANSWER: 3
Rationale: Levothyroxine is a synthetic thyroid hormone used to treat hypothyroidism. It is not used to treat hypotension, hypertension, or hyperthyroidism.

Test-Taking Strategy: Apply the clinical judgment/cognitive skill, *recognize cues.* Note the subject, use of the medication levothyroxine. Focus on the name of the medication. Recalling that most thyroid medications contain the letters *thy* in their name will assist in eliminating options 1 and 2. From the remaining options, eliminate option 4 because it would be harmful to administer thyroid medication to a client who is in a hyperthyroid state. **Review:** **Levothyroxine**.

Tip for the Nursing Student: Hypothyroidism is a condition characterized by decreased activity of the thyroid gland, resulting in

Priority Concepts. Cellular Regulation; Health Promotion
Level of Nursing Student: Intermediate

slowing of the body's metabolic processes. Treatment includes thyroid replacement therapy with thyroid medication.

---

22. The nurse checks the serum digoxin level for a client with heart failure who is taking digoxin and notes that the result is 0.8 ng/mL (1.02 nmol/L). Which action would the nurse take based on this laboratory result?
    1 Notify the primary health care provider.
    2 Withhold the next scheduled dose of digoxin.
    3 Place the report in the client's medical record.
    4 Obtain another serum digoxin level to verify the results.

Level of Cognitive Ability: Applying
Client Needs: Physiological Integrity
Clinical Judgment/Cognitive Skills: Take Action
Integrated Process: Nursing Process/ Implementation
Content Area: Pharmacology
Priority Concepts: Clinical Judgment; Safety
Level of Nursing Student: Intermediate

ANSWER: 3
Rationale: The normal therapeutic range for digoxin is 0.5 to 2.0 ng/mL (0.63 to 2.56 nmol/L). Therefore, the nurse would place the report in the client's medical record. Options 1, 2, and 4 are unnecessary actions.

Test-Taking Strategy: Apply the clinical judgment/cognitive skill, *take action*. Focus on the subject, the normal serum digoxin level. Note the words *result is 0.8 ng/mL (1.02 nmol/L)*, and focus on the client's diagnosis. Recalling that the overall normal therapeutic range for digoxin is from 0.5 to 2.0 ng/mL (0.63 to 2.56 nmol/L) will direct you to the correct option. **Review:** The therapeutic serum **digoxin level**.

Tip for the Nursing Student: Digoxin is a cardiac glycoside used to manage and treat heart failure, control atrial fibrillation, and treat and prevent atrial tachycardia. A concern with the medication is that it can cause toxicity, and an important nursing responsibility is to monitor for signs of toxicity. Before administering this medication, the nurse checks the client's apical heart rate; if the rate is below 60 beats/min, the nurse withholds the medication, collects additional client data, and contacts the primary health care provider for further prescriptions. Some manifestations of digoxin toxicity include gastrointestinal disturbances and ocular disturbances.

---

23. A client with acute kidney injury has been treated with sodium polystyrene sulfonate by mouth. The nurse would evaluate this therapy as **most effective** if which value was noted on follow-up laboratory testing?
    1 Calcium 9.8 mg/dL (2.45 mmol/L)
    2 Sodium 142 mEq/L (142 mmol/L)
    3 Potassium 4.9 mEq/L (4.9 mmol/L)
    4 Phosphorus 3.9 mg/dL (1.26 mmol/L)

Level of Cognitive Ability: Evaluating
Client Needs: Physiological Integrity
Clinical Judgment/Cognitive Skills: Evaluate Outcomes
Integrated Process: Nursing Process/ Evaluation
Content Area: Pharmacology
Priority Concepts: Clinical Judgment; Fluids and Electrolytes
Level of Nursing Student: Intermediate

ANSWER: 3
Rationale: Of all the electrolyte imbalances that accompany acute kidney injury, hyperkalemia is the most dangerous because it can lead to cardiac dysrhythmias and death. If the potassium level rises too high, sodium polystyrene sulfonate may be administered to cause excretion of potassium through the gastrointestinal tract. Each electrolyte level noted in the options falls within the normal reference range for that electrolyte. The potassium level, however, is measured after administration of this medication to note the extent of its effectiveness.

Test-Taking Strategy: Apply the clinical judgment/cognitive skill, *evaluate outcomes*. Focus on the strategic words, *most effective*. Next, focus on the client's diagnosis to assist in answering correctly. **Review: Polystyrene sulfonate.**

Tip for the Nursing Student: Acute kidney injury is the inability of the kidneys to excrete wastes, concentrate urine, and maintain electrolyte balance. Acute kidney injury is characterized by the rapid accumulation of wastes in the blood. Many electrolyte imbalances can occur in acute kidney injury because the kidneys are unable to maintain electrolyte balance. Sodium polystyrene sulfonate is an antihyperkalemic medication used to treat high potassium levels.

24. The nurse notes that the primary health care provider has prescribed sulfasalazine for a client. The nurse checks the nursing history form in the client's medical record for documentation of an allergy to which item?
1 Shellfish
2 Strawberries
3 Sulfonamides
4 Acetaminophen

Level of Cognitive Ability: Analyzing
Client Needs: Physiological Integrity
Clinical Judgment/Cognitive Skills: Recognize Cues
Integrated Process: Nursing Process/Assessment/Data Collection
Content Area: Pharmacology
Priority Concepts: Immunity; Safety
Level of Nursing Student: Intermediate

ANSWER: 3
Rationale: The client who has been prescribed sulfasalazine should be checked for a history of allergy to either sulfonamides or salicylates because the chemical compositions of sulfasalazine and these medications are similar. The other options are incorrect and are unrelated to the administration of this medication.

Test-Taking Strategy: Apply the clinical judgment/cognitive skill, *recognize cues*. Focus on the subject, history of allergy. Note the relationship of *sulfasalazine* in the question and *sulfonamides* in the correct option. **Review: Sulfasalazine.**

Tip for the Nursing Student: Sulfasalazine is a sulfonamide and an anti-inflammatory medication that is used to treat a variety of conditions. An important point to remember about this medication is that it is important to ask the client about allergies to sulfonamides or salicylates, such as aspirin, before administration. Before administering any medication, it is always important to ask the client about allergies.

---

25. A client with a diagnosis of sepsis is receiving tobramycin. The nurse realizes that the client is responding favorably to the medication therapy if which laboratory result is noted?
1 Sodium of 145 mEq/L (145 mmol/L) and chloride of 106 mEq/L (106 mmol/L)
2 Sodium of 140 mEq/L (140 mmol/L) and potassium of 3.9 mEq/L (3.9 mmol/L)
3 White blood cell (WBC) count of 8000 mm^3 (8×10^9/L) and creatinine level of 0.9 mg/dL (80 mcmol/L)
4 WBC count of 15,000 mm^3 (15×10^9/L) and a blood urea nitrogen of 38 mg/dL (13.6 mmol/L)

Level of Cognitive Ability: Evaluating
Client Needs: Physiological Integrity
Clinical Judgment/Cognitive Skills: Evaluate Outcomes
Integrated Process: Nursing Process/Evaluation
Content Area: Pharmacology
Priority Concepts: Cellular Regulation; Safety
Level of Nursing Student: Advanced

ANSWER: 3
Rationale: Tobramycin is an antibiotic that can cause nephrotoxicity and ototoxicity. The medication is effective if the WBC count drops back into the normal range and the kidney function remains normal. Option 4 indicates an elevated WBC count and elevated blood urea nitrogen level, and options 1 and 2 are unrelated to the use of this medication.

Test-Taking Strategy: Apply the clinical judgment/cognitive skill, *evaluate outcomes*. Focus on the subject, the therapeutic effect of tobramycin. Noting the client's diagnosis will assist in determining that this medication is an antibiotic. This will assist in eliminating options 1 and 2. To select correctly from the remaining options, focus on the words *the client is responding favorably*. The correct option is the one that identifies normal laboratory values. **Review: Tobramycin and normal laboratory values.**

Tip for the Nursing Student: Sepsis refers to a systemic infection that can occur as a result of a localized or other type of infection in the body. This serious infection needs to be treated aggressively with antibiotics, and usually blood cultures are done to determine the antibiotic of choice. Tobramycin is an antibiotic (aminoglycoside) that may be used to treat sepsis. As with many antibiotics, it causes nephrotoxicity and ototoxicity. The normal WBC count ranges from 5000 to 10,000 mm^3 (5 to 10×10^9/L). The normal creatinine level ranges from 0.5 to 1.2 mg/dL (44 to 106 mcmol/L), depending on gender. The normal blood urea nitrogen ranges from 10 to 20 mg/dL (3.6 to 7.1 mmol/L). The normal potassium level ranges from 3.5 to 5.0 mEq/L (3.5 to 5.0 mmol/L). The normal sodium level ranges from 135 to 145 mEq/L (135 to 145 mmol/L). The normal chloride level ranges from 98 to 106 mEq/L (98 to 106 mmol/L).

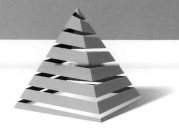

CHAPTER 19

Delegating/Prioritizing Questions

1. A client is being admitted to the neurological unit from the emergency department with a diagnosis of a cervical (C4) spinal cord injury. Which action would the nurse take **first** when admitting the client to the nursing unit?
   1 Listen to breath sounds.
   2 Check peripheral pulses.
   3 Check for muscle flaccidity.
   4 Determine extremity muscle strength.

   Level of Cognitive Ability: Analyzing
   Client Needs: Physiological Integrity
   Clinical Judgment/Cognitive Skills: Take Action
   Integrated Process: Nursing Process/ Assessment/Data Collection
   Content Area: Delegating/Prioritizing
   Priority Concepts: Clinical Judgment; Safety
   Level of Nursing Student: Advanced

ANSWER: 1
Rationale: Because compromise of respiration is a leading cause of death in cervical cord injury, collecting data on the respiratory system is the highest priority. Checking the peripheral pulses and muscle strength can be done after adequate oxygenation is ensured.

Test-Taking Strategy: Apply the clinical judgment/cognitive skill, *take action*. Note the strategic word, *first.* Eliminate options 3 and 4 first because they are comparable or alike options. Next use the ABCs—airway, breathing, and circulation—to direct you to the correct option. Remember that a cord injury, particularly at the level of C4, can affect respiratory status. Breath sounds will be diminished if respiratory muscles are weakened or paralyzed. **Review:** Priority care of the client with a C4 **spinal cord injury.**

Tip for the Nursing Student: A spinal cord injury is caused by a traumatic disruption of the spinal cord occurring from a car crash or another type of violent impact. It is often associated with extensive musculoskeletal injury. Where the injury occurred in the spinal cord (level of injury) determines the effect on the client. A major concern with a cervical spinal cord injury is respiratory status.

2. The nurse notes redness, warmth, and a purulent drainage at the insertion site of a central venous catheter in a client receiving total parenteral nutrition (TPN). The nurse would take which **priority** action?
   1 Change the intravenous tubing.
   2 Slow the rate of infusion of the TPN.
   3 Notify the primary health care provider.
   4 Call the pharmacy for a new bag of TPN solution.

   Level of Cognitive Ability: Analyzing
   Client Needs: Physiological Integrity
   Clinical Judgment/Cognitive Skills: Take Action
   Integrated Process: Nursing Process/ Implementation
   Content Area: Delegating/Prioritizing
   Priority Concepts: Clinical Judgment; Infection
   Level of Nursing Student: Advanced

ANSWER: 3
Rationale: Redness, warmth, and purulent drainage are signs of an infection. Infections of a central venous catheter site can lead to septicemia; therefore, the primary health care provider needs to be notified. Although the nurse may change the intravenous tubing and hang a new bag of TPN solution, these are not priority actions. Adjusting the rate of the infusion is unrelated to the client's complication.

Test-Taking Strategy: Apply the clinical judgment/cognitive skill, *take action.* Note the strategic word, *priority.* Also note the words *redness, warmth, and a purulent drainage,* and recall that these signs indicate infection. Recalling that infections of a central venous catheter site can lead to septicemia (a life-threatening condition) will direct you to the correct option. **Review:** Nursing interventions related to complications associated with **TPN via a central venous catheter.**

Tip for the Nursing Student: TPN involves the administration of nutrients by a route other than orally and is usually administered intravenously. It is administered by means of an intravenous catheter through a central vein, such as the subclavian vein. The tip of the catheter normally rests in the superior vena cava. This type of catheter is known as a *central venous catheter,* and meticulous nursing care is required in the care of the catheter and catheter site to prevent infection.

---

3. A client is brought to the emergency department by emergency medical services after having seriously lacerated both wrists. The nurse would perform which action **first?**
   1 Assess and treat the wound sites.
   2 Contact the crisis intervention team.
   3 Collect data on psychosocial aspects.
   4 Encourage the client to talk about her or his feelings.

Level of Cognitive Ability: Analyzing
Client Needs: Physiological Integrity
Clinical Judgment/Cognitive Skills: Take Action
Integrated Process: Nursing Process/
   Implementation
Content Area: Delegating/Prioritizing
Priority Concepts: Clinical Judgment; Safety
Level of Nursing Student: Intermediate

ANSWER: 1
Rationale: The initial action when a client has attempted suicide is to assess and treat any injuries. Although options 2, 3, and 4 may be appropriate at some point, the initial action would be to treat the wounds.

Test-Taking Strategy: Apply the clinical judgment/cognitive skill, *take action.* Note the strategic word, *first.* Use Maslow's Hierarchy of Needs theory to prioritize. Physiological needs come first. The correct option is the only one that addresses a physiological need. Options 2, 3, and 4 address psychosocial needs. **Review:** Initial care to the client who has attempted **suicide.**

Tip for the Nursing Student: A suicide attempt is an act to intentionally take one's own life. If a client has attempted suicide, it is extremely important to collect data on the injuries as a result of the suicide attempt. Other very important interventions include one-to-one supervision of the client and other therapy.

---

4. The nurse prepares a plan of care for a client receiving a chemotherapy treatment with intravenous bleomycin sulfate. The nurse would document which **priority** intervention in the plan?
   1 Monitor for dyspnea.
   2 Monitor for alopecia.
   3 Monitor for anorexia.
   4 Monitor for a change in bowel patterns.

Level of Cognitive Ability: Analyzing
Client Needs: Physiological Integrity
Clinical Judgment/Cognitive Skills: Prioritize
   Hypotheses
Integrated Process: Nursing Process/Analysis
Content Area: Delegating/Prioritizing
Priority Concepts: Gas Exchange; Safety
Level of Nursing Student: Intermediate

ANSWER: 1
Rationale: Bleomycin sulfate, an antineoplastic medication, can cause interstitial pneumonitis that can progress to pulmonary fibrosis. The nurse needs to monitor for dyspnea and monitor lung sounds for adventitious sounds that indicate pulmonary toxicity. Pulmonary function studies along with hematological, hepatic, and renal function tests need to be monitored. Also, the nurse needs to notify the primary health care provider immediately if pulmonary toxicity occurs. Alopecia (hair loss) can occur, but monitoring for it is not a priority intervention. Monitoring for anorexia and bowel pattern changes are important but are not the priority.

Test-Taking Strategy: Apply the clinical judgment/cognitive skill, *prioritize hypotheses.* Note the strategic word, *priority,* and use the ABCs—airway, breathing, and circulation. Select the option that relates to airway. **Review:** The interventions associated with caring for the client receiving **bleomycin sulfate.**

Tip for the Nursing Student: Chemotherapy is the use of medications that kill cancer cells in the treatment of cancer. A concern with the use of chemotherapy is that it also affects and destroys normal cells. This is what causes the side and adverse effects of the medications. Many chemotherapeutic agents cause nausea, vomiting, and alopecia (hair loss), among other effects. Also, some chemotherapeutic medications affect specific cells in certain organs. Bleomycin sulfate is one of these medications and can cause interstitial pneumonitis that can progress to pulmonary fibrosis. Pneumonitis refers to inflammation of the lungs, and pulmonary fibrosis refers to the formation of scar tissue in the connective tissue of the lungs.

---

5. Quinapril hydrochloride is prescribed as an adjunctive therapy in the treatment of heart failure. After administering the first dose, the nurse would specifically monitor which parameter as the **priority?**
   1 Respirations
   2 Urine output
   3 Lung sounds
   4 Blood pressure

Level of Cognitive Ability: Analyzing
Client Needs: Physiological Integrity
Clinical Judgment/Cognitive Skills: Prioritize Hypotheses
Integrated Process: Nursing Process/Analysis
Content Area: Delegating/Prioritizing
Priority Concepts: Perfusion; Safety
Level of Nursing Student: Intermediate

ANSWER: 4
Rationale: Quinapril hydrochloride is an angiotensin-converting enzyme (ACE) inhibitor. It is used in the treatment of hypertension and as adjunctive therapy in the treatment of heart failure. Excessive hypotension ("first-dose syncope") can occur in clients with heart failure or in clients who are severely salt or volume depleted. Although respirations, urine output, and lung sounds would be monitored, the nurse would specifically monitor the client's blood pressure.

Test-Taking Strategy: Apply the clinical judgment/cognitive skill, *prioritize hypotheses*. Focus on the name of the medication, and note the strategic word, *priority*. This tells you that all options may be correct and that you must prioritize. Options 1 and 3 are comparable or alike options and can be eliminated. Noting that the question is referring to a first dose of a medication and recalling that this medication is an ACE inhibitor will assist in answering correctly. **Review:** The side, adverse, and toxic effects of **quinapril hydrochloride.**

Tip for the Nursing Student: Quinapril hydrochloride is a medication that is primarily used to treat hypertension and manage heart failure. This medication is classified as an ACE inhibitor and antihypertensive. A priority nursing intervention when a medication with antihypertensive effects is administered is to monitor the client's blood pressure. An additional important intervention is client teaching related to safety because of the hypotensive effects of the medication. One important point to teach the client is to rise slowly from a lying to sitting position and to permit the legs to dangle from the bed momentarily before standing.

---

6. The nurse is creating a plan of care for a postoperative client who is receiving morphine sulfate by continuous intravenous infusion for pain. The nurse would include the monitoring of which item as a **priority** nursing action in the plan of care?
   1 Constipation
   2 Urine output
   3 Temperature
   4 Blood pressure

Level of Cognitive Ability: Creating
Client Needs: Physiological Integrity
Clinical Judgment/Cognitive Skills: Prioritize Hypotheses

ANSWER: 4
Rationale: Morphine sulfate suppresses respirations and decreases the client's blood pressure; therefore, monitoring for both decreased respirations and decreased blood pressure are priority nursing actions. Although monitoring of options 1, 2, and 3 may be a component of the plan of care for this client, option 4 identifies the priority nursing action.

Test-Taking Strategy: Apply the clinical judgment/cognitive skill, *prioritize hypotheses*. Note the strategic word, *priority*. Use the ABCs—airway, breathing, and circulation—to direct you to the correct option. Monitoring blood pressure determines the circulatory status of the client. **Review:** The effects of **morphine sulfate.**

Tip for the Nursing Student: Morphine sulfate is an opioid analgesic that is used to alleviate pain in a client. It is used to treat pain that

Integrated Process: Nursing Process/Analysis
Content Area: Delegating/Prioritizing
Priority Concepts: Perfusion; Safety
Level of Nursing Student: Intermediate

occurs in many types of disorders and is frequently used to alleviate pain in the postoperative client or the client with cancer. Because it is an opioid analgesic, it will cause a decrease in vital signs, specifically respirations and blood pressure. Monitoring vital signs, specifically respirations and blood pressure, is a critical nursing intervention.

---

7. A postoperative client who underwent pelvic surgery suddenly develops dyspnea and tachypnea. The nurse suspects that the client has a pulmonary embolism and would prepare to take which action **first**?
   1 Insert a urinary (Foley) catheter.
   2 Administer low-flow oxygen through a nasal cannula.
   3 Obtain an intravenous (IV) infusion pump to administer heparin.
   4 Increase the rate of the IV fluids infusing to prevent hypotension.

Level of Cognitive Ability: Analyzing
Client Needs: Physiological Integrity
Clinical Judgment/Cognitive Skills: Take Action
Integrated Process: Nursing Process/ Implementation
Content Area: Delegating/Prioritizing
Priority Concepts: Clinical Judgment; Gas Exchange
Level of Nursing Student: Intermediate

ANSWER: 2
Rationale: Pulmonary embolism is a life-threatening emergency. Maintenance of cardiopulmonary stability is the first priority. The nurse would prepare to administer low-flow oxygen by nasal cannula first. Hypotension is treated with fluids as prescribed. IV anticoagulation may be initiated. Some clients may require endotracheal intubation to maintain an adequate Pao$_2$. A perfusion scan, among other tests, may be performed, and the electrocardiogram (ECG) is monitored for the presence of dysrhythmias. In addition, a urinary catheter may be inserted. However, the first nursing action is to administer oxygen.

Test-Taking Strategy: Apply the clinical judgment/cognitive skill, *take action*. Note the strategic word, *first*. Use of the ABCs—airway, breathing, and circulation—will direct you to the correct option. **Review:** The immediate nursing actions when **pulmonary embolism** occurs.

Tip for the Nursing Student: Pulmonary embolism is characterized by the blockage of a pulmonary artery by fat, air, tumor tissue, or a thrombus that usually arises from a peripheral vein. It is characterized by dyspnea, tachycardia, anxiety, sudden chest pain, shock, and cyanosis. It is a life-threatening condition and requires immediate and aggressive treatment. Airway is the priority.

---

8. A client returns to the nursing unit from the postanesthesia care unit (PACU) after a transurethral resection of the prostate. The nurse would perform which action **first**?
   1 Check the client's respirations.
   2 Check the color of the client's urine.
   3 Check the urinary (Foley) catheter for patency.
   4 Read the nursing notes written by the PACU nurse.

Level of Cognitive Ability: Analyzing
Client Needs: Physiological Integrity
Clinical Judgment/Cognitive Skills: Take Action
Integrated Process: Nursing Process/ Implementation
Content Area: Delegating/Prioritizing
Priority Concepts: Clinical Judgment; Gas Exchange
Level of Nursing Student: Intermediate

ANSWER: 1
Rationale: The first action of the nurse is to check the patency of the airway, and the nurse would observe the client and monitor the breathing pattern and respirations. If the airway is not patent and the client is not breathing, immediate measures must be taken for the survival of the client. The nurse then checks cardiovascular function, the condition of the surgical site, the tubes or drains for patency and drainage, and function of the central nervous system. The PACU nurse normally provides a verbal report. Even so, reading the nursing notes would not be the first action.

Test-Taking Strategy: Apply the clinical judgment/cognitive skill, *take action*. Note the strategic word, *first*. Use the ABCs—airway, breathing, and circulation. This will direct you to the correct option. Airway patency and respirations are the priorities. **Review:** Priority data collection measures in the **postoperative client**.

Tip for the Nursing Student: A transurethral resection of the prostate is a surgical procedure in which a cystoscope (an instrument used for examining and treating lesions of the urinary tract) is passed through the urethra to resect (remove tissue from) the prostate. An important point to remember is that airway is always the priority in the care of any client.

9. A child with a diagnosis of pertussis (whooping cough) is being admitted to the pediatric unit. As soon as the child arrives on the unit, which action would the nurse perform **first**?
   1 Weigh the child.
   2 Take the child's temperature.
   3 Place the child on a pulse oximeter.
   4 Administer the prescribed antibiotic.

Level of Cognitive Ability: Analyzing
Client Needs: Physiological Integrity
Clinical Judgment/Cognitive Skills: Take Action
Integrated Process: Nursing Process/ Implementation
Content Area: Delegating/Prioritizing
Priority Concepts: Clinical Judgment; Gas Exchange
Level of Nursing Student: Intermediate

ANSWER: 3
Rationale: To adequately determine whether the child is getting enough oxygen, the child is placed on a pulse oximeter. The pulse oximeter will then provide ongoing information on the child's oxygen level. The child is also immediately placed on a cardiorespiratory monitor to provide early identification of periods of apnea and bradycardia. The nurse would then collect data on the client, including taking the child's temperature and weight and asking the parents about the child. An antibiotic may be prescribed, but the child's airway status needs to be checked first.

Test-Taking Strategy: Apply the clinical judgment/cognitive skill, *take action*. Note the strategic word, *first*. Focus on the child's diagnosis, and use the ABCs—airway, breathing, and circulation. This will direct you to the correct option. **Review:** Care of the child with **pertussis**.

Tip for the Nursing Student: Pertussis is an acute, highly contagious respiratory disease that occurs primarily in infants and children and is characterized by coughing and a loud whooping inspiration. Pulse oximetry uses a cliplike device that measures the amount of saturated hemoglobin in the tissue capillaries and thus the percentage of oxygen saturation in the blood. An important point to remember is that airway is always the priority in the care of a client.

---

10. The nurse is preparing to perform oral suctioning on a client who has coughed, resulting in secretions in the mouth, and is unable to expectorate the secretions adequately. The nurse determines that there is a prescription for the procedure and explains the procedure to the client. Which actions would the nurse take to perform this procedure? **Select all that apply.**
   ☐ 1 Washes hands
   ☐ 2 Applies a face shield
   ☐ 3 Removes the client's oxygen mask
   ☐ 4 Tells the client not to cough or breathe during the procedure
   ☐ 5 Applies a clean disposable glove to the dominant hand and attaches the suction catheter to the connecting tubing
   ☐ 6 Inserts the catheter into the client's mouth and moves the catheter around the mouth, pharynx, and gum line until secretions are cleared

Level of Cognitive Ability: Analyzing
Client Needs: Safe and Effective Care Environment
Clinical Judgment/Cognitive Skills: Take Action
Integrated Process: Nursing Process/ Implementation
Content Area: Delegating/Prioritizing
Priority Concepts: Clinical Judgment; Gas Exchange
Level of Nursing Student: Beginning

ANSWER: 1, 2, 3, 5, 6
Rationale: The nurse always washes the hands before performing any procedure, applies a face shield because suctioning may cause splashing of body fluids, and then dons a clean glove to each hand or dominant hand for oropharyngeal suctioning. A clean rather than a sterile glove can be used in this procedure because the oral cavity is not sterile. The nurse then completes preparation by attaching the suction catheter to the connecting suction tubing. The nurse removes the oxygen mask just before implementing the procedure so that the client is oxygenated as much as possible (remember that suctioning can deplete oxygen). The catheter is then inserted into the client's mouth until secretions are cleared. If the client is not tolerating the procedure, then the catheter is removed and the oxygen mask is reapplied. The nurse next encourages the client to cough because coughing moves secretions from the lower to upper airways into the mouth. At this point, suctioning is repeated if necessary. The oxygen mask is then reapplied.

Test-Taking Strategy: Apply the clinical judgment/cognitive skill, *take action*. Focus on the subject, the procedure for oral suctioning. The best strategy to use to answer this question is to first focus on the data in the question and then to visualize the procedure. Read each option carefully, and remember that coughing is important to move secretions from the airways to the mouth. **Review:** The procedure for **oral suctioning**.

Tip for the Nursing Student: Suctioning is a procedure that is used to remove accumulated secretions from the oral cavity or respiratory tract when the client is unable to effectively cough them out. It is a sterile procedure when done to remove secretions from the respiratory tract and is a nonsterile procedure when suctioning secretions from the oral cavity. It requires specific actions to prevent trauma to the mucosa of the oral cavity or respiratory tract and to prevent hypoxia.

11. The nurse hears the alarm sound on the telemetry monitor, quickly looks at the monitor, and notes that a client is in ventricular tachycardia. The nurse rushes to the client's room. Upon reaching the client's bedside, the nurse would perform which action **first**?
    1 Open the airway.
    2 Begin chest compressions.
    3 Determine unresponsiveness.
    4 Deliver two effective breaths.

Level of Cognitive Ability: Analyzing
Client Needs: Physiological Integrity
Clinical Judgment/Cognitive Skills: Take Action
Integrated Process: Nursing Process/ Implementation
Content Area: Delegating/Prioritizing
Priority Concepts: Clinical Judgment; Perfusion
Level of Nursing Student: Intermediate

ANSWER: 3
Rationale: Determining unresponsiveness is the first action to take. When a client is in ventricular tachycardia, there is a significant decrease in cardiac output. However, checking for unresponsiveness determines whether the client is affected by the decreased cardiac output. If the client is unresponsive, the nurse proceeds through CAB—compressions, airway, and breathing—of the cardiopulmonary resuscitation (CPR) sequence, remembering that the nurse would collect data before taking an action.

Test-Taking Strategy: Apply the clinical judgment/cognitive skill, *take action*. Focus on the subject, actions to take in performing CPR, and note the strategic word, *first*. Use the steps of basic life support to answer the question. Remember that determining unresponsiveness is the first action, followed by CAB. Also, use the steps of the nursing process, and remember that data collection comes before implementation. **Review:** The priority nursing actions if a client experiences **ventricular tachycardia.**

Tip for the Nursing Student: Ventricular tachycardia means that the ventricles are beating at a rate greater than 100 beats/min. If the client experiencing ventricular tachycardia is unresponsive, CPR may need to be initiated because ventricular tachycardia can progress to ventricular fibrillation, another life-threatening situation.

---

12. The nurse is collecting data on a client with a diagnosis of bulimia nervosa who has problems with nutrition. The nurse would obtain information from the client about which finding **first**?
    1 Lack of control
    2 Previous and current coping skills
    3 Feelings about self and body weight
    4 Eating patterns, food preferences, and concerns about eating

Level of Cognitive Ability: Analyzing
Client Needs: Physiological Integrity
Clinical Judgment/Cognitive Skills: Recognize Cues
Integrated Process: Nursing Process/ Assessment/Data Collection
Content Area: Delegating/Prioritizing
Priority Concepts: Nutrition; Stress and Coping
Level of Nursing Student: Intermediate

ANSWER: 4
Rationale: The nurse would first identify the client's eating patterns, food preferences, and concerns about eating when collecting data on a client with bulimia nervosa to determine a baseline for further planning and because this information relates to the client's physiological needs. The nurse would also obtain information about lack of control, previous and current coping skills, and the client's feelings about self and body weight, but this information is secondary to eating patterns and food preferences.

Test-Taking Strategy: Apply the clinical judgment/cognitive skill, *recognize cues*. Note the strategic word, *first*. Use Maslow's Hierarchy of Needs theory to prioritize. The correct option is the only one that relates to a physiological need. **Review:** Care for the client with **bulimia nervosa.**

Tip for the Nursing Student: Bulimia nervosa is a disorder characterized by a craving for food and continuous eating followed by purging. It is also known as *binge eating*. The condition can lead to severe nutritional deficiencies, self-deprivation, and depression.

---

13. The community health nurse is assisting residents involved in a hurricane and flood. Many of the older residents are emotionally despondent and refuse to evacuate their homes. With regard to rescue and relocation of the older residents, the nurse would plan to perform which action **first**?

ANSWER: 3
Rationale: Attending to people's basic needs of food, shelter, and clothing is the priority. Options 1, 2, and 4 may or may not be needed at a later time.

Test-Taking Strategy: Apply the clinical judgment/cognitive skill, *generate solutions*. Note the strategic word, *first*, and use Maslow's

1 Contact families.
2 Attend to emotional needs.
3 Attend to nutritional and basic needs.
4 Arrange for transportation to shelters.

Level of Cognitive Ability: Analyzing
Client Needs: Physiological Integrity
Clinical Judgment/Cognitive Skills: Generate Solutions
Integrated Process: Nursing Process/Planning
Content Area: Delegating/Prioritizing
Priority Concepts: Care Coordination; Leadership
Level of Nursing Student: Advanced

Hierarchy of Needs theory. The correct option addresses basic physiological needs. Options 1, 2, and 4 address psychosocial needs and may be appropriate at a later time. **Review:** The nurse's role in the event of a **disaster.**

Tip for the Nursing Student: A disaster is any human-made or natural event that causes destruction and devastation requiring assistance from others. In regard to a health care agency, a disaster can be external or internal. External disasters include those that occur outside the agency, and internal disasters include those that occur inside the agency. A disaster preparedness plan is a formal plan of action for coordinating the response of a health care agency's staff in the event of a disaster in the health care agency or surrounding community.

---

14. An antepartum client at 32 weeks' gestation positioned herself supine on the examination table to await the obstetrician. The nurse enters the examination room, and the client says, "I'm feeling a little light-headed and sick to my stomach." The nurse recognizes that the client may be experiencing vena cava syndrome (hypotensive syndrome) and would take which **immediate** action?
1 Give the client an emesis basin.
2 Place a cool cloth on the client's forehead.
3 Call the obstetrician to see the client immediately.
4 Place a folded towel or sheet under the client's right hip.

Level of Cognitive Ability: Analyzing
Client Needs: Physiological Integrity
Clinical Judgment/Cognitive Skills: Take Action
Integrated Process: Nursing Process/Implementation
Content Area: Delegating/Prioritizing
Priority Concepts: Clinical Judgment; Perfusion
Level of Nursing Student: Intermediate

ANSWER: 4
Rationale: Lying supine (on the back) applies additional gravity pressure on the abdominal blood vessels (iliac vessels, inferior vena cava, and ascending aorta), increasing compression and impeding blood flow and cardiac output. This results in hypotension, dizziness, nausea, pallor, clammy (cool, damp) skin, and sweating. Raising one hip higher than the other reduces the pressure on the vena cava, restoring the circulation and relieving the symptoms. Although an emesis basin and a cool cloth placed on the forehead may be helpful, these are not the immediate actions. It is unnecessary to call the obstetrician immediately unless the client's complaints are unrelieved after repositioning.

Test-Taking Strategy: Apply the clinical judgment/cognitive skill, *take action*. Note the strategic word, *immediate*. Focus on the data in the question and the goals of care. In other words, think about what complications you want to prevent. Remember that if a question requires you to prioritize and one of the options relates to positioning a client, that option may be the correct one. **Review:** Care of the client experiencing vena cava syndrome.

Tip for the Nursing Student: Vena cava syndrome, also known as *supine hypotension*, is a condition in which a fall in blood pressure occurs when a pregnant woman is lying on her back. It is caused by impaired venous return that results from pressure of the large uterus on the vena cava. Therefore, raising one hip higher than the other reduces the pressure on the vena cava, restoring the circulation and relieving the symptoms.

---

15. A client is hospitalized with chest pain, and myocardial infarction is suspected. The client tells the nurse that the chest pain has returned, and the nurse administers one 0.4-mg nitroglycerin tablet sublingually as prescribed. If the pain is not relieved, what would the nurse plan to do **next** before administering another sublingual nitroglycerin tablet?

ANSWER: 2
Rationale: In the hospitalized client, nitroglycerin tablets are usually administered one every 5 minutes, not exceeding three tablets, for chest pain as long as the client maintains a systolic blood pressure of 100 mm Hg or above. The nurse would check the client's blood pressure before administering a second nitroglycerin tablet. The PHCP is notified if the chest pain is not relieved after administering three tablets. If there is a sudden drop in blood pressure, the client is placed in a flat position and the PHCP is notified. Deep breathing will not relieve the chest pain that occurs as a result of myocardial infarction.

1 Place the client in a flat position.
2 Check the client's blood pressure.
3 Encourage the client to deep-breathe.
4 Notify the primary health care provider (PHCP).

Level of Cognitive Ability: Analyzing
Client Needs: Physiological Integrity
Clinical Judgment/Cognitive Skills: Generate Solutions
Integrated Process: Nursing Process/Planning
Content Area: Delegating/Prioritizing
Priority Concepts: Clinical Judgment; Perfusion
Level of Nursing Student: Advanced

Test-Taking Strategy: Apply the clinical judgment/cognitive skill, *generate solutions.* Note the strategic word, *next.* Use the ABCs— airway, breathing, and circulation. This will direct you to the correct option. Checking the blood pressure is a means of collecting data on the client's circulatory status. **Review:** Care of the client experiencing **chest pain.**

Tip for the Nursing Student: A myocardial infarction is also known as a *heart attack* and results in necrosis of cardiac muscle caused by an obstruction in a coronary artery. When a client experiences chest pain and a cardiac problem is suspected, nitroglycerin is administered. Nitroglycerin is a coronary vasodilator that acts by dilating the coronary vessels and thus increased blood flow and oxygenation ensue.

---

16. A client receiving a blood transfusion develops signs of a blood transfusion reaction. The nurse stops the transfusion and maintains the intravenous (IV) line with normal saline. Which action would the nurse take **next**?
1 Document the occurrence.
2 Check the client's vital signs.
3 Send the blood bag and tubing to the blood bank for examination.
4 Check the client's urine output, and obtain a urine specimen for analysis.

Level of Cognitive Ability: Analyzing
Client Needs: Physiological Integrity
Clinical Judgment/Cognitive Skills: Take Action
Integrated Process: Nursing Process/ Implementation
Content Area: Delegating/Prioritizing
Priority Concepts: Clinical Judgment; Immunity
Level of Nursing Student: Intermediate

ANSWER: 2
Rationale: If a transfusion reaction is suspected, the transfusion is stopped and then normal saline is infused with new IV tubing pending further primary health care provider prescriptions. This maintains a patent IV access line and aids in maintaining the client's intravascular volume. The nurse would next check the client's vital signs and notify the primary health care provider and the blood bank about the reaction. The nurse would obtain a urine specimen for analysis to check for hemolysis of red blood cells. The nurse then sends the blood bag and tubing to the blood bank for examination and documents the occurrence on the transfusion report and in the client's chart.

Test-Taking Strategy: Apply the clinical judgment/cognitive skill, *take action.* Note the strategic word, *next,* and visualize the occurrence. Stopping the blood is the first action, and because the IV line needs to remain patent, normal saline solution needs to be infused. Next use the ABCs—airway, breathing, and circulation— to determine that the client's vital signs need to be monitored. Then monitoring urine output and obtaining a urine specimen are done. Documentation is done last because all interventions, including that the nurse sent the blood bag and tubing to the blood bank for examination, need to be documented. **Review:** Interventions if a **transfusion reaction** occurs.

Tip for the Nursing Student: A blood transfusion involves the administration of whole blood or a component of blood, such as packed red blood cells. It is prescribed to replace blood lost as a result of trauma, surgery, or disease. A major concern associated with the administration of blood is a blood transfusion reaction, and the nurse monitors the client very closely for this life-threatening complication. It is important to know the signs of a transfusion reaction and the nursing interventions if a transfusion reaction occurs.

17. A client with a diagnosis of sickle cell crisis is being admitted to the hospital. The nurse anticipates that which **priority** intervention will be prescribed?
    1 Laboratory studies
    2 Genetic counseling
    3 Oxygen administration
    4 Electrolyte replacement therapy

Level of Cognitive Ability: Analyzing
Client Needs: Physiological Integrity
Clinical Judgment/Cognitive Skills: Prioritize Hypotheses
Integrated Process: Nursing Process/Analysis
Content Area: Delegating/Prioritizing
Priority Concepts: Gas Exchange; Perfusion
Level of Nursing Student: Intermediate

ANSWER: 3

Rationale: Oxygen, intravenous fluids, pain medication, and red blood cell transfusions are the priority interventions for treating sickle cell crisis. Laboratory studies may also be prescribed, but are not the priority in the care of the client. Genetic counseling is recommended, but not during the acute phase of illness. Electrolyte replacement therapy may be necessary, but this treatment would be based on the results of laboratory studies.

Test-Taking Strategy: Apply the clinical judgment/cognitive skill, *prioritize hypotheses*. Note the strategic word, *priority*. Option 2 can be eliminated first, using Maslow's Hierarchy of Needs theory, because this option addresses a psychosocial need, not a physiological one. From the remaining options use the ABCs—airway, breathing, and circulation—to direct you to the correct option. Review: Care of the client in **sickle cell crisis.**

Tip for the Nursing Student: Sickle cell anemia is a severe, chronic, and incurable anemic condition characterized by abnormal hemoglobin (Hgb S) that results in distortion and fragility of the erythrocytes (sickle shape). Sickle cell crisis is an acute episodic condition that can occur when an individual has sickle cell anemia and results in the aggregation and clumping of the distorted erythrocytes, leading to occlusion and ischemia of tissue.

18. The nurse is planning the client assignments for the day. Which client would the nurse assign to the assistive personnel (AP)?
    1 A client on strict bed rest
    2 A client scheduled for discharge to home
    3 A client scheduled for a cardiac catheterization
    4 A postoperative client who had an emergency appendectomy

Level of Cognitive Ability: Analyzing
Client Needs: Safe and Effective Care Environment
Clinical Judgment/Cognitive Skills: Generate Solutions
Integrated Process: Nursing Process/ Planning
Content Area: Delegating/Prioritizing
Priority Concepts: Care Coordination; Leadership
Level of Nursing Student: Advanced

ANSWER: 1

Rationale: The nurse is legally responsible for client assignments and must assign tasks based on the guidelines of nurse practice acts and the job descriptions of the employing agency. A client scheduled for discharge to home, a client scheduled for a cardiac catheterization, and a postoperative client who had an emergency appendectomy have both physiological and psychosocial needs that require care by a licensed nurse. The AP has been trained to care for a client on bed rest. The nurse provides instructions to the AP, but the tasks required are within the role description of an AP.

Test-Taking Strategy: Apply the clinical judgment/cognitive skill, *generate solutions*. Focus on the subject, principles of assignment-making. Note that the question asks for the assignment to be delegated to the AP. When asked questions related to delegation, think about the role description of the employee and the needs of the client. This will direct you to the correct option. **Review:** Principles of **assignment-making.**

Tip for the Nursing Student: Delegating and assignment-making are responsibilities of the nurse, and it is important that you assign tasks and activities that are appropriate based on the individual's educational experience, nurse practice acts, and the health care agency's policies and procedures. When you need to assign a task or activity to an AP, one strategy is to think about the word *noninvasive*. Select the task or activity that is a noninvasive one.

19. A hospitalized client with type 1 diabetes mellitus tells the nurse that he feels as if he is having a hypoglycemic reaction. The nurse would complete which action **first?**

1 Obtain a blood glucose reading.
2 Give the client 4 oz (120 mL) of orange juice.
3 Prepare to administer 50% dextrose intravenously.
4 Prepare to administer subcutaneous glucagon hydrochloride.

Level of Cognitive Ability: Analyzing
Client Needs: Physiological Integrity
Clinical Judgment/Cognitive Skills: Take Action
Integrated Process: Nursing Process/
    Implementation
Content Area: Delegating/Prioritizing
Priority Concepts: Clinical Judgment;
    Glucose Regulation
Level of Nursing Student: Intermediate

ANSWER: **1**
Rationale: Management of hypoglycemia depends on the severity of the reaction. To reverse mild hypoglycemia, a 15-g simple carbohydrate is given and works quickly to increase blood glucose levels. However, a blood glucose test (with a glucose meter) would be performed first as soon as manifestations begin. If a meter is unavailable, it is safest to treat the hypoglycemia. Fifty percent dextrose and glucagon hydrochloride are used to treat severe hypoglycemia, particularly in the unconscious client.

Test-Taking Strategy: Apply the clinical judgment/cognitive skill, *take action*. Note the strategic word, *first*, and note that the client is hospitalized. Use the steps of the nursing process, and note that the correct option is the only one that addresses assessment/data collection. **Review:** Care of the client experiencing a **hypoglycemic** reaction.

Tip for the Nursing Student: Diabetes mellitus is a disorder of carbohydrate, fat, and protein metabolism that is primarily the result of a deficiency or complete lack of insulin secretion by the beta cells of the pancreas or resistance to insulin. The client is treated with exogenous insulin, and both hypoglycemia (a low blood glucose level) and hyperglycemia (a high blood glucose level) are complications. It is important to know the signs of each complication and how to treat them. It is also important to teach the client these signs and their treatment. If a low blood glucose level occurs, the client is treated with a 15-g simple carbohydrate to increase blood glucose levels.

20. A client is admitted to the emergency department with complaints of severe, radiating chest pain, and a myocardial infarction is suspected. The nurse immediately applies oxygen to the client and takes which action **next?**

1 Obtain a 12-lead electrocardiogram (ECG).
2 Call radiology to prescribe a chest radiograph.
3 Call the laboratory to prescribe stat blood work.
4 Notify the coronary care unit to inform them that the client will need admission.

Level of Cognitive Ability: Analyzing
Client Needs: Physiological Integrity
Clinical Judgment/Cognitive Skills: Take Action
Integrated Process: Nursing Process/
    Implementation
Content Area: Delegating/Prioritizing
Priority Concepts: Clinical Judgment;
    Perfusion
Level of Nursing Student: Advanced

ANSWER: **1**
Rationale: The initial action is to apply oxygen, because the client may be experiencing myocardial ischemia. Based on the options provided, an ECG will be done next because this test can provide evidence of cardiac damage and the location of myocardial ischemia. Vital signs are also measured and would be done just before obtaining the ECG or quickly thereafter. Nitroglycerin, a coronary artery vasodilator, may also be administered. The nurse would then obtain blood work because it can assist in determining the diagnosis and choice of treatment. Although the chest radiograph may show cardiac enlargement, it does not influence the immediate treatment. Notifying the coronary care unit to inform them that the client will need admission would be done once the diagnosis is confirmed and admission is deemed necessary.

Test-Taking Strategy: Apply the clinical judgment/cognitive skill, *take action*. Note the strategic word, *next*. Remember that the immediate goal of therapy is to prevent myocardial ischemia. Use knowledge regarding the procedures for determining treatment, and visualize the situation to answer this question. **Review:** Care of the client with **chest pain.**

Tip for the Nursing Student: A myocardial infarction is also known as a *heart attack* and results in necrosis of cardiac muscle caused by an obstruction in a coronary artery. Chest pain is a significant characteristic of a heart attack. In fact, whenever a client complains of chest pain, the nurse would suspect the presence of a heart attack and act quickly until this diagnosis can be ruled out.

21. The nurse is caring for a client with an injury to the brainstem. The nurse would monitor which parameter as the **priority?**
1 Urine output
2 Electrolyte results
3 Peripheral vascular status
4 Respiratory rate and rhythm

Level of Cognitive Ability: Analyzing
Client Needs: Physiological Integrity
Clinical Judgment/Cognitive Skills: Prioritize Hypotheses
Integrated Process: Nursing Process/Analysis
Content Area: Delegating/Prioritizing
Priority Concepts: Gas Exchange; Intracranial Regulation
Level of Nursing Student: Advanced

ANSWER: 4
Rationale: The respiratory center is located in the brainstem. Therefore, monitoring the respiratory status is a priority in a client with a brainstem injury. The nurse may also monitor urine output, electrolyte results, and peripheral vascular status, but these are not the priority.

Test-Taking Strategy: Apply the clinical judgment/cognitive skill, *prioritize hypotheses*. Note the strategic word, *priority*, and use the ABCs—airway, breathing, and circulation. Also, recalling the anatomical location of the respiratory center will direct you to the correct option. **Review:** Care of the client with a **brain injury.**

Tip for the Nursing Student: The brainstem is made up of several structures, including the midbrain, pons, and medulla oblongata. The vital centers of cardiac, respiratory, and vasomotor control are located in the medulla oblongata. If injury occurs to the brainstem, the nurse would monitor the respiratory status as a priority, followed by the cardiac status and vasomotor status.

---

22. A client is scheduled for a diagnostic procedure requiring the injection of a radiopaque dye. The nurse would check which **priority** information before the procedure?
1 Intake and output
2 Height and weight
3 Baseline vital signs
4 Allergy to iodine or shellfish

Level of Cognitive Ability: Analyzing
Client Needs: Physiological Integrity
Clinical Judgment/Cognitive Skills: Prioritize Hypotheses
Integrated Process: Nursing Process/Analysis
Content Area: Delegating/Prioritizing
Priority Concepts: Immunity; Safety
Level of Nursing Student: Beginning

ANSWER: 4
Rationale: Procedures that involve the injection of a radiopaque dye require an informed consent. The risk for allergic reaction exists if the client has an allergy to iodine or shellfish. The risk of allergic reaction and possible anaphylaxis must be determined before the procedure. Although options 1, 2, and 3 identify information obtained before the procedure, these items are not the priority.

Test-Taking Strategy: Apply the clinical judgment/cognitive skill, *prioritize hypotheses*. Note the strategic word, *priority*. Use the ABCs—airway, breathing, and circulation. The risk for an allergic reaction and anaphylaxis is the correct option. **Review:** The complications associated with injection of a **radiopaque dye.**

Tip for the Nursing Student: Many diagnostic tests may require injection of a radiopaque dye. This type of dye, which contains properties of iodine, is used for diagnosis to provide better visualization of body structures. Whenever a radiopaque dye is used, the nurse needs to check the client for an allergy to both iodine and shellfish.

---

23. The nurse is caring for a client in Buck's extension traction. The nurse would identify which client problem as the **priority?**
1 Expressed feelings of social isolation
2 Observed inability to distract oneself
3 Verbalized anger about the need for immobility
4 Observed skin redness around the edges of the boot appliance

Level of Cognitive Ability: Analyzing
Client Needs: Physiological Integrity
Clinical Judgment/Cognitive Skills: Prioritize Hypotheses

ANSWER: 4
Rationale: Buck's extension traction is a type of skin traction in which weights are attached to the skin with the use of a boot or elastic bandage. A priority problem for the client in this type of traction is the potential for breaks in skin. The potential for alteration in neurovascular status is also a concern. Options 1, 2, and 3 may be problems for the client in Buck's extension traction, but redness around the edges of the boot appliance presents the greatest risk for skin breakdown.

Test-Taking Strategy: Apply the clinical judgment/cognitive skill, *prioritize hypotheses*. Note the strategic word, *priority*. Use Maslow's Hierarchy of Needs theory. The only option that indicates a physiological need is option 4. Options 1, 2, and 3 indicate psychosocial needs. **Review:** Care for the client in **Buck's extension traction.**

Integrated Process: Nursing Process/Analysis
Content Area: Delegating/Prioritizing
Priority Concepts: Perfusion; Tissue Integrity
Level of Nursing Student: Intermediate

Tip for the Nursing Student: Traction may be used to treat fractures; it provides immobilization to hold the broken bone fragments in contact with each other or in very close approximation until healing takes place. The 2 types of traction are skin and skeletal. Skin traction is achieved by applying a boot, wrap, or commercially prepared device directly to the skin, which is then attached to weights. Skeletal traction is attached directly to bone.

---

24. The nurse is caring for a child with juvenile idiopathic arthritis (JIA). The nurse would identify which problem as the **priority**?
    1 Complaints of acute pain
    2 Unsteadiness when ambulating
    3 Embarrassment about appearance
    4 Inability to perform self-hygienic measures

Level of Cognitive Ability: Analyzing
Client Needs: Physiological Integrity
Clinical Judgment/Cognitive Skills: Prioritize Hypotheses
Integrated Process: Nursing Process/Analysis
Content Area: Delegating/Prioritizing
Priority Concepts: Pain; Stress and Coping
Level of Nursing Student: Intermediate

ANSWER: 1
Rationale: All the problems presented are appropriate for the child with JIA. The priority problem relates to complaints of acute pain. Acute pain needs to be managed before other problems can be addressed.

Test-Taking Strategy: Apply the clinical judgment/cognitive skill, *prioritize hypotheses*. Note the strategic word, *priority*. Use Maslow's Hierarchy of Needs theory, remembering that physiological needs (option 1) receive highest priority. Option 2 addresses safety and would be the second priority. Option 3 addresses self-image needs. Option 4 is also a concern but is a lesser priority as compared with acute pain. **Review:** Care of the child with **JIA.**

Tip for the Nursing Student: Arthritis is an inflammatory condition of the joints characterized by pain, swelling, heat, redness, and limitation of movement. It can affect the client's ability to perform activities of daily living. It can also result in debilitation. It can occur in childhood or adulthood.

---

25. A client has been newly diagnosed with diabetes mellitus. The nurse would perform which action as the **first** step in teaching the client about the disorder?
    1 Decide on the teaching approach.
    2 Plan for the evaluation of the session.
    3 Gather all available resource materials.
    4 Identify the client's knowledge and needs.

Level of Cognitive Ability: Analyzing
Client Needs: Health Promotion and Maintenance
Clinical Judgment/Cognitive Skills: Generate Solutions
Integrated Process: Teaching and Learning
Content Area: Delegating/Prioritizing
Priority Concepts: Client Education; Glucose Regulation
Level of Nursing Student: Intermediate

ANSWER: 4
Rationale: Determining what to teach a client begins with a determination of the client's own knowledge and learning needs. Once these have been determined, the nurse can effectively plan a teaching approach, the actual content, and resource materials that may be needed. The evaluation is done after teaching is completed.

Test-Taking Strategy: Apply the clinical judgment/cognitive skill, *generate solutions*. Note the strategic word, *first*. Use the steps of the nursing process to remember that assessment and data collection are the first step. **Review: Teaching and learning principles.**

Tip for the Nursing Student: Diabetes mellitus is a disorder of carbohydrate, fat, and protein metabolism that is primarily the result of a deficiency or complete lack of insulin secretion by the beta cells of the pancreas or resistance to insulin. Treatment includes diet, medication, and exercise. The client needs to be taught about the disorder and needs to understand how to care for self to maintain normal blood glucose levels and to prevent complications of the disease. Teaching is a very important role of the nurse for all clients.

CHAPTER 20

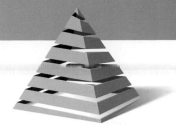

Leadership/Management Questions

1. The charge nurse is observing as a new nursing graduate performs an ear irrigation to remove impacted cerumen from the client's ear. The charge nurse would intervene during the procedure if the new nursing graduate performs which action?
   1 Washes hands before performing the procedure
   2 Positions the client with the affected side up after the irrigation
   3 Warms the irrigating solution to a temperature that is close to body temperature
   4 Directs a slow, steady stream of irrigation solution toward the upper wall of the ear canal

   Level of Cognitive Ability: Applying
   Client Needs: Safe and Effective Care Environment
   Clinical Judgment/Cognitive Skills: Take Action
   Integrated Process: Nursing Process/ Implementation
   Content Area: Leadership/Management
   Priority Concepts: Clinical Judgment; Sensory Perception
   Level of Nursing Student: Advanced

   ANSWER: 2
   Rationale: During the irrigation, the client is positioned sitting with an ear basin under the ear. Irrigation solutions that are not close to the client's body temperature can be uncomfortable and may cause injury, nausea, and vertigo. A slow, steady stream of solution would be directed toward the upper wall of the ear canal and not toward the tympanic membrane. Too much force and a flow directed toward the tympanic membrane could cause tympanic membrane rupture. After the irrigation, the client would lie on the affected side for a time to finish the drainage of the irrigating solution and to allow gravity to assist in the removal of the earwax and solution.

   Test-Taking Strategy: Apply the clinical judgment/cognitive skill, *take action*. Focus on the subject, an indication that the nurse would intervene. This indicates that you are looking for an incorrect nursing action. Visualizing this procedure will assist in directing you to the correct option. **Review: Removal of cerumen** from the ear.

   Tip for the Nursing Student: An ear irrigation is the instillation of water or a saline solution into the ear and is usually done to remove excess cerumen from the ear. Ear irrigations are not done if a perforated tympanic membrane is suspected. It is important for the nurse to know the procedure for performing an ear irrigation to prevent complications of the procedure, such as rupture of the tympanic membrane.

2. The nurse is supervising an assistive personnel (AP) performing mouth care on an unconscious client. The nurse would intervene if the nurse noted the AP performing which actions? **Select all that apply.**
   ☐ 1 Turning the client's head to one side
   ☐ 2 Placing the client in a flat supine position
   ☐ 3 Using small volumes of fluid to rinse the mouth
   ☐ 4 Using a gloved finger to open the client's mouth
   ☐ 5 Placing an emesis basin under the client's mouth

   ANSWER: 2, 4
   Rationale: The client who is unconscious is at a great risk for aspiration. The client would have the head of the bed elevated because a flat supine position presents the risk of aspiration. The AP would either place the client in a side-lying position or turn the client's head to the side. An emesis basin is placed underneath the mouth to collect the small volumes of fluids used to rinse the mouth. A bite stick or a padded tongue blade, not a gloved finger, is used to open the mouth to prevent injury to the caregiver.

   Test-Taking Strategy: Apply the clinical judgment/cognitive skill, *take action*. Focus on the subject, an indication that the nurse would intervene. This indicates that you are looking for the option that is incorrect. Visualize this procedure, and remember that the nurse

Level of Cognitive Ability: Applying
Client Needs: Safe and Effective Care
Environment
Clinical Judgment/Cognitive Skills: Take
Action
Integrated Process: Nursing Process/
Implementation
Content Area: Leadership/Management
Priority Concepts: Caregiving; Safety
Level of Nursing Student: Advanced

never places a finger into a client's mouth or places the client in a flat position. **Review:** The procedure for administering **mouth care** to the client who is unconscious.

Tip for the Nursing Student: Unconsciousness is a state of complete or partial unawareness or lack of response to stimuli. It can be caused by a variety of conditions, such as shock, hypoxia, or stroke (brain attack). The client who is unconscious requires complete care, including mouth care. Depending on the state of unawareness, the client may exhibit some responses to stimuli, such as bearing down with the teeth if an object is placed in the mouth; therefore, you would never insert a finger into a client's mouth, regardless of the state of consciousness. It is extremely important to remember that the flat position places the client at risk for aspiration.

---

3. The nurse is observing as a student dons a pair of sterile gloves and prepares a sterile field. The nurse would intervene if the student performs which actions? **Select all that apply.**
   ☐ 1 Puts the right glove on and then the left glove
   ☐ 2 Dons the sterile gloves without washing the hands
   ☐ 3 Uses the inner wrapper of the gloves as a sterile field
   ☐ 4 Maintains the gloved hands below the level of the waist
   ☐ 5 Touches the gloves on the over-bed table, removes them, and dons another sterile pair

Level of Cognitive Ability: Applying
Client Needs: Safe and Effective Care
Environment
Clinical Judgment/Cognitive Skills: Take Action
Integrated Process: Nursing Process/
Implementation
Content Area: Leadership/Management
Priority Concepts: Infection; Leadership
Level of Nursing Student: Intermediate

ANSWER: 2, 4
Rationale: Hands must always be washed (even though sterile gloves are used) to keep germs from spreading. The hands would be maintained above the level of the waist to keep them and the areas that need to remain sterile exposed to as few contaminated areas as possible. The inside wrapper provides an excellent area for usage because it is sterile. Gloves that touch anything unsterile must be considered contaminated, and a new package of gloves must be obtained and used. The order of placing gloves on is up to the individual as long as sterile technique is not broken.

Test-Taking Strategy: Apply the clinical judgment/cognitive skill, *take action.* Focus on the subject, an indication that the nurse would intervene. This indicates that you are looking for the option that identifies an incorrect action. Visualize each option, keeping the principles of sterile technique in mind. Noting the words *without washing the hands* and *below the level of the waist* will direct you to the correct options. **Review: Sterile technique** for donning gloves.

Tip for the Nursing Student: Sterile technique, also known as *aseptic technique,* is the use of special procedures to prevent contamination of the nurse, object, or area by microorganisms. A sterile field is an area that the nurse prepares that is considered free of microorganisms. Sterile technique and a sterile field are used to perform various procedures, such as changing a wound dressing. Hand washing is always done before any procedure even if the nurse plans to don gloves.

---

4. The nurse reviews the laboratory results of a client receiving chemotherapy and notes that the white blood cell count is extremely low. The nurse asks a nursing student assigned to care for the client to place the client on neutropenic precautions. The nurse determines the **need to review** the procedures for neutropenic precautions if the student nurse takes which action?
   1 Removes the water pitcher from the client's room

ANSWER: 4
Rationale: In the immunocompromised client, a low-bacteria diet is necessary. This includes avoiding fresh fruits and vegetables. Thorough cooking of all food is also required. Anyone who enters the client's room would perform strict and thorough hand washing and wear a mask. Cut flowers or any standing water is removed from the room because it tends to harbor bacteria.

Test-Taking Strategy: Apply the clinical judgment/cognitive skill, *evaluate outcomes.* Note the strategic words, *need to review.* These words indicate a negative event query and that you are looking for the action that is incorrect. Recall that neutropenic precautions

2 Removes fresh cut flowers from the client's room

3 Places a box of face masks at the entrance to the client's room

4 Leaves fresh pears and apples brought to the client by a family member in the client's room

Level of Cognitive Ability: Evaluating
Client Needs: Safe and Effective Care Environment
Clinical Judgment/Cognitive Skills: Evaluate Outcomes
Integrated Process: Teaching and Learning
Content Area: Leadership/Management
Priority Concepts: Immunity; Safety
Level of Nursing Student: Intermediate

are implemented when a client is at high risk for contracting an infection. Next, look for the action that places the client at risk for infection. This will direct you to the correct option. **Review:** Interventions for the client on **neutropenic precautions.**

Tip for the Nursing Student: Neutropenia is an abnormal decrease in the number of neutrophils in the blood that places the client at risk for infection. Therefore, neutropenic precautions are instituted. This type of precaution focuses on protecting the client from infection, and any potential source of infection is avoided in the client's environment or in the care of the client.

---

5. The nurse is observing a nursing student perform nasotracheal suctioning on an adult client. The nurse would intervene if the nursing student performs which actions? **Select all that apply.**

   ☐ 1 Sets the wall suction pressure at 140 mm Hg

   ☐ 2 Encourages the client to cough after suctioning

   ☐ 3 Inserts the suction catheter during client inhalation

   ☐ 4 Inserts the catheter beyond the point at which the client elicits the gag reflex

   ☐ 5 Applies intermittent suction on the catheter during removal for up to 10 to 15 seconds

Level of Cognitive Ability: Applying
Client Needs: Safe and Effective Care Environment
Clinical Judgment/Cognitive Skills: Take Action
Integrated Process: Nursing Process/ Implementation
Content Area: Leadership/Management
Priority Concepts: Gas Exchange; Safety
Level of Nursing Student: Intermediate

ANSWER: **1, 4**
Rationale: When suctioning an adult client, the wall suction would be set at 80 to 120 mm Hg (portable suction is set at 7 to 15 mm Hg). Elevated suction pressure settings can increase the risk of trauma to the mucosa and can induce greater hypoxia. The catheter would be inserted until the gag reflex is elicited. The catheter would not be inserted beyond this point. Suction is applied intermittently during withdrawal afterward. Options 2, 3, and 5 are correct steps in performing this procedure.

Test-Taking Strategy: Apply the clinical judgment/cognitive skill, *take action.* Focus on the subject, an indication that the nurse would intervene. This indicates that you are looking for an incorrect action. Visualizing this procedure will assist in eliminating options 2, 3, and 5 because they are correct actions. **Review: Suctioning** procedures.

Tip for the Nursing Student: Nasotracheal suctioning is a procedure that is used to remove accumulated secretions from the respiratory tract when the client is unable to effectively cough them out. It is a sterile procedure and requires specific actions to prevent trauma to the mucosa of the respiratory tract and to prevent hypoxia.

---

6. The nurse is preparing to administer a medication to a client and notes that the dose prescribed is higher than the recommended dosage. The nurse calls the primary health care provider (PHCP) to clarify the prescription, and the PHCP instructs the nurse to administer the dose as prescribed. Which action would the nurse take?

ANSWER: **2**
Rationale: If the PHCP writes a prescription that requires clarification, it is the nurse's responsibility to contact the PHCP for clarification. If there is no resolution regarding the prescription because the prescription remains as it was written after talking with the PHCP or because the PHCP cannot be located, the nurse would then contact the nurse manager or supervisor for further clarification as to what the next step would be. Under no circumstances would the nurse proceed to carry out the prescription until clarification is obtained. Calling the

1 Call the pharmacy.
2 Contact the nursing supervisor.
3 Administer the dose as prescribed.
4 Contact the medical director on call.

Level of Cognitive Ability: Applying
Client Needs: Safe and Effective Care
  Environment
Clinical Judgment/Cognitive Skills: Take
  Action
Integrated Process: Nursing Process/
  Implementation
Content Area: Leadership/Management
Priority Concepts: Clinical Judgment; Safety
Level of Nursing Student: Intermediate

pharmacy is a resource action that will confirm that the dose of medication prescribed is inappropriate, but this action will not resolve the problem facing the nurse. Option 4 is a premature action.

Test-Taking Strategy: Apply the clinical judgment/cognitive skill, *take action*. Focus on the subject, nursing responsibilities related to prescriptions requiring clarification. Eliminate option 3 first because this is an unsafe action. Option 4 is a premature action and would be eliminated next. Eliminate option 1 next because this action would not resolve the problem. Also recall that the nurse would follow the organizational chain of command and seek assistance from the nursing supervisor. **Review:** Nursing responsibilities related to a discrepancy in PHCP's prescriptions and the associated **ethical and legal responsibilities.**

Tip for the Nursing Student: The client's PHCP will document specific prescriptions regarding the client's care in the medical record, and the nurse needs to follow the prescriptions unless the nurse deems that a prescription may harm the client. If the prescription can cause harm to the client, the nurse needs to contact the PHCP to change the prescription. If the PHCP does not change the prescription or if the nurse is unable to locate the PHCP, the nurse would follow the chain of command in the health care organization. In this situation, the nurse would contact the nursing supervisor. Under no circumstances would the nurse implement a prescription that could cause harm to the client.

---

7. The charge nurse is observing a new nursing graduate insert an indwelling urinary (Foley) catheter. The charge nurse would intervene if the new nursing graduate begins to perform which actions? **Select all that apply.**
   ☐ **1** Lubricates the catheter before inserting it
   ☐ **2** Positions the client in a side-lying position
   ☐ **3** Inflates the balloon to test patency before inserting the catheter
   ☐ **4** Cleans the area around the urinary meatus before inserting the catheter
   ☐ **5** Inflates the balloon as soon as urine begins to flow through the catheter tubing

Level of Cognitive Ability: Applying
Client Needs: Safe and Effective Care
  Environment
Clinical Judgment/Cognitive Skills: Take Action
Integrated Process: Nursing Process/
  Implementation
Content Area: Leadership/Management
Priority Concepts: Elimination; Safety
Level of Nursing Student: Intermediate

ANSWER: 2, 3, 5
Rationale: Before insertion of the catheter, the client (if female) would be positioned on the back with the posterior sides of the feet touching each other and with the knees bent. This allows for optimal visualization and access to the urethral meatus. The balloon is not inflated before insertion of the catheter because this can increase the fragility of the balloon and increase the likelihood of balloon breakage or fragmenting. After urine begins to flow, the catheter is inserted 2.5 cm (1 inch) more. Doing so ensures that the balloon is in the bladder, not in the urethra. Options 1 and 4 identify correct procedure.

Test-Taking Strategy: Apply the clinical judgment/cognitive skill, *take action*. Focus on the subject, an indication that the nurse would intervene. This tells you that you are looking for options that identify incorrect actions by the new nursing graduate. Visualizing this procedure and reading each option carefully will direct you to options 2, 3, and 5. **Review:** The procedure for inserting an **indwelling urinary (Foley) catheter.**

Tip for the Nursing Student: An indwelling urinary (Foley) catheter is a rubber tube with a balloon tip that is filled with a sterile liquid after it is inserted in the bladder. It is connected to a bag that collects urine draining from the bladder. Sterile technique is used to insert this catheter. This type of catheter is used when continuous drainage of the bladder is needed, such as during a surgical procedure.

8. A hospitalized client tells the evening nurse that she received pain medication at 10:00 AM and again at 2:00 PM but that the medication provided no relief from the pain. The client says to the nurse, "Whenever that daytime nurse takes care of me and gives me pain medication, it never works! I am so glad that you are here so that I can get some relief from this pain." The nurse has observed this same occurrence with other clients who were cared for by this same daytime nurse and suspects that the daytime nurse is self-abusing drugs. The nurse would implement which action?
   1 Report the information to the nursing supervisor.
   2 Talk with the daytime nurse who gave the medication to the client.
   3 Call the impaired nurse organization and report the daytime nurse.
   4 Report the information about the day time nurse to the police department.

Level of Cognitive Ability: Applying
Client Needs: Safe and Effective Care Environment
Clinical Judgment/Cognitive Skills: Take Action
Integrated Process: Nursing Process/ Implementation
Content Area: Leadership/Management
Priority Concepts: Communication; Health Policy
Level of Nursing Student: Advanced

ANSWER: 1
Rationale: If the nurse suspects that another nurse is self-abusing drugs, the nurse needs to report the suspicion to the nursing supervisor. Factual information such as that described by the client and specific information related to the nurse's observations need to be reported. The nurse would not confront the nurse who is suspected of self-abusing drugs because this may lead to a conflict or confrontation. The nurse would follow the organizational chain of communication of the institution to report the incident. The suspicion needs to be reported to the nursing supervisor, who will then report to the board of nursing. The board of nursing has jurisdiction over the practice of nursing and may develop plans for treatment and supervision.

Test-Taking Strategy: Apply the clinical judgment/cognitive skill, *take action.* Eliminate options 3 and 4 first because they are comparable or alike options and both relate to reporting the incident to agencies outside the hospital. From the remaining options, recall that agency channels of communication are used when reporting an incident. Also the action in option 2 can lead to a conflict. **Review:** Nursing responsibilities related to **incident reporting.**

Tip for the Nursing Student: Drug abuse is the use of drugs illegally. If a nurse is suspected of drug abuse and is taking drugs intended for use by the client, the suspecting nurse needs to report such suspicion. Failure to provide a client with required and needed treatment is harmful to the client and is illegal.

---

9. The nurse determines that a client with a stroke is experiencing difficulty with fine motor coordination when performing activities of daily living. The nurse would suggest that the client be referred to which member of the health care team?
   1 Physical therapist
   2 Speech pathologist
   3 Recreational therapist
   4 Occupational therapist

Level of Cognitive Ability: Applying
Client Needs: Safe and Effective Care Environment
Clinical Judgment/Cognitive Skills: Generate Solutions
Integrated Process: Nursing Process/ Planning
Content Area: Leadership/Management

ANSWER: 4
Rationale: The occupational therapist helps in developing methods that assist in managing difficulty with fine motor coordination when performing activities of daily living. Although a physical therapist may also address fine motor activities, the focus is primarily on gross motor skills and the development of muscle strength. Speech pathologists and recreational therapists do not address this aspect of care.

Test-Taking Strategy: Apply the clinical judgment/cognitive skill, *generate solutions.* Focus on the subject, fine motor coordination when performing activities of daily living. This will assist in eliminating options 2 and 3. From the remaining options, noting the words *activities of daily living* will direct you to the correct option. **Review:** Roles of health care team members.

Tip for the Nursing Student: A stroke is an abnormal condition of the brain that is characterized by occlusion by a clot, hemorrhage, or vasospasm that results in ischemia of the brain tissues. Paralysis,

Priority Concepts: Care Coordination;
    Mobility
Level of Nursing Student: Intermediate

weakness, sensory changes, speech defects, or even death can occur. The client who experiences a stroke will require rehabilitative services that will assist the client in relearning activities to promote independence.

---

10. The nurse notes that an assistive personnel (AP) dons clean gloves but does not perform hand washing first before taking an oral temperature on a client. The nurse plans to implement a teaching session for APs and would incorporate which principle?
    1 Learning involves a change of behavior.
    2 Learning is a cognitive, passive process.
    3 APs need constant supervision when caring for clients.
    4 Negative rewards reduce undesirable behavior and would be used when an error is seen.

Level of Cognitive Ability: Applying
Client Needs: Safe and Effective Care
    Environment
Clinical Judgment/Cognitive Skills: Generate
    Solutions
Integrated Process: Teaching and Learning
Content Area: Leadership/Management
Priority Concepts: Leadership; Safety
Level of Nursing Student: Advanced

ANSWER: 1
Rationale: The nurse assumes leadership for improving client care by implementing a teaching session that has the potential for changing behavior. Persons who change their behavior have internalized information and apply it to their actions. Options 3 and 4 use negative strategies to change behavior; this is usually unsuccessful. Option 2 views the learner as not being actively involved in the teaching and learning process.

Test-Taking Strategy: Apply the clinical judgment/cognitive skill, *generate solutions*. Eliminate options 3 and 4 first because they are comparable or alike options and do not provide a positive view of learners. Eliminate option 2 because learning would be an active, not a passive, process. **Review: Teaching and learning principles.**

Tip for the Nursing Student: Hand washing is always done before and after every client contact even if the nurse intends to don gloves for client care. If the nurse observes an incorrect action by another health care team member, it is the nurse's responsibility to teach correct procedure to ensure client safety and a safe environment. Learning involves acquiring knowledge about a skill and changing behavior as a result of the training.

---

11. The primary health care provider has prescribed a cleansing enema for an adult client. The nurse provides directions to a nursing student who is trained to administer enemas. As part of the directions, the nurse would tell the student that the maximum volume of fluid that can be administered is which volume?
    1 100 mL
    2 300 mL
    3 500 mL
    4 1000 mL

Level of Cognitive Ability: Applying
Client Needs: Safe and Effective Care
    Environment
Clinical Judgment/Cognitive Skills: Take Action
Integrated Process: Nursing Process/
    Implementation
Content Area: Leadership/Management
Priority Concepts: Elimination; Safety
Level of Nursing Student: Beginning

ANSWER: 4
Rationale: Cleansing enemas promote complete evacuation of feces from the colon. They act by stimulating peristalsis through the infusion of a large volume of solution or through local irritation of the colon's mucosa. For an adult client, 750 to 1000 mL is used. Therefore, the maximum volume of solution for an adult is 1000 mL.

Test-Taking Strategy: Apply the clinical judgment/cognitive skill, *take action*. Focus on the subject, the procedure for administering a cleansing enema. Note the words *maximum volume*, and note that the question addresses an adult client. Recalling the anatomy of the colon in an adult client and the procedure for administering a cleansing enema will direct you to the correct option. **Review: The procedure for administering a cleansing enema.**

Tip for the Nursing Student: An enema is the introduction of solution into the rectum for cleansing the bowel. Cleansing of the bowel may be prescribed to treat constipation or may be prescribed as a preprocedure treatment, such as before a diagnostic test or surgical procedure involving the colon.

12. A client requires a partial bed bath. The nurse gives instructions to an assistive personnel (AP) about the partial bed bath and would tell the AP to perform which action?
1 Wash only the client's hands and face.
2 Provide mouth care and perineal care only.
3 Let the client decide what she or he wants washed.
4 Be sure to bathe the client's body parts that would cause discomfort or odor if left unbathed.

Level of Cognitive Ability: Applying
Client Needs: Safe and Effective Care Environment
Clinical Judgment/Cognitive Skills: Take Action
Integrated Process: Nursing Process/ Implementation
Content Area: Leadership/Management
Priority Concepts: Caregiving; Safety
Level of Nursing Student: Beginning

ANSWER: 4
Rationale: A partial bed bath involves bathing the body parts that would cause discomfort or odor if left unbathed. This may include the axillary areas, perineal areas, and any skinfold areas. Options 1, 2, and 3 do not completely address a partial bed bath.

Test-Taking Strategy: Apply the clinical judgment/cognitive skill, *take action.* Note the words *partial bed bath.* Eliminate options 1 and 2 because of the closed-ended word "only." From the remaining options, recalling the definition of a partial bed bath will direct you to the correct option. **Review:** The components of a **partial bed bath.**

Tip for the Nursing Student: Bathing a client is an important role of the nurse and is necessary for hygienic purposes and to prevent infection, maintain skin integrity, stimulate circulation, and provide comfort. Several types of baths may be given, including a bed bath, tub bath, shower, complete bath, or partial bath.

---

13. The charge nurse is observing as a new nursing graduate inserts a nasal trumpet airway to provide a route for suctioning the client. The nurse would intervene if the new nursing graduate performs which action?
1 Checks the nose for septal deviation
2 Uses a nasal trumpet that is slightly larger than the nares
3 Inserts the nasal trumpet gently following the contour of the nasopharyngeal passageway
4 Lubricates the nasal trumpet with a water-soluble lubricant jelly containing a local anesthetic

Level of Cognitive Ability: Applying
Client Needs: Safe and Effective Care Environment
Clinical Judgment/Cognitive Skills: Take Action
Integrated Process: Nursing Process/ Implementation
Content Area: Leadership/Management
Priority Concepts: Gas Exchange; Safety
Level of Nursing Student: Intermediate

ANSWER: 2
Rationale: The nurse would select a nasal trumpet airway that is slightly smaller than the nares and slightly larger than the suction catheter to be used to suction the client. Options 1, 3, and 4 are correct actions for inserting a nasal trumpet airway.

Test-Taking Strategy: Apply the clinical judgment/cognitive skill, *take action.* Focus on the subject, an indication that the nurse would intervene. This indicates that you are looking for the option that indicates an incorrect action by the new nursing graduate. Noting the words *slightly larger than the nares* and visualizing this procedure will direct you to the correct option. **Review:** The procedure for **suctioning.**

Tip for the Nursing Student: A nasal trumpet is a tube that is inserted into one of the client's nostrils to provide assistance in maintaining the client's airway and to provide a route for suctioning secretions from the client.

14. The nurse is observing as an assistive personnel (AP) measures the blood pressure (BP) of a client. The nurse would intervene if which action was observed that would interfere with accurate measurement of the BP?
    1 Positions the client's arm at heart level
    2 Exposes the extremity fully by removing constricting clothing
    3 Explains the procedure to the client and asks the client to rest for 5 minutes
    4 Palpates the carotid artery and then places the cuff of the sphygmomanometer 1 inch (2.5 cm) above the brachial artery

Level of Cognitive Ability: Applying
Client Needs: Safe and Effective Care Environment
Clinical Judgment/Cognitive Skills: Take Action
Integrated Process: Nursing Process/ Implementation
Content Area: Leadership/Management
Priority Concepts: Perfusion; Safety
Level of Nursing Student: Beginning

ANSWER: 4
Rationale: When taking a BP, the brachial artery (not the carotid artery) is palpated and the cuff of the sphygmomanometer is positioned 1 inch (2.5 cm) above this site of pulsation. Options 1, 2, and 3 are correct actions when taking a BP.

Test-Taking Strategy: Apply the clinical judgment/cognitive skill, *take action*. Focus on the subject, an indication that the nurse would intervene. This indicates that you are looking for the option that identifies an incorrect action by the AP. Visualizing this procedure will assist in eliminating options 1, 2, and 3. **Review:** The principles related to **BP measurement.**

Tip for the Nursing Student: BP is the amount of pressure exerted on the walls of the arteries and veins and the heart chambers by the circulating volume of blood. This pressure is measured by taking the client's BP. To ensure accuracy of the measurement, a specific procedure is followed.

15. The nurse is reviewing the preprocedure care for a client scheduled to have an echocardiogram after a myocardial infarction. The nurse determines that the student nurse understands the preprocedure instructions if the student nurse makes which statement?
    1 "The client needs to sign an informed consent."
    2 "The procedure is painless and takes 30 to 60 minutes to complete."
    3 "The client cannot eat or drink anything for 4 hours before the procedure."
    4 "An allergy to iodine or shellfish is a contraindication to having the procedure."

Level of Cognitive Ability: Evaluating
Client Needs: Safe and Effective Care Environment
Clinical Judgment/Cognitive Skills: Evaluate Outcomes
Integrated Process: Teaching and Learning
Content Area: Leadership/Management
Priority Concepts: Leadership; Safety
Level of Nursing Student: Intermediate

ANSWER: 2
Rationale: Echocardiography uses ultrasound to evaluate the heart's structure and motion. It is a noninvasive risk-free, pain-free test that involves no special preparation. It is commonly done at the bedside or on an outpatient basis. The client must lie quietly for 30 to 60 minutes while the procedure is being performed. Options 1, 3, and 4 are not preprocedure preparations.

Test-Taking Strategy: Apply the clinical judgment/cognitive skill, *evaluate outcomes*. Note the subject, client instructions related to echocardiogram. Focus on the diagnostic test being performed. Recalling that echocardiography uses ultrasound and that ultrasound is noninvasive will assist in eliminating options 1, 3, and 4. **Review:** Client instructions related to **echocardiogram.**

Tip for the Nursing Student: Diagnostic uses of an echocardiogram include the detection of atrial or other tumors, measurement of the heart chambers, and evaluation of valve and chamber function. An important point to remember is that an informed consent is needed only if the test is invasive. Another important point is that the nurse must ensure that the client understands the test to be done and its purpose and teaches the client about the test.

16. A client is scheduled for a cardiac catheterization, and the nurse is reviewing the preprocedure care with a nursing student. The nurse determines that the student **needs further instruction** while preparing the client if the nursing student makes which statement?
    1 "The procedure takes about 5 hours."
    2 "The client may experience flushing feelings during the procedure."
    3 "The blood vessels and flow of blood will be examined with this procedure."
    4 "There is minimal discomfort with catheter insertion because a local anesthetic is used."

Level of Cognitive Ability: Evaluating
Client Needs: Safe and Effective Care Environment
Clinical Judgment/Cognitive Skills: Evaluate Outcomes
Integrated Process: Teaching and Learning
Content Area: Leadership/Management
Priority Concepts: Leadership; Safety
Level of Nursing Student: Intermediate

ANSWER: 1
Rationale: A cardiac catheterization is a diagnostic test that examines the coronary arteries and the flow of blood through them. The procedure is done in a darkened cardiac catheterization room in the radiology department. A local anesthetic is used, so there is minimal discomfort with catheter insertion. The preprocedure preparation and the procedure may take approximately 1 to 3 hours, during which the client may feel various sensations, such as a feeling of warmth or flushing, with catheter passage and dye injection.

Test-Taking Strategy: Apply the clinical judgment/cognitive skill, *evaluate outcomes*. Note the strategic words, *needs further instruction*. These words indicate a negative event query and the need to select the incorrect statement by the nursing student. Recalling the purpose of the procedure will assist in eliminating option 3. Next, recalling that a dye is injected will assist in eliminating options 2 and 4. Also noting the words *5 hours* in option 1 will direct you to this option. **Review:** The procedure for a **cardiac catheterization.**

Tip for the Nursing Student: Cardiac catheterization is a test performed to examine the status of the coronary arteries or the presence of congenital heart disease, stenosis, or valvular disease. Risks associated with the procedure include dysrhythmias (irregular heartbeats), infection, and thrombosis, and the nurse needs to monitor the client closely after the procedure.

---

17. The nurse has instructed an assistive personnel (AP) in the procedure for collecting a 24 hour urine specimen from a client. The nurse determines that the AP understands the directions if the AP makes which statement?
    1 "I need to keep the specimen at room temperature."
    2 "I need to save the first urine specimen collected at the start time."
    3 "I need to discard the last voided specimen at the end of the collection time."
    4 "I need to ask the client to void, discard the specimen, and note the start time."

Level of Cognitive Ability: Evaluating
Client Needs: Safe and Effective Care Environment
Clinical Judgment/Cognitive Skills: Evaluate Outcomes
Integrated Process: Teaching and Learning
Content Area: Leadership/Management
Priority Concepts: Elimination; Safety
Level of Nursing Student: Beginning

ANSWER: 4
Rationale: Because a 24-hour urine specimen is a timed quantitative determination, the test must be started with an empty bladder. Therefore, the first urine is discarded. Fifteen minutes before the end of the collection time, the client would be asked to void, and this specimen is added to the collection. The urine collection would be refrigerated or placed on ice to prevent changes in urine composition.

Test-Taking Strategy: Apply the clinical judgment/cognitive skill, *evaluate outcomes*. Focus on the subject, the procedure for collecting a 24-hour urine specimen. Note that options 2 and 4 are opposite, which is an indication that one of them is likely to be the correct option. Recalling that the 24-hour urine specimen is a timed quantitative determination will assist in directing you to the correct option. **Review:** The procedure for collecting a **24-hour urine specimen.**

Tip for the Nursing Student: Urine specimens may be collected to diagnose various conditions. These specimens may be prescribed to be collected as a random specimen, a sterile specimen, or a 24-hour urine collection. An important point to remember is that the procedure for its collection needs to be followed to ensure accurate results.

18. The nurse is teaching an assistive personnel (AP) how to measure a carotid pulse. The nurse would tell the AP to measure the pulse on only one side of the client's neck for which **primary** reason?
    1 Because the pulse rate will be easier to count
    2 To prevent dizziness and a drop in the heart rate
    3 So that the client will not feel a sense of choking
    4 Because it will provide a more accurate determination of the quality of the pulse

Level of Cognitive Ability: Applying
Client Needs: Safe and Effective Care Environment
Clinical Judgment/Cognitive Skills: Generate Solutions
Integrated Process: Teaching and Learning
Content Area: Leadership/Management
Priority Concepts: Perfusion; Safety
Level of Nursing Student: Beginning

ANSWER: 2
Rationale: Applying pressure to both carotid arteries at the same time is contraindicated. Excess pressure to the baroreceptors in the carotid vessels could cause the heart rate and blood pressure to reflexively drop and cause syncope. In addition, the manual pressure could interfere with the flow of blood to the brain. The remaining options are unrelated to the reason for measuring the pulse on only one side of the client's neck.

Test-Taking Strategy: Apply the clinical judgment/cognitive skill, *generate solutions*. Note the strategic word, *primary*. Note that option 2 describes the greatest danger to the client. **Review:** The function and location of **baroreceptors** in the carotid vessels.

Tip for the Nursing Student: The carotid artery is located in the neck region and is one of the major arteries supplying blood to the head. It is one of the pulse points in the body that can be palpated to check a client's pulse.

---

19. The nurse is supervising a nursing student who is performing a pulse oximetry measurement on a client with peripheral vascular disease. The nurse determines that the nursing student is performing the procedure accurately if the student places the oximetry probe on which anatomical area? **Refer to figure.**

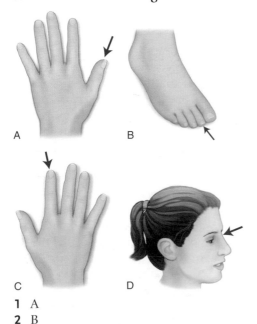

A   B

C   D

    1 A
    2 B
    3 C
    4 D

ANSWER: 4
Rationale: If the client has peripheral vascular disease, the pulse oximetry probe would be placed on the earlobe or bridge of the nose because peripheral vasoconstriction or inadequate blood flow to the peripheral areas of the body will interfere with the oxygen saturation measurement. It is also important to note that the probe would not be attached to a finger, ear, or bridge of the nose if the area is edematous, if the skin integrity is compromised, or if the area is hypothermic. Additionally, the sensor would not be placed on the same extremity as an electronic blood pressure cuff because blood flow is temporarily interrupted when the cuff inflates. Placing the probe on the anatomical areas noted in options 1, 2, and 3 will not provide an accurate measurement of the oxygen saturation.

Test-Taking Strategy: Apply the clinical judgment/cognitive skill, *evaluate outcomes*. Focus on the client's diagnosis—peripheral vascular disease—and recall the pathophysiology associated with the disease. Note that options 1, 2, and 3 are comparable or alike options in that they indicate using a peripheral body area. **Review:** The procedure for **pulse oximetry** measurement.

Tip for the Nursing Student: Peripheral vascular disease is an abnormal condition that affects the blood vessels, leading to decreased blood flow to the body part. Pulse oximetry uses a cliplike device that measures the amount of saturated hemoglobin in the tissue capillaries and thus the percentage of oxygen saturation in the blood.

Level of Cognitive Ability: Evaluating
Client Needs: Safe and Effective Care
Environment
Clinical Judgment/Cognitive Skills: Evaluate
Outcomes
Integrated Process: Teaching and Learning
Content Area: Leadership/Management
Priority Concepts: Perfusion; Safety
Level of Nursing Student: Beginning

---

20. The nursing student is preparing a client who will have spinal anesthesia for surgery. The nurse in charge asks the nursing student to identify which preoperative data would get the **highest priority** to report to the nurse on the next shift who will care for the client postoperatively?

    1 Pulse rate of 78 beats/min
    2 Voided 300 mL preoperatively
    3 Blood pressure of 126/78 mm Hg
    4 Presence of weakness in the left lower extremity

Level of Cognitive Ability: Analyzing
Client Needs: Safe and Effective Care
Environment
Clinical Judgment/Cognitive Skills: Prioritize
Hypotheses
Integrated Process: Nursing Process/Analysis
Content Area: Leadership/Management
Priority Concepts: Clinical Judgment;
Sensory Perception
Level of Nursing Student: Intermediate

ANSWER: 4
Rationale: It is important to document and report any preoperative weakness or impaired movement of a lower extremity in the client who is to have spinal anesthesia because it causes temporary paralysis of the lower extremities. When the client's function returns, the preoperative weakness or impairment will not be misinterpreted as a complication of anesthesia. Options 1, 2, and 3 may be documented and reported, but they are not the highest priority.

Test-Taking Strategy: Apply the clinical judgment/cognitive skill, *prioritize hypotheses*. Note the strategic words, *highest priority.* Note the relationship between the words *spinal anesthesia* and the correct option. Also note that the data in options 1, 2, and 3 are normal findings. **Review:** Care of the **preoperative client.**

Tip for the Nursing Student: Spinal anesthesia is done by an injection into the subarachnoid cerebrospinal fluid space. It produces a state of lack of sensation in the lower part of the body. An important nursing responsibility in the postoperative period is to monitor for the return of sensation in the lower body. If sensation does not return or is altered in any way, the surgeon is notified.

---

21. A client comes to the hospital emergency department with complaints of severe right lower abdominal pain characteristic of appendicitis. The client has no health insurance. The nurse understands that legally the hospital has which obligation?

    1 Refer the client to the nearest public hospital.
    2 Provide uncompensated care in emergency situations.
    3 Have a primary health care provider see the client before admission.
    4 Respect the family's requests to admit their family member to the hospital.

Level of Cognitive Ability: Applying
Client Needs: Safe and Effective Care
Environment
Clinical Judgment/Cognitive Skills: Generate
Solutions

ANSWER: 2
Rationale: Federal law and many state laws require that hospitals must provide emergency care. The client can be transferred only after the client has been medically screened and stabilized. The client must give consent for the transfer, and there must be a facility that will accept the client. Options 1, 3, and 4 do not fully address the legal requirements for emergency care.

Test-Taking Strategy: Apply the clinical judgment/cognitive skill, *generate solutions.* Focus on the subject, legal implications in the care of the client without insurance. Note the words *has no health insurance* and the word *legally.* Noting that the situation presented is an emergency will direct you to the correct option, which addresses the legal scope of providing emergency care. **Review:** The **legal issues.** related to providing **emergency care.**

Tip for the Nursing Student: Remember that the client is the priority. If an emergency condition exists, the health care agency must provide care, regardless of the client's insurance status. Appendicitis is an acute inflammation of the appendix that, if left untreated, can lead to perforation and peritonitis, which is life threatening.

Integrated Process: Nursing Process/Planning
Content Area: Leadership/Management
Priority Concepts: Health Care Economics;
      Health Policy
Level of Nursing Student: Intermediate

---

22. The nurse tells an assistive personnel (AP) that a client recovering from a myocardial infarction requires a complete bed bath. During the bath, the nurse would intervene if the nurse observed the AP performing which action?

    1 Washing the client's chest
    2 Giving the client a back rub
    3 Washing the client's perineal area
    4 Asking the client to wash her or his legs

Level of Cognitive Ability: Applying
Client Needs: Safe and Effective Care
      Environment
Clinical Judgment/Cognitive Skills: Take
      Action
Integrated Process: Nursing Process/
      Implementation
Content Area: Leadership/Management
Priority Concepts: Perfusion; Safety
Level of Nursing Student: Intermediate

ANSWER: 4
Rationale: A complete bed bath is for clients who are totally dependent and require total hygiene care. Total care may be necessary for a client recovering from a myocardial infarction to conserve the client's energy and reduce oxygen requirements. The nurse would intervene if the nurse observed the AP asking the client to wash her or his legs. Options 1, 2, and 3 are components of providing a complete bed bath.

Test-Taking Strategy: Apply the clinical judgment/cognitive skill, *take action.* Focus on the **subject**, an indication that the nurse should intervene. This indicates that you need to select the option that identifies an incorrect action by the AP. Focusing on the words *complete bed bath* will direct you to the incorrect action in option 4 because in this option the nurse asks the client to participate in the bathing process. **Review:** The procedure for giving a **complete bed bath.**

Tip for the Nursing Student: Bathing a client is an important role of the nurse and is necessary for hygienic purposes and to prevent infection, maintain skin integrity, stimulate circulation, and provide comfort. Several types of baths may be given, including a bed bath, tub bath, shower, complete bath, or partial bath.

---

23. The nurse is observing a nursing student auscultating the breath sounds of a client. The nurse would intervene if the nursing student performs which action?

    1 Uses the diaphragm of the stethoscope
    2 Places the stethoscope directly on the client's skin
    3 Asks the client to breathe slowly and deeply through the mouth
    4 Asks the client to lie flat on the right side and then on the left side

Level of Cognitive Ability: Applying
Client Needs: Safe and Effective Care
      Environment
Clinical Judgment/Cognitive Skills: Take Action
Integrated Process: Nursing Process/
      Implementation
Content Area: Leadership/Management
Priority Concepts: Clinical Judgment; Gas
      Exchange
Level of Nursing Student: Intermediate

ANSWER: 4
Rationale: The client ideally would sit up and breathe slowly and deeply through the mouth. The diaphragm of the stethoscope, which is warmed before use, is placed directly on the client's skin, not over a gown or clothing.

Test-Taking Strategy: Apply the clinical judgment/cognitive skill, *take action.* Focus on the **subject**, an indication that the nurse would intervene. This indicates that you are looking for the option that gives an incorrect action by the nursing student. Noting the words *lie flat* will direct you to the correct option. **Review:** The procedure for **auscultating breath sounds.**

Tip for the Nursing Student: A breath sound is the sound of air passing in and out of the lungs as heard with a stethoscope. Normal breath sounds include vesicular, bronchovesicular, and bronchial sounds. Auscultating breath sounds is a part of data collection.

24. The nurse is observing an assistive personnel (AP) talking to a client who is hearing impaired. The nurse would intervene if the AP performs which action during communication with the client?

1 Speaks in a normal tone
2 Speaks clearly to the client
3 Faces the client when speaking
4 Speaks directly into the impaired ear

Level of Cognitive Ability: Applying
Client Needs: Safe and Effective Care Environment
Clinical Judgment/Cognitive Skills: Take Action
Integrated Process: Communication and Documentation
Content Area: Leadership/Management
Priority Concepts: Collaboration; Communication
Level of Nursing Student: Beginning

ANSWER: 4

Rationale: When communicating with a hearing-impaired client, the nurse would speak in a normal tone to the client and would not shout. The nurse would talk directly to the client while facing the client and speak clearly. If the client does not seem to understand what is said, the nurse would express the statement differently. Moving closer to the client and toward the better ear may facilitate communication, but the nurse would avoid talking directly into the impaired ear.

Test-Taking Strategy: Apply the clinical judgment/cognitive skill, *take action*. Focus on the subject, an indication that the nurse would intervene. This indicates that you are looking for the option that gives an incorrect action by the AP. Noting the words *directly into the impaired ear* will direct you to the correct option. **Review:** Care of the **hearing-impaired client.**

Tip for the Nursing Student: Special communication techniques are needed when caring for a hearing-impaired client. For example, the nurse would face the client when speaking; enunciate words slowly, clearly, and in a normal voice; avoid placing the hands over the mouth when speaking so that the client can lip-read; and avoid speaking into the impaired ear. The nurse needs to use these techniques to communicate with the hearing-impaired client to prevent social isolation. In addition, teaching and supervising others are roles of the nurse, and the nurse needs to intervene if she or he observes incorrect communication techniques performed by another health care team member.

---

25. The nurse administers a fatal dose of morphine sulfate to a client. During the subsequent investigation of error, it is determined that the nurse did not check the client's respiratory rate before administering the medication. Failure to adequately assess the client is addressed under which function of the nurse practice act?

1 Defining the specific educational requirements for licensure in the state
2 Describing the scope of practice of licensed and unlicensed care providers
3 Identifying the process for disciplinary action if standards of care are not met
4 Recommending specific terms of incarceration for nurses who violate the law

Level of Cognitive Ability: Analyzing
Client Needs: Safe and Effective Care Environment
Clinical Judgment/Cognitive Skills: Take Action
Integrated Process: Nursing Process/Implementation
Content Area: Leadership/Management
Priority Concepts: Clinical Judgment; Safety
Level of Nursing Student: Intermediate

ANSWER: 3

Rationale: In this situation, acceptable standards of care were not met (the nurse failed to adequately check the client before administering a medication). Option 3 refers specifically to the situation described in the question, whereas options 1, 2, and 4 do not.

Test-Taking Strategy: Apply the clinical judgment/cognitive skill, *take action*. Focus on the subject, nursing implications and legal implications for medication errors. Note the relationship between the words *failure to adequately assess the client* in the question and *standards of care are not met* in the correct option. **Review:** The legal implications related to **medication errors.**

Tip for the Nursing Student: A nurse practice act is a statute enacted by the legislation of a state. Nurse practice acts may vary from state to state, but they generally include the educational requirements of the nurse, a distinction between nursing practice and medical practice, and a definition of the scope of practice for the nurse. Additional issues that may be covered in the act include grounds for disciplinary action and the rights of the nurse if disciplinary action is taken. All nurses are responsible for knowing the provisions of the act in the state in which they work.

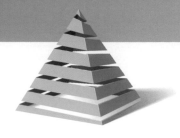

References and Bibliography

Dickison, P., Haerling, K. A., & Lasater, K. (2019). Integrating the National Council of State Boards of Nursing Clinical Judgment Model into Nursing Educational Frameworks. *Journal of Nursing Education, 58*(2), 72–78.

Gahart, B., Nazareno, A., & Ortega, M. (2021). *2021 Intravenous medications* (37th ed.). St. Louis, MO: Mosby.

Hockenberry, M., & Wilson, D. (2019). *Wong's nursing care of infants and children* (11th ed.). St. Louis, MO: Mosby.

Huether, S., & McCance, K. (2020). *Understanding pathophysiology* (7th ed.). St. Louis, MO: Mosby.

Ignatavicius, D. D., Workman, M. L., Rebar, C., & Heimgartner, N. M. (2021). *Medical-surgical nursing: Concepts for interprofessional collaborative care.* (10th ed.). St. Louis, MO: Elsevier.

Jarvis, C. (2020). *Physical examination and health assessment* (8th ed.). St. Louis: Saunders.

Keltner, N., & Steele, D. (2019). *Psychiatric nursing* (8th ed.). St. Louis, MO: Mosby.

Kizior, R., and Hodgson, B. (2022). *Saunders nursing drug handbook 2022*. St. Louis, MO: Saunders.

Lewis, S., Bucher, L., Heitkemper, M., et al. (2020). *Medical-surgical nursing: Assessment and management of clinical problems* (11th ed.). St. Louis, MO: Mosby.

Lilley, L., Rainforth Collins, S., & Snyder, J. (2020). *Pharmacology and the nursing process* (9th ed.). St. Louis, MO: Mosby.

Lowdermilk, D., Perry, S., Cashion, M., Alden, K., & Olshansky, E. (2020). *Maternity and women's health care* (12th ed.). St. Louis, MO: Mosby.

National Council of State Boards of Nursing. (2019). *2020 NCLEX-PN® detailed test plan*. Chicago: National Council of State Boards of Nursing. Retrieved from http://www.ncsbn.org.

National Council of State Boards of Nursing. (2018). *2019 NCLEX-RN® detailed test plan*. Chicago: National Council of State Boards of Nursing. Retrieved from http://www.ncsbn.org.

Nix, S. (2021). *Williams' basic nutrition and diet therapy* (15th ed.). St. Louis, MO: Mosby.

Pagana, K., Pagana, T., & Pagana, T. N. (2021). *Mosby's diagnostic and laboratory tests reference* (15th ed.). St. Louis, MO: Mosby.

Petersen, E., Betts, J., & Muntean, W. (2020). *Next Generation NCLEX® (NGN) Webinar*. Chicago: NCSBN.

Potter, P., Perry, A., Stockert, P., & Hall, A. (2021). *Fundamentals of nursing* (10th ed.). St. Louis, MO: Mosby.

ProEdit. (2019). *Understanding Bloom's and Anderson and Krathwohl's Taxonomy*. Retrieved from http://www.proedit.com/understanding-blooms-and-anderson-and-krathwohls-taxonomy/.

Skidmore-Roth, L. (2021). *Mosby's 2021 nursing drug reference* (34th ed.). St. Louis, MO: Mosby.

Stromberg, H. (2021). *deWit's medical-surgical nursing: Concepts & practice* (4th ed.). St. Louis, MO: Saunders.

Varcarolis, E., & Fosbre, C. (2021). *Essentials of psychiatric-mental health nursing: A communication approach to evidence-based care* (4th ed.). St. Louis, MO: Mosby.

Yoost, B., & Crawford, L. (2020). *Fundamentals of nursing: Active learning for collaborative practice* (2nd ed.). St. Louis, MO: Elsevier.

Index

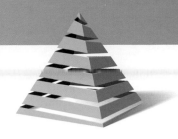

Note: Page numbers followed by "f" indicate figures, "t" indicate tables, and "b" indicate boxes.

Heparin sodium, 204
Hepatitis, @140, 151
  viral, 165
Herbal therapy, 138
High-fat food groups, 141
Hip spica cast, 194
Hirschsprung's disease, 191
Histamine H$_2$ receptor antagonists, 116
HIV. *See* Human immunodeficiency virus
Homonymous hemianopsia, after stroke, 166
Hospitalized toddler, 194
Hot spot question, 57b
Human chorionic gonadotropin (hCG), increased levels of,
    in morning sickness, 184
Human immunodeficiency virus (HIV), 143–144, 153
Human-made disasters, 132b
  definition of, 132
  sample question for, 132b–133b
Humulin N, 200
Humulin R, 200
Hunger, type 1 diabetes mellitus and, 151
Hydatidiform mole, 179
Hydroxyzine hydrochloride, calculation for, 142–143
Hyperemesis gravidarum, 179
Hypertension, 199, 201
  metoprolol for, 205
  quinapril hydrochloride for, 199
Hypoglycemia, 151, 196
  management of, 220
Hypoglycemic reaction, 220
Hypospadias, 191
Hypotension
  excessive, 213
  supine, 217
Hypothyroidism, 208–209
Hypotonic uterine dysfunction, 181

I

Ice, apply, for eye injury, 160
Illustration/figure question, 35
  ingredients of, 57b
  sample of, 40b–41b
  strategies for, 39–41, 40b
Immunization, 193
Implementation questions, 87–88, 87b–89b
  sample of, 88b–89b
Incident reporting, 227
Indwelling urinary (Foley) catheter, 226
Ineffective grieving, 180
Infection
  of central venous catheter site, 211
  urinary tract, 197
Informed consent, 145
Informing, 103t
Infusion, intravenous, 192
Infusion pump, for volume infusion irregularities, 192
Inhaled medications, spacer with, 162
Injury
  brain, 221
  eye, 195
  head, 198
  spinal cord, 211

Insulin, 200
  regular and NPH, 17b
  for type 1 diabetes mellitus, 151
Intended effects, of medication, 112, 112b
  sample question about, 112b–113b
Interactive learning, 16
Internal cervical, radiation implant, 164
Internal disasters, 132, 217
Internships, 93b
Interventions, sleeping, difficulty, 136
Intraocular pressure, normal, 161
Intrauterine fetal demise, 179
Intravenous calculation questions, 109–120
  sample question, 120b
  strategies for, 118–120
Intravenous infusion, 192
Involution, 186
Iron, deficiency anemia, 138
Iron-rich foods, for iron-deficiency anemia, 138
Irrigation, ear, 223
IV insertion, 142

J

JIA. *See* Juvenile idiopathic arthritis
Juvenile idiopathic arthritis (JIA), 222

K

Kegel exercises, for urinary frequency, 184
Key points, in textbook, 8
Knowledge, lack of, 180

L

Labor
  normal, 182
  precipitate, 181
  total duration of, 182
Laboratory values, 126–127, 127b, 210
  NCLEX exam and, 126–127
  sample question for, 127b
Laceration, right finger, 158
Lansoprazole, 200
Lasix (furosemide), 115
Last menstrual period (LMP), 178
Leadership questions, 91–100, 223–235
Learning principles, 222, 228
Leg, right, pallor and coolness of, 157
Legal issues, 233
Legal responsibilities, 226
Levothyroxine, 208
Licensed practical nurse, delegation to, 91, 95–96
Licensed vocational nurse, delegation to, 91, 95–96
Lifestyle planning, 5b, 8b
Listening skills, 15
Lithium carbonate, 203
Low-fat diet, 141

M

Magnesium sulfate, for preeclampsia, 179
Malnutrition, 169
Management questions, 91–100, 223–235
Mania, 173
Manic-depressive disorder, 203

⚠ Test-Taking Strategy Guide

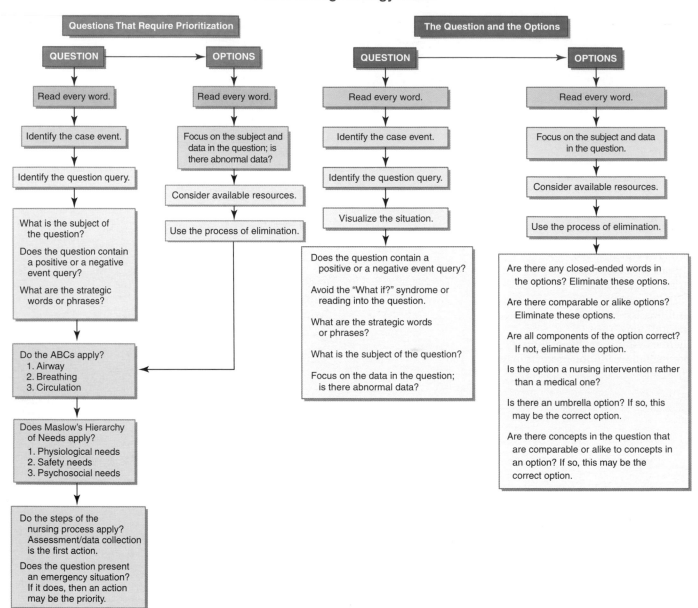

Questions That Require Prioritization

QUESTION → **OPTIONS**

QUESTION
- Read every word.
- Identify the case event.
- Identify the question query.
- What is the subject of the question?
- Does the question contain a positive or a negative event query?
- What are the strategic words or phrases?
- Do the ABCs apply?
  1. Airway
  2. Breathing
  3. Circulation
- Does Maslow's Hierarchy of Needs apply?
  1. Physiological needs
  2. Safety needs
  3. Psychosocial needs
- Do the steps of the nursing process apply? Assessment/data collection is the first action.
- Does the question present an emergency situation? If it does, then an action may be the priority.

OPTIONS
- Read every word.
- Focus on the subject and data in the question; is there abnormal data?
- Consider available resources.
- Use the process of elimination.

The Question and the Options

QUESTION → **OPTIONS**

QUESTION
- Read every word.
- Identify the case event.
- Identify the question query.
- Visualize the situation.
- Does the question contain a positive or a negative event query?
- Avoid the "What if?" syndrome or reading into the question.
- What are the strategic words or phrases?
- What is the subject of the question?
- Focus on the data in the question; is there abnormal data?

OPTIONS
- Read every word.
- Focus on the subject and data in the question.
- Consider available resources.
- Use the process of elimination.
- Are there any closed-ended words in the options? Eliminate these options.
- Are there comparable or alike options? Eliminate these options.
- Are all components of the option correct? If not, eliminate the option.
- Is the option a nursing intervention rather than a medical one?
- Is there an umbrella option? If so, this may be the correct option.
- Are there concepts in the question that are comparable or alike to concepts in an option? If so, this may be the correct option.

⚠ Use these strategies for multiple choice and alternate item questions. For Next Generation NCLEX®(NGN) test items, you will need to consider many aspects of the case situation and think beyond what is presented in the case situation in order to correctly answer test items. Cognitive Skills, which include Recognize Cues, Analyze Cues, Prioritize Hypotheses, Generate Solutions, Take Action, and Evaluate Outcomes are measured in these NGN test items.